250 SHORT CASES IN CLINICAL MEDICINE

Second Edition

250 SHORT CASES IN CLINICAL MEDICINE

Second Edition

Ragavendra R. Baliga
MBBS, MD, DNB, MRCP(UK)

Cardiovascular Division
Brigham and Women's Hospital
Harvard Medical School
Boston, Massachusetts
USA

(Formerly, Hammersmith Hospital and Royal
Postgraduate Medical School, London, UK)

WB SAUNDERS

Edinburgh   London   New York   Philadelphia   Sydney   Toronto

WB SAUNDERS
An imprint of Harcourt Publishers Limited

First published 1997
Reprinted 1997
Reprinted 1999
Reprinted 2000

ISBN 0-7020-2205-5

British Library Cataloguing in Publication Data
A catalogue record for this book is available from the British Library

Library of Congress Cataloging in Publication Data
A catalog record for this book is available from the Library of Congress

Printed in China
GCC/05

CONTENTS

RESPIRATORY SYSTEM   257

Examination of the chest   257

Contents ix

MISCELLANEOUS

PREFACE

Since the previous edition of this book was published in 1993, many spectacular advances have been made in medicine, particularly in the understanding of the origins of disease and, consequently, often in the treatment of these conditions. Although these advances have required revision of this book, the goals remain the same: to provide strategies to satisfy the requirements of a clinical examination in general internal medicine. Each candidate will have to mix and match these strategies depending on a given examination situation. In writing this book, I have assumed that readers will have a background knowledge in general medicine and will frequently consult textbooks of medicine and books on clinical methods. It does not serve to replace such books or bedside clinical examination.

As before, the book is particularly useful for the MBBS, PLAB, LRCP, MRCP(UK), MRCPI, postgraduate clinical examinations in Australia (FRACP), Canada (FCCP) and MD (New Zealand, Malaysia, Singapore, India, Pakistan, Sri Lanka and Bangladesh). In this edition the number of cases has been increased to 250 and each case has been discussed in more detail.

Salient features of the book include the following:

- A total of 250 cases (not including the schemes provided for examination of each system) are arranged in the frequency with which they are seen in the ward and, consequently, the clinical examination.
- Almost all chapters begin with a suggested scheme for the examination of that particular system.
- Cases that are seen commonly in the ward and the clinical examination are discussed in greater detail than others.
- Cases for examinations are drawn from the same pool for both undergraduate and postgraduate examinations, although in the latter the candidate's performance has to be faultless and he or she will be expected to know certain aspects in greater detail.

Each short case is discussed under the following headings:

- **Instruction.** This allows the candidate to know what sort of instruction or command may be expected from an examiner.

- **Salient features.** This section highlights the important features in each case and provides guidelines on how to proceed when faced with these signs (under the heading 'Proceed as follows') and what to tell the examiner in order to satisfy the examiner that the candidate is 'safe and sound' to be a junior doctor.
- **Diagnosis.** Many candidates are unable to present their diagnosis in a succinct manner, although they are able to elicit the clinical signs. This heading has been included to help candidates present their diagnosis in a crisp and confident fashion. The candidate must endeavour to present the diagnosis so that it includes three features: the lesion, the underlying aetiology and the functional status of the patient. It might not always be possible to determine the aetiology and functional status in the examination situation.
- **Questions.** This section supplies the questions (with answers) that a candidate can expect in a given case. These are also useful for the viva component of examination. The advanced-level questions are for postgraduates.
- **Footnotes.** Many of the cases have footnotes giving historical facts relevant to that particular case. Although examiners will not deduct marks for ignorance of things that have little relevance to patient welfare, candidates who know the facts can expect a congratulatory glow to pervade the examiner, so that the rest of the questions may be softened accordingly.
- **References.** The list of references will be invaluable for the medical student, postgraduate and house officer.

Learning is enhanced if this book is used soon after examining the patient. This also allows the candidate to go back to the patient and confirm classical clinical features. I would encourage candidates to take this book to the wards at least 6 months before the clinical examinations.

I thank my mentor Professor Thomas W Smith, Chief of the Cardiovascular Division of Brigham and Women's Hospital, and Dr Ralph A Kelly, the Co-director of our laboratory, for their support.

I also thank Mr Seàn Duggan, Editor-in-Chief, WB Saunders, UK, for his continuing support for this book and for inviting to me to write this second edition. Once again, I thank my wife Jayashree for doing my share of the domestic chores while I worked on this book.

Dedicated to
Thomas W Smith MD
Chief, Cardiovascular Division,
Brigham and Women's Hospital,
Professor of Medicine,
Harvard Medical School
who developed the radioimmunoassay for digitalis and made
several contributions to the understanding and treatment of
heart failure.

ACKNOWLEDGEMENTS

Dr Baliga is a recipient of the National Research Service Award from the National Institutes of Health, USA.

I wish to thank the following for their support.

Hammersmith Hospital, London
Prof. James Scott, FRCP
Dr. J.S. Kooner, MD, FRCP
Prof. P.G. Camici, FACC, FESC

Aberdeen Royal Infirmary, Aberdeen
Prof. J.C. Petrie, FRCP
Dr. P.W. Brunt, OBE, FRCP
Dr. John Webster, MD, FRCP

Royal London Hospital
Prof. N. Benjamin, MD, MRCP

St. Mary's Hospital, Portsmouth
Prof. H.A. Lee, FRCP

St. Mary's Hospital Medical School, London
Prof. C.J. Mathias, DPHIL, FRCP, DSC

Stoke Mandeville Hospital, Aylesbury
Dr. H.L. Frankel, OBE, FRCP

Brigham and Women's Hospital, Boston
Prof. T.W. Smith, MD
Dr. R.A. Kelly, MD

CARDIOVASCULAR SYSTEM

EXAMINATION OF THE CARDIOVASCULAR SYSTEM

1. Introduce yourself: 'I am Dr/Mr/Ms .... May I examine your heart?'.

2. Ensure adequate exposure of the precordium: 'Would you take your top off, please?'. However, be sensitive of the feelings of female patients.

3. Get the patient to sit at 45 degrees – use pillows to support the neck.

4. Inspection: comment on the patient's decubitus (whether he or she is comfortable at rest or obviously short of breath); comment on malar flush (seen in mitral stenosis).

5. Examine the pulse: rate (count for 15 s), rhythm, character, volume; lift the arm to feel for the collapsing pulse. Feel the other radial pulse simultaneously.

6. Comment on the scar at antecubital fossa (cardiac catheterization scars).

7. Look at the tongue for pallor, central cyanosis.

8. Look at the eye for pallor, Argyll Robertson pupil.

9. Examine the jugular venous pulse: comment on the wave form and height from the sternal angle. Check the abdominojugular reflux.

10. Comment on any carotid pulsations (Corrigan's sign of aortic regurgitation).

11. Examine the precordium: comment on surgical scars (midline sternotomy scars, thoracotomy scars for mitral valvotomy may be missed under the female breast).

12. Feel the apex beat – position and character.

13. Feel for left parasternal heave and thrills at the apex and on either side of the sternum.

14. Listen to the heart, beginning from the apex: take care to palpate the right carotid pulse simultaneously so that the examiner notices that you are timing the various cardiac events.

    Always comment on the first and second heart sounds. Mention any additional heart sounds.

    If you do not hear the mid-diastolic murmur of mitral stenosis, make sure you listen to the apex in the left lateral position with the bell of the stethoscope.

    If you hear a murmur at the apex, ensure that you get the patient to breathe in and out – the examiner will be observing whether or not you are listening for the variation in intensity with respiration.

    If you hear a pansystolic murmur, listen at the axilla (mitral regurgitant murmurs are conducted to the axilla).

15. Using the diaphragm of your stethoscope listen at the apex, below the sternum, along the left sternal edge, the second right intercostal space and the neck (for ejection systolic murmur of aortic stenosis, aortic sclerosis).

16. Request the patient to sit forward and listen with the diaphragm along the left sternal edge in the 3rd intercostal area with the patient's breath held in expiration for early diastolic murmur of aortic regurgitation.

17. Tell the examiner that you would like to do the following:
    - Listen to lung bases for signs of cardiac failure.
    - Check for sacral and leg oedema.
    - Examine the liver (tender liver of cardiac failure), splenomegaly (endocarditis).
    - Check the blood pressure.
    - Check the peripheral pulses and also check for radiofemoral delay.

René Theophile Hyacinthe Laennec invented the stethoscope in 1816 and reported his early experience with auscultation in a two-volume book published 3 years later. British physician Sir John Forbes (1787–1861) is best remembered for popularizing the stethoscope among English-speaking doctors. Forbes was born in Banff in the north east of Scotland. He studied at Marischal College, Aberdeen, before he went to Edinburgh where he received his medical education. Forbes translated Laennec's monograph in English in 1821 and published his own book on the subject in 1824. The latter included a brief biographical sketch of the Austrian physician Leopald Auenbrugger and the first English translation of his essay (which was in Latin) on percussion. It also contained a summary of Parisian physician Victor Collin's recent manual on cardiac physical diagnosis.

References

Bruns DLA (1959) A general theory of the causes of murmurs in the cardiovascular system. *Am J Med* 27:360.

Forbes J (1824) *Original Cases with Dissections and Observations Illustrating the Use of the Stethoscope and Percussion in the Diagnosis of the Diseases of the Chest.* London: T and G Underwood.

Laennec RTH (1821) *A Treatise on the Diseases of the Chest.* London: T and G Underwood (Translated by and with a preface and notes by John Forbes).

CASE 1 Mitral Stenosis

Instruction

Listen to this patient's heart.
Examine this patient's cardiovascular system.

Salient features

- Pulse regular or irregularly irregular (due to atrial fibrillation).
- Jugular venous pressure (JVP) may be raised.
- Malar flush.
- Tapping apex beat in the 5th intercostal space just medial to midclavicular line.
- Left parasternal heave (indicating right ventricular enlargement).
- Loud first heart sound.
- Opening snap (often difficult to hear; a high-pitched sound that can vary from 0.04 to 0.10 s after the second sound, and is heard best at the apex with the patient in the lateral decubitus position).
- Rumbling, low-pitched, mid-diastolic murmur – best heard in the left lateral position on expiration. In sinus rhythm there may be presystolic accentuation of the murmur. If you are not sure about the murmur, tell the examiner that you want the patient to perform sit-ups or hopping on one foot to increase the heart rate. This will increase the flow across the mitral valve and the murmur is better heard.

- Pulmonary component of second sound (P_2) is loud.

Note. In patients with valvular lesions the candidate would be expected to comment on rhythm, the presence of heart failure and signs of pulmonary hypertension.

In atrial septal defect, large flow murmurs across the tricuspid valve can cause mid-diastolic murmurs. The presence of wide, fixed splitting of second sound, absence of loud first heart sound, and an opening snap and incomplete right bundle branch block should indicate the correct diagnosis. However, about 4% of the patients with atrial septal defect have mitral stenosis, a combination called Lutembacher's syndrome.

Diagnosis

This patient has mitral stenosis (lesion) which is almost always due to rheumatic heart disease (aetiology), and has atrial fibrillation, pulmonary hypertension and congestive cardiac failure (functional status).

Questions

What is the commonest cause of mitral stenosis?

Rheumatic heart disease.

What is the mechanism of tapping apex beat?

It is due to an accentuated first heart sound.

What does the opening snap indicate?

The opening snap is caused by the opening of the stenosed mitral valve and indicates that the leaflets are pliable. The opening snap is usually accompanied by a loud first heart sound. It is absent when the valve is diffusely calcified. When only the tips of the leaflets are calcified, the opening snap persists.

What is the mechanism of a loud first heart sound?

The loud first heart sound occurs when the valve leaflets are mobile. The valve is open during diastole and is suddenly slammed shut by ventricular contraction in systole.

What is the mechanism of presystolic accentuation of the mumur?

In sinus rhythm it is due to the atrial systole which increases flow across the stenotic valve from the left atrium to the left ventricle; this causes accentuation of the loudness of the murmur. This may also been seen in atrial fibrillation and is explained by the turbulent flow caused by the mitral valve starting to close with the onset of ventricular systole. This occurs before the first heart sound and gives the impression of falling in late diastole. It is, however, due to the start of ventricular systole.

What are the complications?

- Left atrial enlargement and atrial fibrillation.
- Systemic embolization, usually cerebral hemispheres.
- Pulmonary hypertension.
- Tricuspid regurgitation.
- Right heart failure.

How does one determine clinically the severity of the stenosis?

- The narrower the distance between the second sound and the opening snap, the greater the severity. The converse is not true. (**Note.** This time interval between the second sound and opening snap is said to be inversely related to the left atrial pressure.)
- The longer the duration of the diastolic murmur, the greater the severity. Note that in tight mitral stenosis the murmur may be less prominent or inaudible and the findings may be primarily those of pulmonary hypertension.

What are the radiological features of mitral stenosis?

- Congested upper lobe veins.
- Double silhouette due to enlarged left atrium.
- Straightening of the left border of the heart due to prominent pulmonary conus and filling of the pulmonary bay by the enlarged left atrium.
- Kerley B lines (horizontal lines in the regions of the costophrenic angles).

Uncommonly:

- Left bronchus may be horizontal due to an enlarged left atrium.
- Mottling due to secondary pulmonary haemosiderosis.

Advanced-level Questions

What are the indications for cardiac catheterization in such patients?

- Concomitant coronary artery disease.

- Technically difficult and inconclusive echocardiogram.
- Associated valvular lesions such as mitral regurgitation (in which case commissurotomy is untenable) or aortic regurgitation.

What is the normal cross-sectional area of the mitral valve?

It ranges from 4 to 6 cm^2 and turbulence of the flow occurs when this area is less than 2 cm^2.

What is the area in 'tight' mitral stenosis?

It is usually less than 1 cm^2.

What are the indications for surgery?

- Patients with severe symptoms of pulmonary congestion and significant mitral stenosis.
- Patients with pulmonary hypertension or haemoptysis even if minimally symptomatic.
- Recurrent thromboembolic events despite therapeutic anticoagulation.

Which surgical procedures are used to treat mitral stenosis?

- Closed commissurotomy.
    Closed mitral valvotomy – involves the use of mechanical dilators, inserted through the apex of the left ventricle. It is complicated by mitral regurgitation, systemic embolization and restenosis.
    Balloon valvuloplasty (a form of closed commissurotomy) – percutaneous trans-septal balloon mitral valvotomy (or valvuloplasty). Remember percutaneous balloon dilatation of the mitral valve is a useful option in patients who are unable to undergo cardiac surgery, as in late pregnancy or when too ill (severe respiratory disease, non-mitral cardiac disease, multiorgan failure).
- Open commissurotomy – requires cardiopulmonary bypass and allows surgical repair of the valve under direct vision resulting in more effective and safer valvotomy than the closed procedure.
- Valve replacement – entails risks including thromboembolism, endocarditis and primary valve failure.

What factors determine the success of balloon valvuloplasty?

- Good mobility of the valves.
- Little calcification.
- Minimal subvalvular disease.

- Mild mitral regurgitation.

In which trimester do patients with mitral stenosis usually become symptomatic?

Patients usually become symptomatic in the second trimester of pregnancy, when blood volume increases significantly and increases pulmonary pressures. As the blood volume diminishes late in third trimester, the symptoms might slightly improve.

Mention some rarer causes of mitral stenosis.

- Calcification of mitral annulus and leaflets.
- Rheumatoid arthritis.
- Systemic lupus erythematosus.
- Malignant carcinoid.
- Congenital stenosis.

Which conditions simulate mitral stenosis?

- Left atrial myxoma.
- Ball valve thrombus in the left atrium.
- Cor triatriatum (a rare congenital heart condition).

Have you heard of Ortner's syndrome?

It refers to the hoarseness of voice caused by left vocal cord paralysis associated with enlarged left atrium in mitral stenosis.

What are the main pathological types of rheumatic stenosis?

- Commissural type, in which there is fusion of commissures with little involvement of the chordae and/or cusps.
- Chordae type, in which there is fusion and thickening of the chordae, resulting in shortening and diminished mobility of the leaflets.
- Leaflet type, in which the leaflets become stiff, rigid and calcified.

N. Ortner (1865–1935), Professor of Medicine, Vienna, described the syndrome in 1897. He believed in laboratory research and its application to bedside clinical work and he said that the clinician's motto ought to be 'übers laboratorium dauernd zur Klinik' (translated: 'always via the laboratory to the clinic').
PJ Kerley (1900–1978), British radiologist.
Paul Wood was a cardiologist at the Hammersmith and National Heart Hospitals. His clinical skills are legendary and he had a profound influence on British cardiology.

Elliott Cutler, in 1923 in Boston, was the first to attempt surgical treatment of mitral stenosis by inserting a knife through the apex of the left ventricle and blindly cutting the valve at right angles to its natural orifice.

Henry Souttar, in 1925, relieved mitral stenosis with a finger inserted through the atrial appendage.

In 1948, four surgeons working independently performed successful valvotomies: Horace Smithy, Charles Bailey, Dwight Harken and Russell Brock.

In 1984, Kanji Inoue from Japan and in 1985, James E Lock, contemporary Professor of Pediatric Cardiology, Harvard Medical School, and colleagues introduced balloon valvuloplasty for mitral stenosis.

References

Bonchek LI (1980) Indications for surgery of the mitral valve *Am J Cardiol* **46**: 155.

Chen C & Cheng TO (1994) Percutaneous balloon mitral valvuloplasty using Inoue technic: a multicenter study of 4832 patients in China. *Circulation* **90**: I65.

Lock JE, Khalilullah M, Shrivastava S, Bahl V & Keane JF (1985) Percutaneous cutaneous catheter commissurotomy in rheumatic mitral stenosis. *N Engl J Med* **313**: 1515–1518.

Selzer A & Cohn KE (1972) Natural history of mitral stenosis: a review. *Circulation* **45**: 878.

Turi ZG, Reyes VP & Raju BSL et al (1991) Percutaneous balloon versus surgical closed commissurotomy for mitral stenosis: a prospecive, randomized trial. *Circulation* **83**: 1179–1185.

Wood P (1954) An appreciation of mitral stenosis. *BMJ* **1**: 1051–1113.

CASE 2 Mitral Regurgitation

Instruction

Examine this patient's heart.

Salient features

- Peripheral pulse may be normal or jerky (i.e. rapid upstroke with a short duration).
- Apex beat will be displaced downwards and outwards and will be forceful in character.
- First heart sound will be soft.
- Third heart sound is common (left ventricular gallop sound).
- Pansystolic murmur (Hope murmur) conducted to the axilla, best detected with the diaphragm and on expiration. (**Note.** It is important to be sure that there is no associated tricuspid regurgitation.)

Note. When mitral regurgitation is caused by left ventricular dilatation and diminished cardiac contractility, the systolic murmur may be mid, late or pansystolic. Other causes of short systolic murmurs at the apex include mitral valve prolapse, papillary muscle dysfunction and aortic stenosis. In calcific aortic stenosis of the elderly, the murmur may be more prominent in the apex and may be confused with mitral regurgitation. In such instances try to listen to the murmur after a pause with premature beat or listen to the beat after a pause with atrial fibrillation. The murmur of aortic stenosis becomes louder, whereas that of mitral regurgitation shows little change.

Diagnosis

This patient has mitral regurgitation (lesion) as evidenced by grade III–VI pansystolic murmur, which is probably due to ischaemic or rheumatic heart disease (aetiology), and is in cardiac failure as evidenced by bibasal crackles (functional status).

Questions

Mention some causes of chronic mitral regurgitation.

- Mitral valve prolapse.
- Rheumatic heart disease.
- Left ventricular dilatation.
- Coronary artery disease.
- Annular calcification.
- Infective endocarditis.
- Papillary muscle dysfunction.
- Cardiomyopathy.
- Connective tissue disorders.

Mention a few causes of acute mitral regurgitation.

- Acute myocardial infarction (rupture of the papillary muscle).
- Endocarditis (due to perforation of the mitral valve leaflet or the chordae).
- Trauma.
- Myxomatous degeneration of the valve.

How would you investigate this patient?

- Electrocardiography (ECG), looking for left ventricular hypertrophy, atrial fibrillation. When coronary artery disease is the cause, there is often evidence of inferior or posterior wall myocardial infarction.

- Chest radiography, looking for large heart, left atrial enlargement.
- Echocardiography to determine the anatomy of the mitral valve apparatus, left atrial and left ventricular size and function.
- Cardiac catheterization, useful to determine coexistent coronary artery or aortic valve disease.

How would you differentiate between mitral regurgitation and tricuspid regurgitation?

	Mitral regurgitation	**Tricuspid regurgitation**
Pulse	Jerky or normal pulse	Normal pulse
JVP		Prominent 'v' wave
Palpation	Left ventricular heave	Left parasternal heave
Auscultation	Pansystolic murmur	Pansystolic murmur
	Intensity increases with	Intensity increases with
	expiration	inspiration
	Radiates to the axilla	
Other signs		Hepatic pulsations

Why may these patients have a jerky pulse?

Because of reduced systolic ejection time, secondary to a large volume of blood regurgitating into the left atrium.

When does the murmur of mitral regurgitation radiate to the neck (i.e. base of the heart)?

Rarely, due to involvement of the posterior mitral leaflet or to ruptured chordae tendinae, the regurgitant jet strikes the left atrial wall adjacent to the aortic root and the murmur radiates to the base of the heart, and therefore may be confused with the murmur of aortic stenosis.

How do you grade systolic murmurs?

Levine's grading of systolic murmurs:

- Grade 1: Murmur is so faint that it is heard only with special effort.
- Grade 2: Murmur is faint but readily detected.
- Grade 3: Murmur is prominent but not loud.
- Grade 4: Murmur is loud.
- Grade 5: Murmur is very loud.
- Grade 6: Murmur is loud enough to be heard with the stethoscope just removed from contact with the chest wall.

What are the causes of pansystolic murmur over the precordium?

- Mitral regurgitation.
- Tricuspid regurgitation.
- Ventricular septal defect (this generally radiates to the right of the sternum).

Advanced-level Questions

Which congenital cardiac conditions can be associated with mitral valve regurgitation?

- Ostium primum atrial septal defect (due to cleft mitral valve).
- Partial atrioventricular canal.
- Corrected transposition of the great arteries.

How would you determine the severity of the lesion?

- The larger the left ventricle on clinical examination, the greater the severity.
- Colour Doppler ultrasonography quantifies the severity of the regurgitant jet, usually into three grades.

What is the significance of third heart sounds in mitral regurgitation?

The prevalence of third heart sounds increases with the severity of mitral regurgitation. However, in patients with mitral regurgitation, the third heart sound is due to rapid ventricular filling and does not necessarily reflect left ventricular systolic dysfunction or increased filling pressure.

What is the medical management of such patients?

- Asymptomatic patients – antibiotic prophylaxis for endocarditis.
- When atrial fibrillation develops – digitalis to slow ventricular response.
- Heart failure – diuretics and inotropes, but major consideration should be given to surgery.

What are the indications for surgery in this patient?

- Moderate to severe symptoms despite medical therapy, provided that left ventricular function is adequate.
- Patients with minimal or no symptoms should be followed up every 6 months by echocardiographic or radionuclide assessment of left

ventricular size and systolic function. When the ejection fraction falls to 55%, or when left ventricular dimension is greater than 60 mm, mitral valve repair or replacement should be considered.

Samuel A Levine was Professor of Cardiology at Harvard Medical School and Peter Bent Brigham Hospital in Boston.
James Hope (1801–1841) was an English physician who worked at St George's Hospital, London, and wrote a book in 1831 entitled *Diseases of the Heart and Great Vessels*.

Reference

Freeman AR & Levine SA (1933) The clinical significance of the systolic murmur. A study of 1000 consecutive 'non-cardiac' cases. *Ann Intern Med* **6**: 1371.

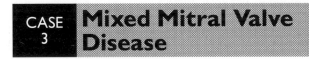

CASE 3 **Mixed Mitral Valve Disease**

Instruction

Listen to this patient's heart.

Salient features

- Patient will have signs of both mitral stenosis and regurgitation.
- The candidate will be expected to indicate the dominant lesion (see below).

Proceed as follows:

- Look carefully for surgical scars of mitral valvotomy in all patients (scars under the left breast in female patients are often missed). Patients with previous valvotomy may have regurgitation and restenosis.

	Dominant mitral stenosis	Dominant mitral regurgitation
Apex beat	Tapping, not displaced	Heaving and displaced
First heart sound	Loud	Soft
Third heart sound	Absent	Present

A third heart sound in mitral regurgitation indicates that any associated mitral stenosis is insignificant.

Note. There may be patients who do not have clear-cut signs such as a loud first heart sound with a displaced apex; in such cases you must say that it is difficult to ascertain clinically the dominant lesion and that cardiac catheterization should resolve the issue.

Diagnosis

This patient has mitral stenosis with mitral regurgitation (lesion), with the dominant lesion being stenosis due to rheumatic heart disease (aetiology), and is in cardiac failure (functional status).

Questions

What is the cause of mitral stenosis with regurgitation?

Mixed mitral valve disease is usually due to chronic rheumatic heart disease.

What are the approximate frequencies with which various valves are affected by rheumatic heart disease?

- Mitral valve disease, 80%.
- Aortic valve, 50%.
- Combined mitral and aortic valve lesion, 20%.
- Tricuspid valve, 10%.
- Pulmonary valve, < 1%.

In patients with mitral regurgitation and a diastolic rumble, what does the presence of a giant left atrium indicate?

It indicates that there is no significant mitral stenosis.

Joseph K Perloff is contemporary Professor of Cardiology, Los Angeles; his chief interest is congenital heart disease.
William C Roberts is contemporary US cardiac pathologist and Editor of the *American Journal of Cardiology.*

References

Ellis LB, Singh JB, Morales DD et al (1973) Fifteen to twenty years' study of one thousand patients undergoing closed mitral valvuloplasty. *Circulation* **48**: 357.
Roberts WC & Perloff JK (1972) Mitral valvular disease: a clinicopathological survey of the conditions causing the mitral valve to function abnormally. *Ann Intern Med* **77**: 939.

CASE 4 Aortic Regurgitation

Instruction

Examine this patient's cardiovascular system.
Examine this patient's heart.

Salient features

- The pulse may be large in volume and collapsing.
- Head nodding in time with the heart beat (de Musset's sign) may be present.
- Visible carotid pulsation may be obvious in the neck – dancing carotids or Corrigan's sign.
- Apex beat will be displaced outwards and forceful.
- Early diastolic, high-pitched murmur is heard at the left sternal edge with the diaphragm – if not apparent, it is important to sit the patient forward and auscultate with the patient's breath held at the end of expiration. When the ascending aorta is dilated and displaced to the right, the murmur may be heard along the right sternal border as well.
- An ejection systolic murmur may be heard at the base of the heart in severe aortic regurgitation. This murmur may be as loud as grade 5 or 6, and underlying organic stenosis can be ruled out only by investigations.

Proceed as follows:

- Tell the examiner you would like to do the following:
  Check the blood pressure (wide pulse pressure).
  Look for signs of hyperdynamic circulation – auscultate over the femoral arteries for 'pistol shots' (Traube's sign) and to-and-fro murmur (Duroziez's sign), and look for capillary pulsations in the nail bed (Quincke's sign).
  Look for systolic pulsations of the uvula (Muller's sign).
  Check pupils for Argyll Robertson pupil of syphilis.
  Look for stigmata of Marfan's syndrome – high arched palate, arm span greater than height.
  Check joints for ankylosing spondylitis and rheumatoid arthritis.

Diagnosis

This patient has pure aortic regurgitation (lesion), which is due to associated ankylosing spondylitis (aetiology), and is in cardiac failure (functional status).

Questions

Mention a few causes of chronic aortic regurgitation.

- Rheumatic fever.
- Hypertension (accentuated tambour quality of second sound).
- Atherosclerosis.
- Bacterial endocarditis.
- Idiopathic dilatation of the aortic root and annulus.
- Syphilis.
- Marfan's syndrome.
- Rheumatoid arthritis.
- Cystic medial necrosis.
- Seronegative arthritis (ankylosing spondylitis, Reiter's syndrome).
- Bicuspid aortic valve.

Advanced-level Questions

What is the prevalence of aortic regurgitation in the elderly?

According to the Helsinki Ageing Study, 13% of persons aged 75–86 years have moderate to severe aortic regurgitation.

What are the clinical signs of severity?

- Wide pulse pressure.
- Soft second heart sound.
- The duration of the decrescendo diastolic murmur.
- Presence of the left ventricular third heart sound.
- Austin Flint murmur.
- Signs of left ventricular failure.

What do you know of Hill's sign?

Hill's sign is the presence of higher systolic pressure in the leg than in the arm, and is said to be an indicator of the severity of aortic regurgitation:

In mild aortic regurgitation the difference is less than 20 mmHg, in moderate regurgitation it is between 20 and 40 mmHg and in severe regurgitation it is over 60 mmHg.

Do characteristics of the early diastolic murmur correlate with severity?

Yes. In mild aortic regurgitation the murmur is short but, as the severity of the regurgitation increases, the murmur becomes longer and louder. In very severe regurgitation the murmur may extend throughout diastole.

What is an Austin Flint murmur?

It is an apical, low-pitched, diastolic murmur due to vibration of the anterior mitral cusp in the regurgitant jet, and is heard at the apex.

Mention a few causes of acute aortic regurgitation.

- Infective endocarditis.
- Aortic dissection.
- Trauma.
- Failure of prosthetic valve.
- Rupture of sinus of Valsalva.

What do you know about the natural history of asymptomatic aortic regurgitation?

About 4% of patients develop symptoms, left ventricular dysfunction, or both, every year.

What do you understand by the term cor bovinum?

In chronic aortic regurgitation there is slow and progressive left ventricular dilatation and hypertrophy in an attempt to normalize wall stress. The heart may thus become larger and heavier than in any other form of chronic heart disease – cor bovinum (bovine or ox heart).

What is the role of nifedipine in aortic regurgitation?

- Long-term vasodilator therapy with nifedipine reduces or delays the need for aortic valve replacement in asymptomatic patients with severe aortic regurgitation.
- Patients in whom left ventricular dysfunction developed when treated with nifedipine respond favourably to valve replacement in terms of both survival and normalization of ejection fraction.
- Long-term vasodilator therapy should not be recommended for patients with left ventricular dysfunction.
- Patients with subnormal left ventricular ejection fractions should be considered candidates for aortic valve replacement rather than vasodilator therapy, since valve replacement remains the more definitive therapy to reduce volume overload.

How is aortic regurgitation treated?

Aortic regurgitation is usually treated surgically. The timing of surgery is important and depends on severity of symptoms and extent of left ventricular dysfunction. Valve replacement should be performed as soon as possible after the onset of ventricular dysfunction. Indications for surgery include:

- Symptoms of heart failure and diminished left ventricular function (an ejection fraction of less than 50% but more than 20–30%).
- A reduction in exercise ejection fraction (as estimated with radio-nuclide ventriculography and exercise testing) of 5% or more is considered by some an indication for surgery, even in the absence of symptoms.
- Several investigators have suggested an end-systolic dimension of 55 mm to represent the limit of surgically reversible dilatation of the left ventricle, so that aortic valve replacement is performed before this chamber size is exceeded. Others have challenged the validity of the 55-mm systolic limit, as postoperative reduction in chamber size remains variable.

Note.

1. Patients with severe symptoms but normal left ventricular size and systolic function should be followed at 6-monthly intervals with echocardiography or radionuclide ventriculography. In the young, mechanical prostheses are used as the valves are more durable.

2. Tissue valves are prone to calcification and degeneration. In the elderly and in those for whom anticoagulants are contraindicated, tissue valves are preferred.

Alfred de Musset was a French poet whose nodding movements were described by his brother in a biography. When told of this, Alfred put his thumb and forefinger on his neck and the head stopped bobbing.

Austin Flint (1812–1886) was one of the founders of Buffalo Medical College, New York, and reported the murmur in two patients with aortic regurgitation, confirmed by autopsy. He also held chairs at New Orleans, Chicago, Louisville and New York.

HI Quincke (1842–1922) was a German physician who described angioneurotic oedema and benign intracranial hypertension.

PI Duroziez (1826–1897), a French physician, was widely acclaimed for his articles on mitral stenosis.

L Traube (1818–1876), a German physician, was the first to describe pulsus bigeminus.

Antonio Maria Valsalva (1666–1723) was an Italian anatomist and surgeon who discovered the labyrinth and developed the Valsalva manoeuvre to remove foreign bodies from the ear.

References

Lindroos M, Kupari M, Heikkila J et al (1993) Prevalence of aortic valve abnormalities in the elderly: an echocardiographic study of a random population sample. *J Am Coll Cardiol* **21**: 1220–1225.

Nishimura RA, McGoon MD, Schaff HV & Giuliani ER (1988) Chronic aortic regurgitation. Indications for operation. *Mayo Clin Proc* **63**: 270.

O'Brien MF, McGiffin DC & Stafford EG (1989) Allograft aortic valve implantation: techniques for all types of aortic valve and root pathology. *Ann Thorac Surg* **48**: 600–609.

Orsinelli DA, Aurigemma GP, Battista S et al (1993) Left ventricular hypertrophy and mortality after aortic valve replacement for aortic stenosis. A high risk subgroup identified by preoperative relative wall thickness. *J Am Coll Cardiol* **22**: 1679–1683.

Scognamiglio R, Rahimtoola SH, Fasoli G, Nistri S & Dalla-Volta SD (1994) Nifedipine in asymptomatic patients with severe aortic regurgitation and normal left ventricular function. *N Engl J Med* **331**: 689.

Siemienczuk D, Greenberg B, Morris C et al (1989) Chronic aortic insufficiency. Factors associated with progression to aortic valve replacement. *Ann Intern Med* **110**: 587.

CASE 5 Aortic Stenosis

Instruction

Examine this patient's heart.

Salient features

- Low volume pulse.
- Apex beat is heaving in nature but is not displaced. (A displaced apex beat indicates left ventricular dilatation and severe disease.)
- Palpable systolic vibrations over the primary aortic area, with the patient in the sitting position during full expiration (often correlates with a gradient of more than 40 mmHg).
- Systolic thrill over the aortic area and the carotids.
- Soft second heart sound.
- Ejection click heard 0.1 s after first heart sound, along the left sternal border (indicates valvular stenosis). An ejection sound that moves with respiration is not aortic in origin.
- An atrial (S4) sound may be heard.
- Ejection systolic murmur at the base of the heart conducted to the carotids. (Listen carefully for an early diastolic murmur as mild aortic regurgitation often accompanies aortic stenosis.)

Proceed as follows:

- Tell the examiner that you would like to:
    Check the blood pressure, keeping in mind that the pulse pressure is low in moderate to severe stenosis.
    Ask the patient about syncope, angina and dyspnoea.

Diagnosis

This patient has pure aortic stenosis (lesion) which may be due to rheumatic aetiology or a bicuspid aortic valve (aetiology); he has severe aortic stenosis as he gives a history of recurrent syncope (functional status).

Questions

How would you differentiate aortic stenosis from aortic sclerosis?

Aortic sclerosis is seen in the elderly; the pulse is normal volume, the apex beat is not shifted and the murmur is localized.

Mention some causes of aortic stenosis.

- Under the age of 60 years: rheumatic, congenital.
- Between 60 and 75 years: calcified bicuspid aortic valve, especially in men.
- Over the age of 75 years: degenerative calcification.

How would you describe the pulse in aortic stenosis?

It is reduced in volume with a delayed upstroke (pulsus parvus et tardus). This is due to a reduction in systolic pressure and a gradual decline in diastolic pressure.

What does the second heart sound tell us in this condition?

- A soft second heart sound indicates valvular stenosis (except in calcific stenosis of the elderly, where the margins of the leaflets usually maintain their mobility).
- A single second heart sound may be seen when there is fibrosis and fusion of the valve leaflets.
- Reversed splitting of the second sound indicates mechanical or electrical prolongation of ventricular systole.
- A perfectly normal second heart sound (i.e. normal splitting with A2 of normal intensity) is strong evidence against the presence of critical aortic stenosis.

What is the significance of the third heart sound in aortic stenosis?

In patients with aortic stenosis, third heart sounds are uncommon but usually indicate the presence of systolic dysfunction and raised filling pressures.

What do you understand by the term ejection systolic murmur?

It is a crescendo–decrescendo murmur which begins after the first heart sound (or after the ejection click when present), peaks in mid or late systole and ends before the second heart sound. This peak is delayed with increasing severity of aortic stenosis.

Advanced-level Questions

Does the loudness of the murmur reflect the severity of the aortic stenosis?

No, the loudness of the murmur is related more to the cardiac output and the systolic turbulence surrounding the valve than to the severity of the stenosis. Thus, a loud murmur may be associated with trivial stenosis and, in severe heart failure, it may be soft because of decreased flow across the valve from the diminished cardiac output.

Mention other causes of ejection systolic murmur at the base of the heart.

- Pulmonary stenosis.
- Hypertrophic obstructive cardiomyopathy.
- Supravalvular aortic stenosis.

How may this patient present?

- Fatigue
- Angina (average survival 5 years).
- Dyspnoea (heart failure reduces life expectancy to less than 2 years).
- Syncope (average survival 3 years).
- Sudden death.

What is the prevalence of aortic stenosis in the elderly?

According to the Helsinki Ageing Study, almost 3% of the individuals aged between 75 and 86 years have critical aortic stenosis.

What is the mechanism of syncope in aortic stenosis?

- The left ventricle is suddenly unable to contract (transient electro-mechanical dissociation) against the stenosed valve.
- Cardiac arrhythmias (bradycardia, ventricular tachycardia or fibrillation).
- Marked peripheral vasodilatation without a concomitant increase in cardiac output, particularly after exercise.

What investigations would you do?

- ECG looking for left ventricular hypertrophy, ST–T changes.
- Chest radiography looking for valve calcification and post-stenotic dilatation of aorta (a bicuspid valve should be suspected if the proximal aorta is greatly enlarged).
- Echocardiography looking for valve gradient, left ventricular hypertrophy, calcified valves.
- Cardiac catheterization, looking for coronary arteries, mitral and aortic valves.

What is the role of exercise stress testing in aortic stenosis?

It should not be undertaken in the symptomatic patient with aortic stenosis, as it may be fatal. However, it has a definite role in asymptomatic patients with high-grade aortic stenosis and gives valuable information with respect to identifying the level of physical activity the patient can attain. It is useful in deciding the role of surgery in these patients.

What are the complications of aortic stenosis?

- Left ventricular failure.
- Infective endocarditis (in 10% of cases).

What are the clinical signs of severity of aortic stenosis?

- Narrow pulse pressure.
- Soft second sound.
- Narrow or reverse split second sound.
- Systolic thrill and heaving apex beat.
- Fourth heart sound.
- Cardiac failure.

How would you manage this patient?

- If the patient is asymptomatic and the valvular gradient is less than

50 mmHg, then observe the patient. Surgery is not recommended in asymptomatic patients.

- Valve replacement in the following circumstances:
  The patient is symptomatic or the valvular gradient is more than 50 mmHg.
  The valve area is less than 0.8 cm² (normal area 2.5–3.0 cm²).
- Often, patients require coronary artery bypass grafts during aortic valve replacement.
- Balloon valvuloplasty should be limited to moribund patients requiring emergency intervention or those with a very poor life expectancy due to other pathology. In one study, although inhospital mortality rates were similar to those following conventional surgical replacement, there were more deaths in the valvuloplasty group in the subsequent follow-up period.

What is the genetics of supravalvular stenosis?

Studies suggest that mutation in the elastin gene causes supravalvular stenosis.

If this patient had bleeding per rectum what unusual cause would come to mind?

Angiodysplasia of the colon.

If the patient was icteric and had haemolytic anaemia, what would the mechanism be?

Microangiopathic haemolysis has been described in severe calcified aortic stenosis manifesting with anaemia and icterus.

What do you understand by the term 'Gallavardin phenomenon'?

The high-frequency components of the ejection systolic murmur may radiate to the apex. This, therefore, falsely suggests mitral regurgitation. This is known as the Gallavardin phenomenon.

Williams' syndrome is characterized by elfin facies, supravalvular aortic stenosis and hypercalcaemia (JCP Williams, New Zealand physician).

References

Bernard Y, Etievant J & Mourand JL (1992) Long term results of percutaneous aortic valvuloplasty compared with aortic valve replacement in patients more than 75 years old. *J Am Coll Cardiol* **20**: 796–801.

Curran ME, Atkinson DL, Ewart AR, Morris CA, Leppert MF & Keating MT
  (1993) The elastin gene is disrupted by a translocation associated with
  supravalvular aortic stenosis. *Cell* **73**: 159.
Gallavardin L & Pauper-Ravault P (1925) Le souffle du rétréassesment aortique
  peut changer de timbre et devenir musical dans sa propogatio apexienne.
  Lyons Med **135**: 523.
Galloway SJ, Casarella WJ & Shimkin PM (1974) Vascular malformations of the
  right colon as a cause of bleeding in patients with aortic stenosis. *Radiology*
  113: 11.
Lindroos M, Kupari M, Heikkila J et al (1993) Prevalence of aortic valve
  abnormalities in the elderly: an echocardiographic study of a random
  population sample. *J Am Coll Cardiol* **21**: 1220–1225.
Lombard JT & Selzer A (1987) Valvular aortic stenosis: a clinical and
  hemodynamic profile of patients. *Ann Intern Med* **106**: 292.
Marsh GW & Lewis SM (1969) Cardiac hemolytic anemia. *Semin Hematol* **6**: 133.
Wood P (1958) Aortic stenosis. *Am J Cardiol* **1**: 533.

CASE 6 — Mixed Aortic Valve Lesion

Instruction

Examine this patient's heart.
Examine this patient's cardiovascular system.
Examine this patient's pulse.

Salient features

- Pulse may be bisferious, small volume or large volume depending on
  the dominant lesion.
- Displaced apex beat.
- Early diastolic murmur of aortic regurgitation.
- Ejection systolic murmur of aortic stenosis.

Proceed as follows:

- Tell the examiner that you would like to check the blood pressure, in
  particular to determine the pulse pressure (systolic minus diastolic
  pressure).

Diagnosis

This patient has mixed aortic stenosis with aortic regurgitation (lesion) due
to rheumatic heart disease (aetiology). He has a dominant stenosis and is
in cardiac failure (functional status).

Note.

In *dominant aortic stenosis*:

    Pulse volume is small.

    Blood pressure is normal and pulse pressure is narrow.

In *dominant aortic regurgitation*:

    Pulse is collapsing.

    Pulse pressure is wide.

Questions

What are common causes of mixed aortic lesions?

- Rheumatic heart disease.
- Bicuspid aortic valve.

CASE 7 Mixed Mitral and Aortic Valve Disease

Instruction

Examine this patient's precordium.

Examine this patient's cardiovascular system.

Examine this patient's heart.

Salient features

- Pulse may be small volume (due to either dominant aortic stenosis or mitral stenosis), regular or irregularly irregular.
- Apex beat may be displaced.
- Left parasternal heave.
- Mid-diastolic murmur of mitral stenosis.
- Pansystolic murmur of mitral regurgitation.
- Ejection systolic murmur of aortic stenosis at the base of the heart.
- Early diastolic murmur of aortic regurgitation heard with the patient sitting forward on end expiration.

Note.

- If the apex beat is not displaced in such mixed lesions then mitral stenosis is the dominant lesion. (However, if the mitral stenosis developed earlier it can mask the signs of a significant stenosis.)
- In aortic stenosis, the murmur of mitral stenosis may be diminished or absent. The presence of the following features should alert the clinician to a coexisting mitral stenosis because they are not commonly associated with isolated aortic stenosis:

Atrial fibrillation.

Absence of left ventricular hypertrophy in patients with left heart failure.

Female sex.

Giant-sized left atrium.

Calcification of the mitral valve.

Absence of aortic valve calcification in the symptomatic patient.

- Severe mitral stenosis and low cardiac output may mask moderate to severe aortic stenosis. Suspect the presence of aortic stenosis if there is a history of angina, syncope or ECG evidence of left ventricular hypertrophy or calcification of the aortic valve on the chest radiograph.
- The murmur of aortic stenosis is occasionally better heard at the apex than at the base, particularly in the elderly. When this occurs in younger individuals with a coexisting mitral stenosis, the murmur of aortic stenosis may be mistaken for mitral regurgitation.

Diagnosis

This patient has mixed mitral valve and aortic valve disease (lesion) of rheumatic aetiology with a dominant mitral regurgitation as evidenced by the hyperdynamic circulation. The patient is in cardiac failure (functional status).

Questions

Mention a few causes of combined aortic and mitral valve disease.

- Rheumatic valvular disease.
- Infective endocarditis.
- Collagen degenerative disorder, e.g. Marfan's syndrome.
- Calcific changes in the aortic and mitral valve apparatus.

What are the indications for surgery?

- New York Heart Association (NYHA) class III status.
- Class II status where there is volume overload of the left ventricle, e.g. in severe aortic regurgitation with moderate mitral valve disease or severe mitral regurgitation with moderate aortic stenosis and regurgitation.

Note. The NYHA grading of cardiac status is:

Grade I – uncompromised.

Grade II – slightly compromised.

Grade III – moderately compromised.
Grade IV – severely compromised.

Robert Frye is contemporary Professor and Chair of the Department of Medicine, Mayo Clinic; his chief interest is cardiovascular diseases.

References

Stephenson LW, Edie RN, Harken AH & Edmunds LH, Jr (1984) Combined aortic and mitral valve replacement: changes in practice and prognosis. *Circulation* **69**: 640.
Terazi AK, Cokkinos DV, Leachman RD et al (1970) Combined mitral and aortic valve disease. *Am J Cardiol* **25**: 588.

CASE 8   Hypertension

Instruction

This patient has hypertension; would you like to examine her?

Salient features

Proceed as follows:

- Comment on cushingoid facies if present.
- Look for radiofemoral delay of coarctation of aorta.
- Palpate the apex for left ventricular hypertrophy.
- Look for signs of cardiac failure.
- Examine the fundus for changes of hypertensive retinopathy.
- Listen for renal artery bruit of renal artery stenosis.

- Tell the examiner that you would like to check urine for protein (renal failure) and sugar (associated diabetes).

Diagnosis

This patient has retinopathy (lesion) due to hypertension, which is probably renovascular (aetiology) as evidenced by the renal artery bruit. She probably has damage to other target organs (functional status).

Questions

How would you investigate a patient with hypertension in outpatients?

- Full blood count (FBC).

- Urine for sugar, albumin and specific gravity.
- Urea, electrolytes and serum creatinine.
- Fasting lipids, serum uric acid.
- ECG.
- Chest radiograph.

What are causes of hypertension?

- Unknown or idiopathic (in 90% of cases).
- Renal: glomerulonephritis, diabetic nephropathy, renal artery stenosis, pyelonephritis.
- Endocrine: Cushing's syndrome, steroid therapy, phaeochromocytoma.
- Others: coarctation of aorta, contraceptives, toxaemia of pregnancy.

How would you manage a patient with mild hypertension?

- General measures
    Diet: weight reduction in obese patients, low cholesterol diets for associated hyperlipidaemia, salt restriction.
    Stop smoking.
    Reduce alcohol consumption.
- Drug treatment
    Beta-blockers in non-smoking males.
    Bendrofluazide in women and male smokers.

What special investigations would you do to screen for an underlying cause?

- Renal digital subtraction angiography.
- 24-hour urinary catecholamines – at least three samples (phaeochromocytoma).
- Overnight dexamethasone suppression test.

Sir Stanley W Peart, Emeritus Professor of Medicine at St Mary's Hospital Medical School, London, purified and sequenced angiotensin II and was involved in pioneering work in the field of hypertension.
Victor Dzau, Professor of Cardiology at Stanford University, who has made major contributions to the genetics of cardiovascular disease and the pharmacology of angiotensin. In September 1995 he became Chairman of Medicine at Brigham and Women's Hospital.

References

Swales JD (1991) First line treatment in hypertension. *Br Med J* **301**: 1172.
Turnbull JM (1995) Is listening for abdominal bruits useful in the evaluation of hypertension. *JAMA* **274**: 1299–1301.

CASE 9   Atrial Fibrillation

Instruction

Examine this patient's pulse.

Salient features

- Irregularly irregular pulse (patients are often digitalized and in slow atrial fibrillation).

Proceed as follows:

- Look for:
  Malar flush (mitral stenosis).
  Mitral valvotomy scar.
  Warm hands, goitre, pretibial myxoedema (thyrotoxicosis).
- If you are not sure tell the examiner that you would like to differentiate from ventricular ectopics by exercising the patient – after exercise, ventricular ectopics diminish in frequency whereas there is no change in the rhythm of atrial fibrillation.
- Tell the examiner that you would like to look for the underlying cause:
  Examine the heart for mitral valvular lesion.
  Check the blood pressure for hypertension.
  Ask the patient for history of ischaemic heart disease.
  Check the patient's thyroid status for thyrotoxicosis.

Diagnosis

This patient has fast atrial fibrillation (lesion) which is commonly due to ischaemic heart disease (aetiology). The patient is short of breath, indicating that he may be in cardiac failure (functional status).

Questions

What are the common causes of atrial fibrillation?

- Mitral valvular disease in the young and middle aged.
- Ischaemic heart disease or hypertension in the elderly.
- Thyrotoxicosis (atrial fibrillation may be the only clinical feature in the elderly).
- Constrictive pericarditis.

Mention common sites of systemic embolization.

Brain, leg, kidney, superior mesenteric artery, coronary artery and spleen.

At the bedside how would you differentiate atrial fibrillation from multiple ventricular ectopics?

If the patient is not in heart failure, exercise the patient: after exercise ventricular ectopics tend to diminish in frequency whereas there is no change in the rhythm of atrial fibrillation.

Advanced-level Questions

Mention a few causes of irregularly irregular pulse.

- Atrial fibrillation.
- Multiple ventricular ectopics.
- Atrial flutter with varying block.
- Complete heart block (there is associated bradycardia).

In which congenital disorders is atrial fibrillation common?

Atrial septal defect, Ebstein's anomaly.

What do you understand by the term atrial fibrillation?

Lone atrial fibrillation occurs in the absence of cardiopulmonary disease or a history of hypertension and before the age of 60 years. Such patients have a low risk of stroke (0.5% per year).

How would you treat a patient with atrial fibrillation?

- Attempt to restore slow ventricular rate:
    In the hypertensive patient use calcium antagonists (verapamil, diltiazem).
    In thyroid disease use a beta-blocker (e.g. propranolol).
    In ischaemic heart disease use a beta-blocker or diltiazem, verapamil.
    In heart failure use digoxin or verapamil.
    In hypertrophic cardiomyopathy use a beta-blocker or calcium antagonists.
- Attempt to restore sinus rhythm by cardioversion if the following conditions apply:
    Left atrial size by echocardiogram is less than 4.5 cm (left atrial size greater than 4.5 cm is not associated with long-term maintenance of sinus rhythm).

Duration of the arrhythmia (acute atrial fibrillation is likely to remain in sinus rhythm).
- Anticoagulation with warfarin is advised for certain patients:
  Undergoing cardioversion (electrical or drug).
  With underlying mitral valve disease.
  In left ventricular failure.
  With cardiomyopathy.
  Above the age of 60 years.

Mention a few drugs used to restore sinus rhythm.

Procainamide, disopyramide or quinidine for 2–3 days restores sinus rhythm in up to 30% of patients.

What is the role of oral anticoagulants in chronic atrial fibrillation?

Non-rheumatic atrial fibrillation is an important risk factor for stroke, even though it is recognized that only 80% of strokes in such patients are due to embolism from the heart. Most patients with non-rheumatic atrial fibrillation should be anticoagulated with warfarin.

Is there any surgical method to restore sinus rhythm in atrial fibrillation?

A novel surgical technique, the Maze procedure, has recently been described in which multiple incisions are made in the atria to prevent re-entrant loops. This procedure is highly effective in preventing atrial fibrillation with only one patient out of 65 suffering a clinical recurrence of the arrhythmia 3 or more months after the procedure. Although the long-term outcome is not known, it remains a promising procedure when atrial fibrillation is not controlled by medical therapy or in those complicated by recurrent thromboembolism.

What do you know about holiday heart syndrome?

It is the occurrence of supraventricular arrhythmias, usually atrial fibrillation and atrial flutter, following an acute alcoholic binge in chronic alcoholics. These are usually transient.

It was James Mackenzie, a Scottish general practitioner working in Burnley, England, utilizing an ink-polygraph to record and label jugular venous pulses, who would pioneer the deciphering of normal and abnormal cardiac rhythms. His key observation that the jugular 'a' wave lost in a patient who went from a normal to an irregular rhythm provided the first insight into the mechanism of atrial fibrillation. In 1924, Willem Einthoven (1860–1927) of Leyden University, The Netherlands, was awarded the Nobel Prize for his discovery of the mechanism of electrocardiography.

In 1909, Lewis in England and Rothberger and Winterberg in Vienna, taking advantage of Einthoven's newly developed string galvanometer, were the first to establish electrocardiographically that auricular fibrillation was the cause of pulsus irregularis perpetuus.

References

Baliga RR & Webster J (1993) Preventing strokes in non-rheumatic atrial fibrillation. *Br J Hosp Med* **50**: 452–457.

Cox JL, Boineau JP, Schuessler RB et al (1991) Operations for atrial fibrillation. *Clin Cardiol* **14**: 827–834.

Pritchett ELC (1992) Management of atrial fibrillation. *N Engl J Med* **326**: 1264–1270.

Silverman ME (1994) From rebellious palpitations to the discovery of auricular fibrillation: contributions of Mackienzie, Lewis and Einthoven. *Am J Cardiol* **73**: 384–389.

CASE 10 Palpitations

Instruction

This patient has palpitations: would you like to ask her a few questions?

Salient features

Proceed as follows:

Ask the following questions:

- Are the palpitations regular or irregular?
- Is the onset abrupt (paroxysmal tachyarrhythmias)?
- How frequent are the palpitations?
- What is the duration of each episode?
- Is each episode followed by polyuria (seen in supraventricular tachycardia)?
- Is there any relation to exercise?
- What happens on standing (postural hypotension)?
- Are there any precipitating factors such as coffee, tea, alcohol or medications such as thyroid extract, ephedrine, aminophylline, monoamino oxidase inhibitors?
- Are there any associated symptoms such as chest pain or shortness of breath?

Note. Palpitations are a common complaint in up to 16% of outpatients. They are non-specific and in only 15% of patients do they correlate with cardiac arrhythmia.

Diagnosis

This patient has palpitations (lesion) accompanied by polyuria, indicating a supraventricular tachycardia (aetiology).

Questions

What are the causes?

- Extrasystole.
- Tachycardia or bradycardia.
- Drugs (see above).
- Other: thyrotoxicosis, hypoglycaemia, unaccustomed exertion, phaeo-chromocytoma, fever.
- Anxiety state (also known as da Costa's syndrome or cardiac neurosis).

How would you investigate a patient suspected of having a disorder of cardiac rhythm?

- 12-lead ECG (look for evidence of a rhythm disturbance and pre-excitation syndrome).
- Continuous ambulatory (Holter) echocardiography (many patients with palpitations may have stable sinus rhythm).

JM da Costa (1833–1900) was Professor of Medicine at Jefferson Medical College, Philadelphia.

References

Brugada P, Gursoy S, Bruguda J & Andries E (1993) Investigation of palpitations. *Lancet* **341**: 1254–1258.

Kopp DE & Wilber DJ (1992) Palpitations and arrhythmias. Separating the benign from the dangerous. *Postgrad Med* **91**: 241–244, 247–248, 251.

Weitz HH & Weinstock PJ (1995) Approach to the patient with palpitations. *Med Clin North Am* **79**: 449–456.

CASE 11 Slow Pulse Rate

Instruction

Examine this patient's pulse.

Salient features

- Pulse rate of less than 60 beats per minute.
- Pulse rate may be either regular or irregular.

Proceed as follows:

- If the pulse is irregular, tell the examiner that you would like to do the following:
    Get the patient to stand and then count his pulse rate (in complete heart block there is no increase in rate).
    Look at the JVP for cannon 'a' waves.
    Auscultate the heart for cannon first heart sound.
- Tell the examiner that you would like to take a drug history: beta-blockers, digoxin, verapamil.

Diagnosis

This patient has a complete heart block (lesion) probably due to ischaemic heart disease (aetiology) and is disabled by syncopal attacks (functional status).

Questions

What are the causes of sinus bradycardia?

- Physical fitness in athletes.
- Acute myocardial infarction.
- Drugs (beta-blockers, digitalis).
- Myxoedema.
- Obstructive jaundice.
- Increased intracranial pressure.
- Hypothermia.
- Hyperkalaemia.

Advanced-level Questions

What are the indications for temporary cardiac pacing in bradyarrhythmias?

- Symptomatic second- or third-degree heart block due to transient drug intoxication or electrolyte disturbance.
- Complete heart block, Mobitz II or bifascicular block in the setting of an acute myocardial infarct.
- Symptomatic sinus bradycardia, atrial fibrillation with slow ventricular response.

What are the indications for permanent pacing in bradyarrhythmias?

- Symptomatic congenital heart block.
- Symptomatic sinus bradycardia.
- Symptomatic second- or third-degree heart block.

Which drug would you use to treat sinus bradycardia seen in the setting of an acute myocardial infarction?

Intravenous atropine.

What you know about Stokes–Adams syndrome?

It refers to syncope or fits occurring during complete heart block.

W Stokes (1804–1878), Regius Professor of Medicine in Dublin, graduated from Edinburgh.
R Adams (1791–1875), Professor of Surgery in Dublin, was an authority on gout and arthritis.

CASE 12 Gallop Rhythm

Instruction

Listen to the precordium.
Examine this patient's heart.

Salient features

- Presence of an abnormal third or fourth heart sound with tachycardia (the presence of a normal third or fourth heart sound does not connote a gallop rhythm unless there is associated tachycardia).

Proceed as follows:

- Auscultate with the bell as third and fourth heart sounds are low pitched.

- Gallop rhythm due to third heart sound seems to sound like 'Kentucky', whereas that due to the fourth heart sound sounds like 'Tennessee'.

Note.
- A left ventricular third heart sound is best heard at the apex, whereas the right ventricular third heart sound is best heard along the left sternal border.
- In emphysematous patients the gallop is better heard when listening over the xiphoid or epigastric area.

Diagnosis

This patient has gallop rhythm (lesion) which indicates that he is in cardiac failure (functional status).

Questions

What is the expression used when both the third and fourth heart sounds are heard with tachycardia?

This is known as the summation gallop. It can sometimes be confused for a diastolic rumbling murmur.

Advanced-level Questions

What is the mechanism of production of the third heart sound?

It is due to rapid ventricular filling in early diastole.

What is the mechanism of production of the fourth heart sound?

It is due to vigorous contraction of the atria (atrial systole) and is hence heard towards the end of diastole.

How do you differentiate between the fourth heart sound, a split first heart sound and an ejection click?

The fourth heart sound is not heard when pressure is applied on the chest piece of the stethoscope, but pressure does not eliminate the ejection sound or the splitting of the first heart sound.

What are the causes of a third heart sound?

- Physiological: in normal children and young adults
- Pathological:

Heart failure.
Mitral regurgitation.

What are the implications of a third heart sound in patients with valvular heart disease?

- In patients with mitral regurgitation, they are common but do not necessarily reflect ventricular systolic dysfunction or increased filling pressure.
- In patients with aortic stenosis, third heart sounds are uncommon but usually indicate the presence of systolic dysfunction and raised filling pressure.

What are the causes of a fourth heart sound?

- Normal: in the elderly.
- Pathological:
    Acute myocardial infarction.
    Aortic stenosis.
    Hypertension (it is a constant finding in hypertension).

Note. The fourth heart sound does not denote heart failure unlike the S_3 gallop.

Potain credited Jean Baptiste Bouillaud (1786–1881), Professor of Medicine in Paris, as being the first person to describe gallop rhythm.
Pierre Carl Edouard Potain (1825–1901), Parisian physician, was the first to distinguish between various types of gallop in a short account titled 'Théorie du Bruit de Gallop' in 1885.

References

Folland ED, Kriegel BJ, Henderson WG, Hammermeister KE, Sethi GK & The Veterans Affairs Cooperative Study on Valvular Heart Disease (1992) *N Engl J Med* **327**: 458–462.
Rolleston JD (1931) Jean Baptiste Bouillaud. *Proc R Soc Med* **24**: 1253–1931.

CASE 13 **Angina Pectoris**

Instruction

This patient is suspected to have angina pectoris. Would you like to ask her a few questions to confirm these suspicions.

Salient features

Proceed as follows:

- Have you ever had any pain or discomfort in the chest?
- How would you describe the chest discomfort (heavy, burning, tightness, stabbing, pressure)?
- Do you get this on walking at ordinary pace on the level or does it come when you walk uphill or hurry?
- When you get the pain/discomfort, do you stop, slow down or continue at the same pace?
- Does the pain/discomfort go away when you stand still? (It is typically relieved by rest or nitroglycerin within 10 minutes.)
- Where do you get this pain? (Because angina is a visceral sensation, it is poorly localized and, therefore, patients rarely point to the location of their discomfort with one finger.)
- Does it radiate elsewhere (e.g. arms, jaw, epigastrium)?
- Does food or cold weather bring on the pain?
- Tell the examiner that you would like to ask about risk factors such as smoking, diabetes, hypertension, family history of ischaemic heart disease?

Diagnosis

This patient has angina pectoris (lesion) which is due to atherosclerotic coronary artery disease (aetiology). She is in Canadian Cardiovascular Society functional class II (functional status).

Questions

How is angina graded by the Canadian Cardiovascular Society?

There are four functional classes:

- Class I: Angina occurs only with strenous or rapid or prolonged exertion.
- Class II: There is slight limitation of ordinary activity (e.g. climbing more than one flight of ordinary stairs at a normal pace and in normal conditions).
- Class III: There is marked limitation of ordinary activity (e.g. climbing more than one flight in normal conditions).
- Class IV: Inability to carry out any physical activity without discomfort – anginal syndrome may be present at rest.

What is the mechanism of angina pectoris?

It is commonly due to increased myocardial oxygen demand triggered by physical activity, but it can also be caused by transient decreases in oxygen delivery due to coronary vasospasm. Unstable angina is due to non-occlusive intracoronary thrombi.

How would you treat a patient with chronic stable angina pectoris?

- Aspirin has been shown to reduce the incidence of non-fatal myocardial infarction and the overall incidence of cardiac events, although overall death rate and the incidence of fatal myocardial infarction were similar to those obtained with placebo in the Swedish Angina Pectoris Aspirin Trial (SAPAT) study.
- Antianginal agents: nitroglycerin, beta-blockers.

Advanced-level Questions

What is the role of percutaneous transluminal coronary angioplasty (PTCA) in the management of patients with chronic stable angina?

- The ACME (Angioplasty Compared to Medicine) study showed that PTCA can offer better symptomatic relief than medical therapy in patients with single-vessel coronary artery disease, but is a much more expensive procedure and is associated with complications (including emergency and elective coronary bypass and second PTCA).
- The RITA (Randomized Intervention Treatment of Angina) study compared PTCA with coronary artery bypass graft (CABG) and found that both procedures have similar prognostic implications with risk of death or myocardial infarction similar in the two groups, but more patients in the PTCA group required a second revascularization procedure and more antianginal therapy.

What is the significance and the mechanism of postprandial angina?

The presence of postprandial angina indicates severe coronary artery disease; one mechanism is 'intramyocardial steal' with blood being distributed from the stenotic territories to the normal territories. It is due to the carbohydrate content of the meal and can be ameliorated by prior treatment with octreotide, which prevents postprandial vasodilatation of the superior mesenteric artery.

What do you understand by the term unstable angina?

This includes patients with more severe or frequent angina superimposed on chronic stable angina, angina at rest or minimal exertion, or angina of new onset (within 1 month) which is brought about by minimal exertion.

It is a potentially dangerous condition and patients should be admitted to a coronary care unit and begun on antianginal therapy including beta-blockers, aspirin and intravenous nitrates. Intravenous heparin should be started in patients with rest angina of 48 hour's duration and in those with chest pain and ischaemic ECG changes on admission. Most patients stabilize with this treatment, although some may require intra-aortic balloon counterpulsation before cardiac catheterization. A monoclonal antibody $7E_3$ against platelet glycoprotein IIb/IIIa, which prevents platelet adhesion and degranulation, is undergoing evaluation in the treatment of unstable angina.

What is Prinzmetal's angina?

It is angina occurring at rest, unpredictably, and associated with transient ST segment elevation on the ECG. Coronary vasospasm is the cause often in the presence of atherosclerosis.

How is exercise testing useful in determining the prognosis of chest pain?

A study at Duke University used exercise testing to determine high- and low-risk subsets in patients with chest pain suggestive of ischaemic heart disease:

- Low-risk subset: subjects who could complete 9 minutes of exercise using the Bruce protocol without evidence of ischaemic ST segment changes and achieve a maximal sinus heart rate in excess of 160 beats per minute. These were found to have a 1-year survival rate of 99% and a 4-year survival rate of 93%. This means that cardiac catheterization and CABG can be deferred.
- High-risk subset: those who were forced to stop exercising in stages I or II (under 6 minutes); survival rate was 85% at 1 year and 63% at 4 years.

What do you understand by the term syndrome X?

- Syndrome X, or microvascular angina, is the presence of classic angina and ST depression on exercise stress testing and a normal coronary angiogram in the absence of any other demonstrable cardiac abnormalities.
- Reaven's syndrome or 'endocrine' syndrome X is the association of insulin resistance, hypertension, and increased very low density lipoprotein (VLDL) and decreased high density lipoprotein (HDL) cholesterol concentrations in the plasma.

L David Hillis, contemporary Professor of Cardiology and Vice-Chair, Department of Medicine, University of Texas Southwestern Medical School, Dallas, whose chief interest is coronary artery disease.

Coronary artery bypass grafting was introduced by RG Favalaro in 1969.

Balloon angioplasty was introduced by Arthur Gruntzig, a Swiss cardiologist, in 1977.

References

Baliga RR, Rosen SD, Camici PG, Oakley CM & Kooner JS (1994) Regional myocardial blood flow in response to food ingestion in post-prandial angina. *Circulation* **90**: I448.

Baliga RR, Burden LJ & Kooner JS (1995) Reduction in exercise threshold to post-prandial angina occurs after carbohydrate, but not fat or protein, and independently of myocardial oxygen consumption. *J Am Coll Cardiol* **25**: 210A.

Favalaro RG (1969) Saphenous vein graft in the surgical treatment of coronary artery disease: operative technique. *J Thorac Cardiovasc Surg* **58**: 178–185.

Gruntzig A (1978) Transluminal dilatation of coronary artery stenosis. *Lancet* **i**: 263.

 Myocardial Infarction

CASE 14

Instruction

This patient has had a myocardial infarction; would you like to examine him?

Salient features

Proceed as follows

- Hands: nicotine staining of fingers.
- Pulse: check pulse rate and rhythm.
- JVP may be raised in cardiac failure or right ventricular infarction.
- Eyes: look for arcus senilis, xanthelasma.
- Cardiac apex: look for double apical impulse.
- Auscultate for fourth heart sound, pericardial rub, pansystolic murmur of papillary muscle dysfunction (or ventricular septal defect).

- Tell the examiner that you would like to examine the following:
  The chest for crackles.
  The abdomen for tender liver of cardiac failure.
  The legs for deep vein thrombosis.

Diagnosis

This patient with myocardial infarction (aetiology) has papillary muscle dysfunction (lesion) and is in fast atrial fibrillation (functional status).

Questions

What is Levine's sign?

In acute myocardial infarction the patient often describes the pain by illustrating a clenched fist.

How would you manage a patient with uncomplicated myocardial infarction in the coronary care unit?

- Bed rest.
- Oxygen.
- Pain relief.
- Sedation.
- Soluble aspirin.
- Intravenous thrombolytics if no contraindications.

What are the complications of myocardial infarction?

- Rhythm disorders: tachycardia, bradycardia, ventricular ectopics, ventricular fibrillation, atrial fibrillation, atrial tachycardia.
- Heart failure: acute pulmonary oedema.
- Circulatory failure: cardiogenic shock.
- Infarction of papillary muscle: mitral regurgitation and acute pulmonary oedema.
- Rupture of the interventricular septum.
- Thromboembolism – cerebral or peripheral.
- Venous thrombosis.
- Pericarditis.
- Dressler's syndrome – characterized by persistent **p**yrexia, **p**ericarditis, **p**leurisy. It was first described in 1956 when Dressler recognized that chest pain following myocardial infarction is not due to coronary artery insufficiency.

Advanced-level Questions

What is a silent myocardial infarct?

A painless infarct, common in diabetics and the elderly; it may present with complications of myocardial infarction.

What are the contraindications of streptokinase therapy?

- History of bleeding.
- Stroke.
- Severe hypertension.
- Recent surgery or other invasive procedure within the previous 10 days.
- Proliferative diabetic retinopathy.
- Pregnancy.
- If the patient has received streptokinase in the previous 6 months.
- Concurrent use of anticoagulants.
- Concurrent terminal illness.

Which thrombolytic agent is preferred?

There are three thrombolytic agents (which reduce mortality) commonly available in the UK: streptokinase, anistreplase and tissue plasminogen activator (tPA), of which streptokinase is the cheapest and tPA the most expensive. In ISIS-3 (Third International Study of Infarct Survival) all three agents were found to be equally effective and in the GISSI-2 (Gruppo Italiano per lo Studio della Sopravvivena nell Infarto Micocardioco) study both tPA and steptokinase were equally effective. However, in both these studies there was an increased risk of haemorrhage with tPA. In the GUSTO (Global Utilization of Streptokinase and Tissue Plasminogen Activator) trial, tPA given in an accelerated manner was particularly useful in young men with anterior wall infarction.

What is the use of heparin with thrombolysis?

In the ISIS-3 and GISSI-2 studies heparin therapy was not beneficial with streptokinase or anistreplase, and it is believed that it may even be harmful. The GUSTO trial showed that, with tPA, early intravenous heparin results in a further reduction in the mortality rate compared with that found with a combination of heparin and streptokinase.

What is the benefit of late administration of thrombolytic therapy?

ISIS-2 showed benefit for up to 24 hours (after the onset of symptoms) with thrombolysis, but more recent studies – the LATE (Late Assessment of Thrombolytic Therapy) and EMRAS (Estudio Multicentrico Estrepto-quinasa Repbulicas de America del Sur) – have shown no benefit for treatment given beyond 12 hours.

What is the role of pre-hospital thrombolysis?

Two studies – the GREAT (Grampian Region Early Administration of Thrombolysis) and EMIP (European Myocardial Infarction Project) – showed that a single bolus dose of antistreplase reduced the total mortality rate. These results suggest that early thrombolysis has greater benefit, and hence the importance in many hospitals for 'door to needle time'.

What is the role of angiotensin converting enzyme (ACE) inhibitors following myocardial infarction?

- The AIRE (Acute Infarction Ramipril Efficacy) study showed that ramipril had a beneficial effect as early as 30 days; at 15 months the mortality rate in the study group was lower than in the placebo group.
- In the SAVE (Survival and Ventricular Enlargement) study ACE inhibitors were used in asymptomatic patients with ejection fraction lower than 40% following myocardial infarction. In this study there was no benefit during the first year, but after a mean follow-up of 3.5 years the survival rate in patients receiving enalapril was 25% compared with 20%. The ISIS-4 and GISSI-3 studies have confirmed the results of the AIRE and SAVE studies. The CONSENSUS-2 (Co-operative North Scandinavian Enalapril Survival Study) was stopped because the condition of two patients treated with enalapril worsened compared with that of those in the placebo group, but in this study the drug was started within 24 hours of infarction. It appears that it is not prudent to initiate therapy within the first 24–48 hours.

What is the role of primary angioplasty in acute infarction?

Three recent prospective randomized trials have compared the efficacy of immediate angioplasty as an alternative to thrombolytic therapy. In all these studies angioplasty resulted in both lower mortality rates and a reduction in the incidence of recurrent ischaemic events. Angioplasty also led to shorter hospital stay, fewer re-admissions and lower follow-up costs. However, the major limitation of this approach is the access to both facilities and personnel to carry out the procedure.

Why is the Asian population in Britain susceptible to premature myocardial infarction?

Premature ischaemic heart disease in migrants from the Indian subcontinent is associated with insulin resistance. The site of this defective insulin action has been localized to the skeletal muscle by means of positron emission tomography.

What is the role of troponins in the diagnosis of myocardial infarction?

Raised concentrations of myocardial regulatory protein troponin I are highly specific for myocardial injury. Estimation of troponin I concentration may be particularly useful in patients with acute or chronic skeletal muscle disease or in those with renal failure in whom the CK-MB (MB isoenzyme of creatine kinase) level may be raised in the absence of myocardial infarction. The measurement of troponin I is a sensitive and specific method (more specific than CK-MB) in the setting of perioperative myocardial infarction. Troponin T is also useful because it has a large diagnostic window, as it is increased from 12 hours to 10 days after myocardial infarction.

What do you know about right ventricular infarction?

Right ventricular infarction presents with retrosternal chest discomfort, nausea, vomiting and diaphoresis, unlike left ventricular infarction which presents with dyspnoea. On examination in right ventricular infarction, there is a raised jugular venous pressure with no evidence of pulmonary congestion; the patient often has a low cardiac output with hypotension. The patient typically presents with ST elevation in the inferior leads (II, III and aVF) and in one or more right-sided leads, particularly V_{4R}. The cornerstones of therapy include restoration of infarct artery patency, intravascular volume expansion and inotropic support.

What do you know about the open infarct-related coronary artery hypothesis?

This hypothesis, championed by Braunwald, holds that early reperfusion of the infarct-related coronary artery results in myocardial salvage which preserves left ventricular function and is responsible for improved survival. This idea led to the development of thrombolysis in the treatment of myocardial infarction.

Valentin Fuster is contemporary Professor of Cardiology at Mount Sinai Hospital, New York University. He graduated in Spain, did his PhD in Edinburgh, and was Professor of Cardiology at The Mayo Clinic and Harvard Medical School. His main interests include coronary artery disease.

Reference

Baliga RR, Lammertsma A, Rhodes CJ, Aitman TJ, Scott J & Kooner JS (1995) Positron emission tomography localises insulin resistance to skeletal muscle in premature coronary heart disease. *Circulation* **92**: I16.

CASE 15 Jugular Venous Pulse

Instruction

Examine this patient's neck.
Examine this patient's cardiovascular system.

Salient features

- The JVP is raised . . . cm above the angle of Louis (manubriosternal angle). Remember that the JVP may be raised to the level of the ear lobes.

Proceed as follows:

- Comment on the waveform (timing it with the carotid pulse):
  'v' waves of tricuspid regurgitation.
  Cannon waves of heart block.
  Absent 'a' waves in atrial fibrillation (irregular carotid pulse).
  Large 'a' waves of pulmonary hypertension, pulmonary stenosis, tricuspid stenosis.
- Tell the examiner that you would like to look for other signs of heart failure:
  Basal crackles.
  Dependent oedema (ankle and sacral oedema).
  Tender hepatomegaly.

Diagnosis

This patient has raised jugular venous pulse with 'v' waves (lesion) due to tricuspid regurgitation and is in heart failure (functional status).

Questions

What are the causes of a raised JVP?

- Congestive cardiac failure.
- Cor pulmonale.
- Tricuspid regurgitation (prominent 'v' waves)
- Tricuspid stenosis (prominent 'a' waves).
- Complete heart block (cannon waves).
- Non-pulsatile neck veins seen in superior venal caval obstruction (see page 563).

How do you differentiate jugular venous pulsations from carotid artery pulsations?

Unlike the arterial pulse, the venous pulse has a definite upper level which falls during inspiration and changes with posture. The venous pulse is seen to have a dominant inward motion, towards the midline (the 'y' descent), whereas the arterial pulse exhibits a dominant outward wave. The venous pulse is better seen than felt, whereas the arterial pulse is readily felt by very slight pressure of the clinician's finger.

Advanced-level Questions

What do you know about the waveforms in the jugular pulse?

- The 'a' wave is due to atrial contraction and is presystolic.
- The 'c' wave is due to closure of the tricuspid valve.
- The 'v' wave is due to venous return to the right heart (*not* due to ventricular contraction).
- The 'x' descent is due to atrial relaxation.
- The 'y' descent is produced by opening of the tricuspid valve and rapid inflow of blood into the right ventricle.

What is Kussmaul's sign?

Normally there is an inspiratory decrease in JVP. In constrictive pericarditis there is an inspiratory increase in JVP. Kussmaul's sign is also seen in severe right heart failure regardless of aetiology. It is caused by the inability of the heart to accept the increase in right ventricular volume without a marked increase in the filling pressure.

Adolf Kussmaul (1822–1902) was Professor of Medicine successively at Heidelberg, Enlargen, Freiburg and Strasbourg, and coined the term 'polyarteritis nodosa'. Kussmaul breathing is deep sighing respiration seen when the arterial pH is low.

Reference

Kussmaul A (1873) Uber Schwielige Mediastino-pericarditis und Den Paradoxen Pulse. *Berl Klin Wochnschr* **10**: 433.

CASE 16 Congestive Cardiac Failure

Instruction

Examine this patient's cardiovascular system.

Salient features

- Raised jugular venous pulse.
- Third heart sound.
- Tender hepatomegaly and ascites.
- Pitting leg oedema.

Proceed as follows:

- Tell the examiner that you would like to take a history of:
  Dyspnoea on exertion.
  Past history of hypertension, ischaemic heart disease or cardiomyopathy.

Diagnosis

This patient has congestive cardiac failure due to hypertension and is severely limited with NYHA grade 4 dyspnoea.

Advanced-level Questions

What is diastolic dysfunction?

It is excessive stiffness of the heart resulting in an inability of the heart to fill properly. This is in contrast to systolic dysfunction, where contractility is impaired. Patients have clinical features of left heart failure but normal systolic function by echocardiography or radionuclide ventriculography. It is a feature of hypertrophic cardiomyopathy, severe left ventricular hypertrophy (e.g. aortic stenosis or hypertension) and restrictive cardiomyopathy (e.g. amyloidosis). Treatment is directed towards the underlying cause.

What is the role of vasodilators in the management of chronic heart failure?

Three trials have shown the benefit of vasodilators in heart failure:

- CONSENSUS (Co-operative North Scandinavian Enalapril Survival Study), which showed clear improvement in patients receiving enalapril compared with those who received placebo in severe heart failure.

- SOLVD (Studies of Left Ventricular Dysfunction), which had a 'treatment' wing for patients with mild to moderate heart failure who received enalapril. These patients had increased survival compared with those on placebo. The 'prevention' wing of the study showed no prognostic benefit in patients with asymptomatic left ventricular dysfunction (i.e. with an ejection fraction lower than 35%) for enalapril. However, these patients were less likely to progress to heart failure or to require hospital admission.
- The VeHeFT-II study, which compared enalapril with hydralazine–isosorbide nitrate. Although both were beneficial, enalapril was superior. Hydralazine-isosorbide nitrate is, however, useful when angiotensin converting enzyme (ACE) inhibitors are contraindicated.

What is the role of digoxin in heart failure in sinus rhythm?

Recently it has been shown in two separate studies that withdrawal of digoxin results in a worsening of exercise capacity, a more rapid and more frequent failure of medical therapy, and a fall in left ventricular ejection fraction: PROVED (Prospective Randomized Study of Ventricular Failure and the Efficacy of Digoxin) and the RADIANCE (Randomized Assessment of the Effect of Digoxin on the Inhibitors of Angiotensin Converting Enzyme).

What are the indications for heart transplantation?

When patients are refractory to treatment, both medical and surgical (such as valve replacement), and are in New York Heart Association class IV, then they are unlikely to survive for 1 year and should be considered for heart transplantation. The survival rate is about 69% at 5 years, although most patients have one episode of rejection and 25% have multiple episodes. They are also prone to accelerated coronary atherosclerosis.

What is the role of beta-blockers in heart failure?

Beta-blockers are generally contraindicated in heart failure, but recent evidence suggests they may be beneficial in dilated cardiomyopathy. An intact sympathetic nervous system is required for the 'slipping' of myocardial cells to cause ventricular dilatation. Beta-blockade prevents this dilatation and actually improves left ventricular function in dilated cardiomyopathy; however, its effects on survival are not known.

Thomas W Smith, contemporary Professor of Cardiology at Harvard Medical School and Chief of Cardiology at Brigham and Women's Hospital, first developed the radioimmunoassay for digitalis and has made several contributions to the pharmacology of digitalis and cardiac failure.

In 1967 Christiaan Barnard, a South African surgeon, was the first to perform cardiac transplantation in humans.

CASE 17 Infective Endocarditis

Instruction

This patient is suspected to have endocarditis; would you like to examine him?

Salient features

Proceed as follows:

- Look for the following signs:
    Anaemia.
    Clubbing.
    Splinter haemorrhages in the nails.
    Osler's nodes (see below).
    Janeway lesions (see below).
    Petechiae – conjuctival and skin.
- Listen to the heart for murmurs and look for signs of cardiac failure.
- Tell the examiner that you would like to do the following:
    Examine the fundus for Roth's spots.
    Examine the abdomen for splenomegaly.
    Test urine for microscopic haematuria.
    Take a history of recent dental procedures.
    Remember that ostium secundum atrial septal defects almost never have infective endocarditis.

Diagnosis

This patient has Janeway lesions and Roth's spots (lesions) confirming infective endocarditis, and is in severe heart failure (functional status).

Questions

How would you investigate such a patient?

- Test the urine for microscopic haematuria.
- Take a full blood count (FBC) to show normocytic, normochromic anaemia and raised white cell count.

- Test for raised erythrocyte sedimentation rate (ESR).
- Blood culture: take three samples from different sites in 24 hours.
- Echocardiography may show vegetations. A negative study does not rule out endocarditis as vegetations less than 3–4 mm in size cannot be detected. Furthermore, all the leaflets of the aortic, tricuspid and pulmonary valves may not be visualized in every patient.

What are the major manifestations of bacterial endocarditis?

- Manifestations of a systemic infection: fever, weight loss, pallor, splenomegaly.
- Manifestations of intravascular phenomenon: cardiac failure, changing murmurs, petechiae, Roth's spots, Osler's nodes, Janeway lesions, splinter haemorrhages, stroke, infarction of viscera, mycotic aneurysm.
- Manifestations of immunological reactions: arthralgia, finger clubbing, uraemia.

Name the common organisms found in infective endocarditis?

Streptococcus viridans, Staphylococcus aureus, Strep. faecalis, fungi.

What precautions would you take to prevent bacterial endocarditis?

Antibiotic prophylaxis before any dental, gastrointestinal, urological or gynaecological procedure. It is recommended in rheumatic valvular disease, most congenital heart lesions (except uncomplicated atrial septal defect of secundum type), valvular aortic stenosis, prosthetic heart valve, previously documented infective endocarditis and calcified mitral valve annulus.

How would you treat a patient suspected to have endocarditis?

Until the bacteriology results are available, with intravenous benzylpenicillin and gentamicin. In severely ill patients intravenous cloxacillin would be added to this regimen.

What are splinter haemorrhages caused by?

The probable cause is embolism to linear capillaries in the nail bed.

What are Osler's nodes?

Tender, erythematous, pea-sized nodules seen in the pulp of the fingers.

They are caused by inflammation around the site of the infected emboli lodged in distal arterioles.

What are Janeway lesions?

Flat, non-tender red spots found on the palms and soles; they blanch on pressure.

Advanced-level Questions

Mention a few prognostic factors.

- Heart failure.
- Non-streptococcal endocarditis, especially *Staph. aureus*, fungal endocarditis.
- Infection of prosthetic valve.
- Elderly patients.
- Valve ring or myocardial abscess.

Mention a few conditions that can simulate clinical manifestations of infective endocarditis.

- Atrial myxoma.
- Non-bacterial endocarditis.
- Systemic lupus erythematosus (SLE).
- Sickle cell disease.

What do you know of prosthetic valve endocarditis (PVE)?

About 3% of patients will develop PVE by the end of the first year of valve replacement; thereafter, the incidence is lower. PVE is classified into two groups:

- Early: occurring within 2 months of surgery. It develops as a result of intraoperative contamination of the prosthetic valve or as a consequence of a postoperative nosocomial infection, such as sternotomy infection, postoperative pneumonia, urinary tract infection or intravenous catheter-related insertion. The clinical features may be masked by the ordinary events in the postoperative course or by another infection. Cutaneous signs are not common.
- Late PVE: develops more than 2 months after valve surgery. It can occur after transient bacteraemia as in minor skin or upper respiratory tract infections or following dental or urinary manipulations. The non-cardiac manifestations resemble those of native valve infective endocarditis.

Although this classification is convenient, the high prevalence of *Staph. epidermidis* and diphtheroids among patients suggests that this division is not absolute.

What are the complications of infective endocarditis?

- Cardiac: cardiac failure, conduction disturbances due to abscesses in ventricular septum.
- Renal: flank pain and haematuria.
- Neurological: cerebral embolization.
- Mycotic aneurysms.

What are the indications for surgery?

- Positive blood cultures or relapse after several days of the best available antibiotic therapy indicates the need for valve replacement.
- Drainage of myocardial or valve ring abscesses.
- Patients with aortic valve endocarditis who develop second- or third-degree heart block.
- Prosthetic valve replacement for non-streptococcal endocarditis, valve dysfunction, valve dehiscence or myocardial invasion.
- Development of a new aneurysm of the sinus of Valsalva.
- Fungal endocarditis.

What do you understand by the term 'marantic endocarditis'?

Marantic or Libman–Sacks endocarditis is seen in SLE and is a post-mortem diagnosis. It is rarely clinical significant.

Sir William Osler (1849–1919) was successively a Professor of Medicine in Montreal, Pennsylvania, Baltimore and Oxford. He was reputed to be a brilliant clinician and educationist.
M Roth (1839–1914), Professor of Pathology in Basel, Switzerland.
EG Janeway (1841–1911) followed Austin Flint as Professor of Medicine at Bellevue Hospital, New York.
E Libman (1872–1946), US physician.
B Sacks (1873–1939), US physician who wrote on Hindu medicine.

CASE 18   Prosthetic Heart Valves

Instruction

Listen to this patient's heart.

Salient features

- *Mitral* valve prostheses can be recognized by their site, metallic first heart sound, normal second heart sound and metallic opening snap. Systolic murmurs are often also present and it is important to note that this does *not* indicate valve malfunction. Diastolic flow murmurs may be heard normally over the disc valves.
- *Aortic* valve prostheses may be recognized by their site, normal first heart sound and metallic second heart sound.
- Both *mitral and aortic* valves may be replaced and both the first and second heart sounds will be metallic. The presence of a systolic murmur does not indicate valve dysfunction. However, the presence of an early diastolic murmur indicates a malfunctioning aortic valve.

Note. Comment on the mid-sternal, vertical thoracotomy scar, and state whether or not the metallic valve sounds are audible to the unaided ear (they are most often audible). Some mechanical valves cause so many clicks that it may not be possible to determine which valve has been replaced solely by auscultation. Porcine and cadaveric heterografts do not cause metallic clicking or plopping sounds.

Diagnosis

This patient has both first and second heart sounds with a metallic quality, indicating that both mitral and aortic valves are artificial valves (lesion) and the patient is not in heart failure (functional status).

Questions

What are the complications of prosthetic valves?

- Thromboembolism.
- Valve dysfunction, including valve leakage, valve dehiscence and valve obstruction due to thrombosis and clogging.
- Bleeding (such as upper gastrointestinal haemorrhage) due to anti-coagulants.
- Haemolysis at valve, causing anaemia.
- Endocarditis which carries a mortality rate of up to 60%; patients

should be urgently referred to a tertiary cardiothoracic centre (see
page 51).
- Structural dysfunction: fracture, poppet escape, cuspal tear, calcification.
- Non-structural dysfunction: paravalvular leak, suture/tissue entrapment,
  noise.

What are causes of anaemia in such a patient?

- Bleeding due to anticoagulants.
- Haemolytic anaemia.
- Secondary to bacterial endocarditis.

What are the advantages of a porcine heart valve?

There is no need for chronic anticoagulation and hence it is safe in women
of childbearing age and in the elderly.

What are the complications of a porcine heart valve?

- Degeneration with time.
- Calcification.

Advanced-level Questions

What are the indications for valve replacement?

- Mitral stenosis (see page 6).
- Mitral regurgitation (see page 11).
- Aortic regurgitation (see page 17).
- Aortic stenosis (see page 22).

What are the different kinds of mechanical valves?

Mechanical valves:

- The Starr–Edwards valve is a caged ball device and, because blood
  flows around the ball, there is a high incidence of haemolysis. This
  valve was introduced in 1960.
- The Bjork–Shiley pivoted single-tilting disc valve has laminar flow and
  hence a lower incidence of haemolysis. It was introduced in 1969.
- The St Jude valve is a double-tilting disc valve.

Xenografts:

- Porcine valves (Carpentier–Edwards, Hancock and Wessex).

- Pericardial valves mounted on a frame (Ionescu–Shiley, Hancock).

Homografts:

- These are cadaveric aortic or pulmonary valves. Homografts are considered the valve of first choice in a young patient requiring aortic valve replacement. They are useful in replacing infected aortic valves as they are more resistant to re-infection than other prosthetic valves.

What kind of valve would you use to replace the mitral valve?

Mechanical prosthesis. However, patients in whom the risk posed by anticoagulants is unacceptably high may receive a bioprosthesis, but at the increased risk of further operation at a later date.

What kind of valve would you use to replace the aortic valve?

Mechanical valves in younger patients in whom the risk of porcine valve failure is higher and for whom durability of the valve is of paramount importance. Porcine valves may be considered for elderly patients whose life expectancy may not exceed that of the prosthesis used.

Why are mechanical valves increasingly preferred over bioprosthetic valves?

Two randomized controlled trials have shown a lower rate of reoperation with mechanical prostheses than with porcine prostheses, and a smaller increased risk of anticoagulant-related bleeding.

What do you know about the convexo-concave model for the Bjork–Shiley prosthesis?

This was a modification of the previously reliable design which resulted in the strut retaining the tilting disc becoming liable to fracture several years after implantation, causing fatality. All Bjork–Shiley valves manufactured after 1975 have a radio-opaque ring marker in the edge of a tilting disc. This ring marker is missing if the strut is fractured. The disc may be spotted in the peripheral circulation. About two-thirds of the patients with strut fracture die acutely. The risk of strut fracture is 7 per 10 000 per year, but the risk of another mitral valve replacement exceeds this. This risk is greatest in patients with a large-size mitral prosthesis (31 and 33 mm) and a weld date between 1 January 1981 and 30 July 1982.

Is there any difference between the lifespan of a porcine mitral prosthesis and a porcine aortic prosthesis?

Porcine mitral bioprostheses usually fail after about 7 years whereas those in the aortic position fail in about 10 years owing to degeneration of the valve leaflets. In younger patients, these prostheses tend to degenerate more rapidly.

Which patients should receive a bioprosthetic valve?

- Those unable to take anticoagulants and those not expected to live longer than the predicted lifespan of the prosthesis.
- Patients over the age of 70 years who require an aortic valve replacement as the rate of degeneration is relatively slow in these patients.

In a woman of childbearing age, which kind of valve – bioprosthetic or mechanical – do you prefer?

Until recently, bioprosthetic valves were advocated in women of childbearing age to avoid the risks of warfarin on the fetus. More recently, it has been found that the risk of fetal abnormalities is very low in pregnant women receiving warfarin, although there is an increased risk of spontaneous abortion. Also there appears to be an accelerated risk of bioprosthetic valve degeneration during pregnancy. Thus the risks of spontaneous abortion have to be weighed against the operative mortality rate of 10% during reoperation following valve failure. Increasingly it is believed that, if valve replacement is needed, a mechanical prosthesis should be used.

If a patient with atrial fibrillation requires a prosthetic mitral valve, which kind of valve would you prefer?

A mechanical valve, as these patients need warfarin treatment for atrial fibrillation.

Note. The first aortic valve replacement (caged ball device) was performed by Dr Dwight Harken in March 1960 at Peter Bent Brigham Hospital in Boston. Shortly thereafter, Dr Nina Braunwald, at the National Institutes for Health, USA, performed a total mitral valve replacement with an artificial flexible leaflet valve. A Starr and ML Edwards, both US physicians.

References

Bloomfield P, Wheatley DJ, Prescott RJ & Miller HC (1991) Twelve year comparison of Bjork–Shiley mechanical heart valve with porcine bioprosthesis. *N Engl J Med* **324**: 573–579. (This study concluded that survival with an intact valve was better in patients with the Bjork–Shiley spherical tilting disc valve than in those with porcine valves, but use of the former carries an increased risk of bleeding due to anticoagulants.)

Hammermeister KE, Sethi GK, Henderson WG, Oprian C, Tai K & Rahimtoola S (1993) A comparison of outcomes in men 11 years after heart valve replacement with a mechanical valve or bioprosthesis. *N Engl J Med* **328**: 1289–1296.

Sbarouni E & Oakley SM (1994) Outcome of pregnancy in women with valve prostheses. *Br Heart J* **71**: 196–201.

Turpie AG, Gent M, Laupacis A et al (1993) A comparison of aspirin with placebo in patients treated with warfarin after heart-valve replacement. *N Engl J Med* **329**: 524–529.

CASE 19   Tricuspid Regurgitation

Instruction

Examine this patient's heart.
Examine this patient's cardiovascular system.

Salient features

- Peripheral cyanosis.
- Large 'v' waves in the jugular venous pulse.
- Left parasternal heave.
- Palpable or loud P_2.
- Pansystolic murmur at the left lower sternal border which increases in inspiration – Carvallo's sign.
- Right ventricular third heart sound may be present.
- Atrial fibrillation may be present.

Proceed as follows:

Look for:

- Mid-diastolic murmur of mitral stenosis.
- Systolic pulsations of an enlarged liver.
- Ascites and ankle oedema.

Diagnosis

This patient has tricuspid regurgitation (lesion) secondary to chronic lung disease and cor pulmonale (aetiology of the lesion) and is in cardiac failure (functional status).

Questions

What are the causes of tricuspid regurgitation?

- Functional:
    Pulmonary hypertension.
    Congestive cardiac failure.
- Rheumatic (associated with mitral and/or aortic valve disease).
- Right heart endocarditis as in drug addicts.
- Uncommon causes: carcinoid syndrome, Ebstein's anomaly, endomyo-cardial fibrosis, infarction of right ventricular papillary muscles, tricuspid valve prolapse, blunt trauma to the heart.

How would you treat organic tricuspid regurgitation?

Surgically:
    Valve plication or annuloplasty.
    Valve replacement.

JMR Carvallo, Mexican cardiologist who worked in Mexico City.

References

McMichael J & Shillingford JP (1957) The role of valvular incompetence in heart failure. *Br Med J* **1**: 537.

Rivero-Carvallo JM (1946) Signo para el diagnostico de las insuficiencias tricuspideas. *Arch Inst Cardiol Mex* **16**: 531.

York PG & Popp RL (1984) Non-invasive estimation of right ventricular systolic presssure by Doppler ultrasound in patients with tricuspid regurgitation. *Circulation* **70**: 657.

CASE 20 Mitral Valve Prolapse

Instruction

Examine this patient's heart.

Salient features

- Mid-systolic click followed by late or mid-systolic mumur.

Note. Squatting will bring the click closer to the second heart sound and decrease the duration of the murmur. A Valsalva manoeuvre and standing have the opposite effect.

Proceed as follows:

- Tell the examiner that you would like to look for features of Marfan's syndrome (high arched palate, arm span greater than height).

Diagnosis

This patient has mitral valve prolapse (lesion) and a long pansystolic murmur, indicating significant mitral regurgitation which will require prophylaxis for infective endocarditis (functional status).

Questions

What are eponyms for mitral valve prolapse (MVP)?

Barlow's syndrome, click-murmur syndrome, floppy mitral valve.

What is the prevalence in the normal population?

The exact prevalence is not known but is between 2 and 10% of the population. It is present in about 7% of females aged between 14 and 30 years.

What are the complications of MVP?

- Severe mitral regurgitation.
- Arrhythmias – ventricular premature contractions, ventricular tachy-cardia, paroxysmal supraventricular tachycardia.
- Atypical chest pain.
- Transient ischaemic attacks (TIAs), embolism.
- Infective endocarditis in those with mitral regurgitation.
- Sudden death.

Mention a few associated conditions.

- Marfan's syndrome.
- Chronic rheumatic heart disease.
- Ischaemic heart disease.
- Cardiomyopathies.
- 20% of patients with arial septal defects – secundum type.
- Ehlers–Danlos syndrome.
- Psoriatic arthritis.
- Ebstein's anomaly.
- SLE.

How would you manage such patients?

- Reassure the asymptomatic patient.
- Advise prophylaxis for infective endocarditis in those with the murmur.
- Relief of atypical chest pain with analgesics or beta-blockers (empiric treatment).
- Aspirin or anticoagulants in those with TIAs.
- Antiarrhythmics in those with frequent tachyarrhythmias or ventricular premature contractions.

Advanced-level Questions

What are the echocardiographic features of MVP?

- M-mode: abrupt posterior displacement of the posterior or sometimes both valve leaflets in mid or late systole.
- 2-D: systolic displacement of one or both mitral valve leaflets into the left atrium.

John Barlow, South African Professor of Cardiology.
Celia Oakley, Professor of Cardiology, Hammersmith Hospital, London.

References

Barlow JB, Bosman CK & Pocock WA (1968) Late systolic murmurs and non-ejection (mid-late) systolic clicks: an analysis of 90 patients. *Br Heart J* **30**: 203.
Oakley C (1985) Mitral valve prolapse. *Q J Med* **219**: 317.
Perloff JK, Child JS & Edwards JE (1986) New guidelines for the clinical diagnosis of mitral valve prolapse. *Am J Cardiol* **57**: 1124.
Procacci PN, Savran SV, Schreiter SL et al (1976) Prevalence of clinical mitral valve prolapse in 1169 young men. *N Engl J Med* **294**: 1986.

CASE 21 Ventricular Septal Defect

Instruction

Listen to this patient's heart.

Salient features

- Normal pulse.
- Normal findings on palpation (there may be either left or right ventricular enlargement).

- Loud pansystolic murmur at the left lower sternal area.
- The second sound may be normal when the defect is small. A_2 is obscured by the pansystolic murmur of large defects. A single second sound indicates that the ventricular pressures are equal and a loud P_2 indicates pulmonary hypertension.

Proceed as follows:

Listen for the following:

- Mid-diastolic flow murmur at the apex.
- Loud P_2 of pulmonary hypertension.
- Signs of cardiac failure.

Note. VSD is the most common congenital cardiac anomaly, occurring in 2 per 1000 births. VSD is a feature of Down's syndrome (see page 561).

Diagnosis

This patient has a ventricular septal defect (lesion) of congenital origin (aetiology) and has pulmonary hypertension (functional status).

Questions

Is the loudness of the murmur related to the size of the VSD?

No; in fact, very small defects (maladie de Roger) cause loud murmurs.

What are causes of a VSD?

- Congenital.
- Rupture of the interventricular septum as a complication of myocardial infarction.

Where is the defect usually situated?

In the membranous portion of the interventricular septum.

Can such defects close spontaneously?

Spontaneous closure usually occurs in a small defect, early childhood in about 50% of the patients.

What are complications of a VSD?

- Congestive cardiac failure.

- Right ventricular outflow tract obstruction (muscular infundibular obstruction develops in about of 5% of VSDs).
- Aortic regurgitation.
- Infective endocarditis.
- Pulmonary hypertension and reversal of shunt (Eisenmenger complex).

Advanced-level Questions

What types of VSD do you know?

- The supracristal type (above the crista supraventricularis) is a high defect just below the pulmonary valve and the right coronary cusp of the aortic valve. The latter may not be adequately supported, resulting in aortic regurgitation. In Fallot's tetralogy this defect is associated with a rightward shift of the interventricular septum, and in double-outlet left ventricle with subaortic stenosis the supracristal defect is associated with a leftward shift of the septum.
- The infracristal defect, which may be in either:
  Upper membranous portion of the interventricular septum, or
  The lower muscular part (less than 5% of the defects):
    Small defects (maladie de Roger).
    Swiss cheese appearance (multiple small defects).
    Large defects.
    Gerbode defect (defect opening into the right atrium).

Note. The crista supraventricularis is a muscular ridge that separates the main portion of the right ventricular cavity from the infundibular or outflow portion.

Mention other cardiac lesions that may be associated with a VSD.

- Conditions in which VSD is an essential part of the syndrome:
  Fallot's tetralogy.
  Truncus arteriosus.
  Double-outlet right ventricle.
  AV canal defects.
- Conditions frequently associated with a VSD but not an essential part of the syndrome:
  Patent ductus arteriosus.
  Pulmonary stenosis.
  Secundum atrial septal defects.
  Coarctation of aorta.
  Tricuspid atresia.
  Transposition of the great arteries.
  Pulmonary atresia.

Which patients merit surgical attention?

Usually, in an adult, VSD is small enough to be safely ignored, or the patient has Eisenmenger's syndrome. However, there are exceptions to this and these patients may benefit from surgery:

Recurrent endocarditis.

Development of aortic regurgitation due to prolapse of the right coronary cusp through the septal defect.

Progressive left ventricular dilatation due to volume overload imposed by the shunt (pulmonary to systemic ratio is 3:1).

When the defect is due to an acute rupture of the ventricular septum.

Note. If the VSD is large enough to cause heart failure or pulmonary hypertension, it usually manifests in the first few years of life.

Henri Roger (1809–1891), a French paediatrician, described maladie de Roger in 1879 in a paper entitled 'Clinical researches on the congenital communication of the two sides of the hearts, but failure of occlusion of the interventricular septum'.

References

Gerbode F, Hultgren H, Melrose D & Osborn J (1958) Syndrome of left ventricular–right atrial shunt. Successful surgical repair of defect in 5 cases, with observation of bradycardia on closure. *Ann Surg* **148**: 433.

Roger H (1879) Recherches cliniques sur la communication congenitale des deux coeurs par inocclusion du septum interventriculaire. *Bulletin de l'Académie de Médicine, 2 Meserie, Tome VIII* 1074–1094.

Weidman WH, Blount SG, DuShane JW et al (1977) Clinical course in ventricular septal defect. *Circulation* **56**(suppl 1): I-56.

CASE 22 Atrial Septal Defect

Instruction

Examine this patient's heart.
Listen to her heart.

Salient features

- Diffuse or normal apical impulse.
- Left parasternal heave.
- Ejection systolic flow murmur in the left second and third intercostal space.
- Wide, fixed, split second heart sound (occasionally a slight movement of P_2 occurs).

- Infrequently, a mid-diastolic murmur may be heard in the tricuspid area (indicating a large left-to-right shunt).

Proceed as follows:

Look for signs of:
Pulmonary hypertension (Eisenmenger's syndrome).
Congenital defects of the thumb (Holt–Oram syndrome).

Note. Atrial secundum defect is often confused with pulmonary stenosis (P_2 is soft, delayed and moves with respiration).

Diagnosis

This patient has atrial septal defect (lesion) which is congenital in origin (aetiology); she is not in cardiac failure and there is no reversal of shunt (functional status).

Advanced-level Questions

What are the types of atrial septal defect (ASD)?

- Ostium secundum defect accounts for 70% of the cases. The defect is in the middle portion of the atrial septum and is usually 2–4 cm in diameter (incomplete right bundle branch block pattern, QRS axis rightward).
- Sinus venosus type is a defect in the septum just below the entrance of the superior vena cava into the right atrium (leftward P wave axis so that P waves are inverted in at least one inferior lead).
- Ostium primum type is a defect in the lower part of the septum and clefts may occur in the mitral and tricuspid valves (QRS axis leftward).

What do you understand by the term patent foramen ovale?

In the fetus, the right and left atria communicate with each other through an oblique valvular opening, which is called the foramen ovale. The foramen ovale persists throughout fetal life. After birth, the left atrium receives blood from the lungs and the pressure in this chamber becomes greater than that in the right atrium; this causes the closure of the foramen ovale.

What is the importance of patent foramen ovale?

The prevalence of patent formen ovale is signficantly higher in patients with stroke.

What is Holt – Oram syndrome?

This is an ostium secundum ASD with a hypoplastic thumb and an accessory phalanx. In addition, the thumb lies in the same plane as the other digits. The inheritance is autosomal dominant and is associated with mutations to chromosome 12q2.

At what age does the reversal of shunt occur?

Usually after the end of the second decade.

What is the mechanism of fixed split second sound?

In normal individuals on inspiration there is a widening of the split between the two components of the second sound due to a delay in closure of the pulmonary valve. In ASD the effect of respiration is eliminated due to the communication between the left and right sides of the heart.

In which conditions is an abnormally widely split second sound present?

- ASD, VSD, pulmonary regurgitation (due to increased right ventricular volume).
- Pulmonary stenosis (due to increased right ventricular pressure).
- Right bundle branch block (due to right ventricular conduction delay).
- Mitral regurgitation, VSD (due to premature left ventricular emptying).

What do you know about the embryology of atrial septal defect?

There are seven septa involved in the partitioning of the heart: three form passively (i.e. when an area of tissue forms a septum because of the rapid growth of contiguous tissue) and these include septum secundum at the atrial septum, the muscular portion of the ventricular septum and the aorticopulmonary septum. The actively formed portions of the septums of the heart include the septum of the atrioventricular canal, the conal septum and the truncal septum.

The atrial septum begins as a passively formed septum; however, active growth from the endocardial cushions completes the septum.

What is Lutembacher syndrome?

ASD with an acquired rheumatic mitral stenosis.

What is Fallot's triology?

ASD, pulmonary stenosis and right ventricular enlargement.

What are the chest X-ray findings?

- Small aortic knob.
- Large pulmonary conus.
- Very large hilar arteries.
- Enlarged right ventricle and right atrium.
- Increased pulmonary vasculature.
- 'Hilar dance' on fluoroscopy.

What are the ECG findings?

- Right bundle branch block pattern in ostium secundum type.
- Left axis deviation in ostium primum type.

What is the commonest arrhythmia seen in ASD?

Atrial fibrillation. It is usually accompanied by the appearance of tricuspid regurgitation.

How would you manage an uncomplicated atrial septal defect?

Early childhood:

- When detected in early childhood surgical closure is recommended between the age of 5 and 10 years to prevent the late onset of either right ventricular failure, atrial arrhythmias or right heart failure.

In adults:

- Small ASDs can be left alone, although many believe all ASDs must be closed. Those operated on before the age of 25 years have an excellent prognosis and one may anticipate normal long-term survival, but older patients require regular supervision. In a recent study surgical repair of atrial septal defects in middle-aged and elderly patients was found to improve longevity and reduce functional limitation due to heart failure, and is therefore superior to medical treatment. However, the risk of atrial arrhythmias, especially fibrillation and flutter, and the attendant risk of thromboembolic events were not reduced by closure of the defect.
- Left-to-right shunt saturations of 2:1 or more require surgical closure.
- Closure in adults results in a reduction in right ventricular size and improves symptoms.

More recently, ASDs are being occluded by transcatheter button or 'clam-shell devices'.

Leonardo da Vinci's description in 1513 of a 'perforating channel' in the atrial septum is believed to be the first recorded account of a congenital malformation of the human heart.

Rene Lutembacher, a French physician, described the Lutembacher syndrome in 1916.

Mary Holt, cardiologist, King's College Hospital, London.

Samuel Oram, cardiologist, King's College Hospital, London.

References

Basson G, Cowley GS, Solomon D et al (1994) The clinical and genetic spectrum of the Holt–Oram syndrome (heart–hand syndrome). *N Engl J Med* **330**: 885–891.

Borow KM & Karp R (1990) Atrial septal defect – lessons from the past, directions for the future. *N Engl J Med* **323**: 1698.

Campbell M (1970) Natural history of atrial septal defect. *Br Heart J* **32**: 820–826.

Holt M & Oram S (1960) Familial heart disease with skeletal malformation. *Br Heart J* **22**: 236.

Konstantinides S, Geibel A, Olschewski M et al (1995) A comparison of surgical and medical therapy for atrial septal defects in adults. *N Engl J Med* **333**: 469–473.

Lechat P, Mas JL, Lascault G et al (1988) Prevalence of patent foramen ovale in patients with stroke. *N Engl J Med* **318**: 1148–1152.

Lutembacher R (1916) De la stenose mitrale avec communication interauriculaire. *Arch Mal Coeur* **9**: 237.

Murphy JG, Gersh BJ, McGoon MD et al (1990). Long term outcome after surgical repair of isolated atrial septal defect: follow up at 27 to 32 years. *N Engl J Med* **323**: 1645–1650.

Rocchini AP (1990) Transcatheter closure of atrial septal defects: past, present and future. *Circulation* **82**: 1044–1045.

CASE 23 Hypertrophic Cardiomyopathy

Instruction

Examine this patient's cardiovascular system.

Salient features

- Carotid pulse is bifid.
- 'a' wave in the JVP.
- *Double apical impulse* (left ventricular heave with a prominent presystolic pulse).
- Pansystolic murmur at the apex, accentuated by standing and Valsalva manoeuvre and softer on squatting.

- Ejection systolic murmur along the left sternal border.
- Fourth heart sound.

Proceed as follows:

- Tell the examiner that you would like to take a family history of the following:
  Similar cardiomyopathy.
  Sudden death.

Diagnosis

This patient has hypertrophic cardiomyopathy (aetiology) as evidenced by a double apical impulse and ejection systolic murmur along the left sternal border which is heard better on standing (lesion); the patient is in cardiac failure.

Questions

How may such a patient present?

- Dyspnoea.
- Syncope.
- Sudden death.
- Angina pectoris.
- Palpitations.

Advanced-level Questions

What single investigation would you do to confirm the diagnosis?

Echocardiography; the features are as follows:

- Asymmetrical septal hypertrophy (ASH).
- Systolic anterior motion of the mitral valve (SAM).
- Mitral regurgitation using Doppler ultrasonography.

What are the ECG findings in hypertrophic cardiomyopathy?

Left ventricular hypertrophy, deep Q waves and conduction defects.

How would you manage such a patient?

- Relief of symptoms.
- Prevention of arrhythmias and sudden death by adminstration of amiodarone.

- Improvement of ventricular function using beta-blocker (propranolol up to 640 mg per day), verapamil, amiodarone and diuretics.
- Prevention of infective endocarditis.
- Dual-chamber pacing or DDD pacing (see page 89) is considered by some as the initial procedure in symptomatic patients resistant to treatment with drugs. DDD pacing causes depolarization from the right ventricular apex, resulting in altered motion of the interventricular septum and diminished subaortic gradient.
- Surgery – such as myotomy or myectomy – relieves symptoms but does not alter the natural history of the disease. Mitral valve replacement may be done simultaneously for severe mitral regurgitation.
- Counselling of sufferers and relatives is essential and they should be encouraged to contact the Hypertrophic Cardiomyopathy Association.

What is the most characteristic pathophysiological abnormality in hypertrophic cardiomyopathy?

Diastolic dysfunction.

What ECG abnormalities may be seen?

- ST segment and T-wave abnormalities.
- Tall R waves due to left ventricular hypertrophy.
- Prominent abnormal Q waves in the inferior and lateral leads (in 20% of cases).

Which condition has the most common association with hypertrophic cardiomyopathy?

Friedreich's ataxia.

What do you know about the genetics of hypertrophic cardiomyopathy?

Implication of β-myosin heavy chain gene, α-tropomyosin or cardiac troponin T.

What do you know about the Brockenbrough – Braunwald – Morrow sign?

Diminished pulse pressure in post-extrasystolic beat occurs in hypertrophic cardiomyopathy/aortic stenosis.

The pathology of hypertrophic cardiomyopathy was first described by two French pathologists in the mid 19th century and by a German pathologist in the early 20th century. The simultaenous reports of Sir Russel Brock, thoracic surgeon at Guy's and Brompton Hospitals, and of Teare in 1958 brought this to modern medical attention.

Eugene Braunwald (b. 1929) was consecutively Chair and Professor of Medicine in San Diego and Harvard Medical School, Boston. His research interests included heart failure, factors influencing cardiac contraction, hypertrophic cardiomyopathy and was responsible for the idea that late patency of an occluded artery can lead to clinical benefit. His wife, Nina H Starr Braunwald, was a cardiothoracic surgeon who made important contributions to heart valve replacement.

References

Brock RC (1957) Functional obstruction of the left ventricle. *Guy's Hosp Rep* **106**: 221–238.

Brockenbrough EC, Braunwald E & Morrow AG (1961) A hemodynamic technic for the detection of hypertrophic subaortic stenosis. *Circulation* **23**: 189–194.

McKenna WJ, Oakley M, Krikler DM & Goodwin JF (1985) Improved survival with amiodarone in patients with hypertrophic cardiomyopathy and ventricular tachycardia. *Br Heart J* **53**: 412–416.

Teare RD (1958) Asymmetrical hypertrophy of the heart in young adults. *Br Heart J* **20**: 1.

CASE 24 Patent Ductus Arteriosus

Instruction

Examine this patient's heart.
Examine this patient's cardiovascular system.

Salient features

- Collapsing pulse (due to an aortic diastolic run-off).
- Heaving apex beat.
- Systolic and/or diastolic thrill in the left second interspace.
- Loud, continuous 'machinery' murmur, i.e. pansystolic and extending into early diastole – known as Gibson murmur – is heard along the left upper sternal border and outer border of the clavicle. The murmur begins after the first heart sound, peaks with the second sound, and trails off in diastole.
- The second sound is not heard.

Proceed as follows:

- Tell the examiner that you would like to:

Take a maternal history of rubella, particularly in the first trimester.
Know whether the patient was a premature baby.
Know whether the patient was born in a place located at a high
   altitude.

Diagnosis

This patient has a patent ductus arteriosus (lesion) which is probably
congenital in origin (aetiology); the patient is not in heart failure
(functional status).

Questions

Mention a few causes of a collapsing pulse.

Hyperdynamic circulation due to:

- Aortic regurgitation.
- Thyrotoxicosis.
- Severe anaemia.
- Paget's disease.
- Complete heart block.

Advanced-level Questions

Mention a few causes of continuous murmurs.

- Venous hum.
- Mitral regurgitation murmur with aortic regurgitant murmur.
- VSD with aortic regurgitation.
- Pulmonary arteriovenous fistula.
- Rupture of the sinus of Valsalva.
- Coronary arteriovenous fistula.
- Arteriovenous anastomosis of intercostal vessels following a fractured
   rib.

*What happens to the continuous murmur of patent ductus arteriosus (PDA) in
pulmonary hypertension?*

First the diastolic murmur, then the systolic murmur, becomes softer and
shorter, and P_2 increases in intensity.

How would you investigate this patient?

- ECG may be normal or shows left ventricular hypertrophy.
- Chest X-ray (CXR) may be normal, or there may be left ventricular and left atrial enlargement.
- Cardiac catheterization establishes the presence and severity of the shunt.
- Angiography defines its anatomy.

Mention a few associated lesions.

- Ventricular septal defect.
- Pulmonary stenosis.
- Coarctation of aorta.

What are complications?

- Congestive cardiac failure is the commonest complication.
- Infective endocarditis or endarteritis.
- Pulmonary hypertension and reversal of shunt (causes differential cyanosis and clubbing, i.e. toes – *not* fingers – are clubbed and cyanosed).

How would you manage such patients?

- Within 1–3 weeks of birth: administer a prostglandin E synthesis inhibitor such as indomethacin.
- A Rashkind PDA occluder can be inserted percutaneously without the need for a thoracotomy. It consists of a series of minature back-to-back umbrellas which are positioned across the duct.
- In children or adults with large shunts: perform surgery, i.e. ligation or division of the PDA.

Note. Pulmonary hypertension is a contraindication for surgery.

Which congenital cardiac lesions are dependent on a PDA?

Hypoplastic left heart syndrome, complex coarctations of aorta and critical congenital aortic stenosis.

Collapsing pulse is also called Corrigan's pulse after Sir Dominic J Corrigan (1802–1880), a Dublin-born physician who graduated from Edinburgh.
RE Gross was the first to report surgical closure of the PDA in 1939.

References

Campbell M (1968) Natural history of persistent ductus arteriosus. *Br Heart J* **30**: 4.
Gibson GA (1890) Persistence of the arterial duct and its diagnosis. *Edinb Med* **8**: 1.

Heymann MA, Rudolph AM & Silerman NH (1976) Closure of the ductus arteriosus by prostaglandin inhibition. *N Engl J Med* **295**: 530.

Krovetz LJ & Rowe RD (1972) Patent ductus, prematurity and pulmonary disease. *N Engl J Med* **287**: 513.

CASE 25 Pulmonary Stenosis

Instruction

Examine this patient's heart.

Salient features

- Round plump facies.
- Normal pulse.
- Prominent 'a' wave in the JVP.
- Left parasternal heave.
- Ejection click (valvular stenosis).
- Soft P_2, with a wide split second sound.
- Ejection systolic murmur in the left upper sternal border, best heard on inspiration. The murmur radiates to the left shoulder and left lung posteriorly. The more severe the stenosis, the longer is the murmur, obscuring the second aortic sound A_2.

Proceed as follows:

- Tell the examiner that you would like to do the following:
  Look for central cyanosis and clubbing (Fallot's tetralogy).
  Ask for a history of maternal rubella.

Questions

What is the underlying cause of pulmonary stenosis?

- Congenital (commonest cause).
- Carcinoid tumour of the small bowel.

Advanced-level Questions

What are the radiological features?

- Normal aortic knuckle.
- Normal or enlarged pulmonary conus (due to post-stenotic dilatation of the valvular stenosis).

● Large left atrium.

What are the complications of this condition?

● Cardiac failure.
● Infective endocarditis: blood cultures are rarely positive; the emboli are entirely in the pulmonary circulation and not systemic.

What are the types of pulmonary stenosis?

● Valvular.
● Subvalvular – infundibular and subinfundibular.
● Supravalvular.

Do you know of any eponymous syndromes linked to pulmonary stenosis?

● Noonan's syndrome: short stature, ptosis, downward slanting eyes, wide-spaced eyes (hypertelorism), low-set ears, webbed neck, mental retardation; low posterior hairline and pulmonary stenosis.
● Watson's syndrome: café-au-lait spots, mental retardation and pulmonary stenosis.

What is the role of balloon valvuloplasty in pulmonary stenosis?

Balloon dilatation is now the treatment of choice in pulmonary valvular stenosis. In a series of 100 patients, balloon dilatation resulted in a significant reduction in the trans-valvular gradient, which was maintained at 12 months' follow-up.

What is Erb's point?

The third left intercostal space adjacent to the sternum is Erb's point, and the murmur of infundibular pulmonary stenosis is best heard in this space and in the left fourth intercostal space.

References

Abrahams DG & Wood P (1951) Pulmonary stenosis with normal aortic root. *Br Heart J* **13**: 519.
Brock RC (1957) *The Anatomy of Congenital Pulmonary Stenosis.* London: Cassel.
Fontes VF, Eduardo J, Sousa MR et al (1988) Pulmonary valvuloplasty – experience of 100 cases. *Int J Cardiol* **21**: 335–342.
Mody MR (1975) The natural history of uncomplicated valvular pulmonic stenosis. *Am Heart J* **90**: 317.

CASE 26 Dextrocardia

Instruction

Examine this patient's precordium.
Listen to this patient's heart.

Salient features

- Apex beat is absent on the left side and present on the right.
- Heart sounds are better heard on the right side of the chest.

Proceed as follows:

- Tell the examiner that you would like to perform the following checks:
    Ascertain whether the liver dullness is present on the right or left
        side.
    Examine the chest for bronchiectasis.
    Obtain a CXR (look for right-sided gastric bubble).
    Obtain an ECG (inversion of all complexes in lead I).

Note. Dextrocardia without evidence of situs inversus is usually associated
with cardiac malformation. It may occur with cardiac malformation in
Turner's syndrome.

Diagnosis

This patient has dextrocardia (lesion) of congenital aetiology.

Advanced-level Questions

What is Kartagener's syndrome?

A type of immotile cilia syndrome in which there is dextrocardia or situs
inversus, bronchiectasis and dysplasia of the frontal sinuses.

Which other abnormality has been associated with dextrocardia?

Asplenia (blood smear may show Heinz bodies, Howell–Jolly bodies).

What do you understand by the term 'situs inversus'?

Right-sided cardiac apex, right stomach, right-sided descending aorta. The
right atrium is on the left. The left lung has three lobes and the right lung
has two.

What do you understand by the term 'dextroversion'?

Right-sided cardiac apex, left-sided stomach and left-sided descending aorta.

What do you understand by the term 'levoversion'?

Left-sided apex, right-sided stomach and right descending aorta.

M Kartagener (b. 1897), a Swiss physician, described this condition in 1933.

References

Kartagener M (1933) Zür pathogenese der Bronchiektasient; Bronchiektasien bei Situs Viscerum Inversus. *Beitr Klin Tuberk* **83**: 489.

Katz M, Benzier EE, Nangeroni L & Sussman B (1953) Kartagener's syndrome (situs inversus, bronchiectasis and chronic sinusitis). *N Engl J Med* **248**: 730.

Rose V, Izukawa I & Moes CAF (1975) Syndromes of asplenia and polysplenia. A review of cardiac and non-cardiac malformations in 60 cases with special reference to diagnosis and prognosis. *Br Heart J* **37**: 840.

CASE 27 Coarctation of Aorta

Instruction

Examine this patient's cardiovascular system.

Salient features

- The upper torso is better developed than the lower part.
- Scapular collaterals are visible (listen over these collaterals for murmur).
- Radial pulse on the left side may be less prominent.
- Heaving apex due to left ventricular hypertrophy.
- Short systolic murmur is present in the chest and back (there may also be an ejection systolic murmur of bicuspid aortic stenotic valve or continuous murmur of a patent ductus arteriosus). The aortic valve is bicuspid in more than 50% of cases.
- Radiofemoral delay (simultaneous palpation of the brachial and femoral arteries using the thumbs is the most convenient method of comparing pulsations in the upper and lower limbs).

Proceed as follows:

- Tell the examiner that you would like to look for the following:
    Turner's syndrome (female, webbing of the neck, increased carrying angle).
    Berry aneurysms (extraocular movements impaired due to third cranial nerve involvement).

Diagnosis

This patient has coarctation of the aorta (lesion) with left ventricular failure (functional status).

Advanced-level Questions

What are the types of aortic coarctation?

Common:
- Infantile or preductal where the aorta between the left subclavian artery and patent ductus arteriosus is narrowed. It manifests in infancy with heart failure. Associated lesions include patent ductus arteriosus, aortic arch anomalies, transposition of the great arteries, ventricular septal defect.
- Adult type: the coarctation in the descending aorta is juxtaductal or slightly postductal. It may be associated with biscuspid aortic valve or patent ductus arteriosus. It commonly presents between the ages of 15 and 30 years.

Rare:
- Localized juxtaductal coarctation.
- Coarctation of the ascending thoracic aorta.
- Coarctation of the distal descending thoracic aorta.
- Coarctation of the abdominal aorta.
- Pseudocoarctation is of no haemodynamic significance and is a 'kinked' appearance of the aorta in the juxtaductal region without stenosis.

What radiological findings may be seen in such patients?

- Rib notching.
- The characteristic '3' sign on a chest radiograph or a reverse '3' sign on the barium swallow. The upper bulge is formed by dilatation of the left subclavian artery high on the left mediastinal border; the sharp indentation is the site of the coarctation and the lower bulge is called the poststenotic dilatation of the aorta.

What causes rib notching?

Collateral flow through dilated, tortuous and pulsatile posterior intercostal arteries typically causes notching on the undersurfaces of the posterior portions of the ribs. The anterior parts of the ribs are spared because the anterior intercostal arteries do not run in the osteal grooves. Notching is seldom found above the third or below the ninth rib and rarely appears before the age of 6 years.

Mention a few conditions in which rib notching is seen.

- Coarctation of aorta.
- Pulmonary oligaemia.
- Blalock–Taussig shunt
- Subclavian artery obstruction.
- Superior vena caval syndrome.
- Neurofibromatosis.
- Arteriovenous malformations of the lung or chest wall.

At what age does the condition manifest?

It is particularly likely to produce significant symptoms in early infancy (presenting as cardiac failure) or between the ages of 20 and 30 years.

How would you manage this patient?

- FBC, urea and elecrolytes.
- CXR, ECG.
- Echocardiography.
- Cardiac catheterization and aortic coronary angiography.

What are the complications of aortic coarctation?

- Severe hypertension and resulting complications:
    Stroke.
    Left ventricular failure.
    Rupture of aorta.
- Infective endocarditis endarteritis (at the site of the coarctation or on a congenitally bicuspid aortic valve).
- Intracranial haemorrhage (combination of hypertension and ruptured berry aneurysm).

What are the fundal findings in coarctation of aorta?

Hypertension due to coarctation of aorta causes retinal arteries to be tortuous with frequent 'U' turns; curiously, the classical signs of hypertensive retinopathy are rarely seen.

What is the treatment of such patients?

Surgical resection and end-to-end anastomosis, although a tubular graft may be required if the narrowed segment is too long.

What happens to the hypertension after surgery?

Despite surgery, some patients may continue to have hypertension and will require monitoring for hypertension and premature coronary artery disease.

Reference

Baron MG (1971) Obscuration of the aortic knob in coarctation of the aorta. *Circulation* **43**: 311.

CASE 28 Eisenmenger Syndrome

Instruction

Examine this patient's heart.
Examine this patient's cardiovascular system.

Salient features

- Clubbing of fingers and central cyanosis.
- 'a' waves in the JVP, 'v' wave if tricuspid regurgitation is also present.
- Left parasternal heave and palpable P_2.
- Loud P_2, pulmonary ejection click, early diastolic murmur of pulmonary regurgitation (Graham Steell murmur).
- Loud pansystolic murmur of tricuspid regurgitation.

Proceed as follows:

Listen carefully to the second sound.
- The clinical findings due to the underlying defect are as follows:
    VSD – single second sound.

ASD – fixed, wide split second sound.

PDA – reverse split of second sound and differential cyanosis where lower-limb cyanosis is marked.

Diagnosis

This patient has Eisenmenger syndrome with a shunt at the atrial level (lesion) which is congenital in origin (aetiology), and severe pulmonary hypertension (functional status).

Questions

What do you understand by the term Eisenmenger syndrome?

Pulmonary hypertension with a reversed or bidirectional shunt. It matters very little where the shunt happens to be (e.g. VSD, ASD, patent ductus arteriosus, persistent truncus arteriosus, single ventricle or common atrioventricular canal).

Advanced-level Questions

What do you understand by the term Eisenmenger complex?

Eisenmenger complex is a VSD with a right-to-left shunt in the absence of pulmonary stenosis.

Mention some cyanotic heart diseases of infancy.

Tetralogy of Fallot, Transposition of the great vessels, Tricuspid regurgitation, Total anomalous pulmonary venous connection.

What is the age of onset of Eisenmenger syndrome?

In the case of patent ductus arteriosus and VSD, about 80% occur in infancy, whereas in the case of ASD over 90% occur in adult life.

What are the symptoms of Eisenmenger syndrome?

Angina, syncope, haemoptysis and congestive cardiac failure.

What are the radiological features of Eisenmenger syndrome?

- Conspicuous dilatation of the pulmonary artery with slight to moderate enlargement of the heart (predominantly right ventricle).
- Peripheral markings are oligaemic.

How do these patients succumb?

- Haemoptysis.
- Cerebral abscess.
- Bacterial endocarditis.
- Heart failure.
- Cerebral thrombosis.

What treatment is available for end-stage Eisenmenger syndrome?

Combined heart–lung transplantation.

Victor Eisenmenger was a German physician who described this condition in an infant in 1897. His patient had cyanosis since infancy and a fairly good quality of life until he succumbed at the age of 32 years.

References

McCarthy PM, Starnes VA, Theodore J, Stinson EB, Oyer PE & Shumway NE (1990) Improved survival after heart–lung transplantion. *J Thorac Cardiovasc Surg* **99**: 54–60.

McCarthy PM, Kirby TJ, White RD et al (1992) Lung and heart–lung transplantation: the state of the art. *Cleve Clin J Med* **59**: 307–316.

Wood P (1958) The Eisenmenger syndrome. *Br Med J* **2**: 701, 709.

CASE 29 **Fallot's Tetralogy**

Instruction

Examine this patient's heart.

Salient features

- Clubbing
- Central cyanosis.
- Left parasternal heave.
- Ejection systolic murmur heard in the pulmonary area.

Signs indicating Blalock–Taussig shunt:

- The left radial pulse is not as prominent as the right.
- The arm on the side of the anastomosis (usually the left) may be smaller than the other arm.
- Blood pressure is difficult to obtain because of the narrow pulse pressure in the arm supplied by the collateral vessels.
- Thoracotomy scar.

Diagnosis

This patient has Fallot's tetralogy with a Blalock–Taussig shunt and is mildy cyanosed, indicating a right to left shunt (functional status).

Questions

What are the constituents of Fallot's tetralogy?

- VSD with a right-to-left shunt.
- Pulmonary stenosis (infundibular or valvular).
- Right ventricular hypertrophy.
- Dextroposition of the aorta with it overriding the septal defect.

How may a patient with Fallot's tetralogy present?

- Syncope (in 20% of cases).
- Squatting.
- Shortness of breath.
- Growth retardation.

What are the complications of Fallot's tetralogy?

- Cyanotic and syncopal spells.
- Cerebral abscess (in 10% of cases).
- Endocarditis (in 10% of cases).
- Strokes – thrombotic secondary to polycythaemia.
- Paradoxical emboli.

Advanced-level Questions

What do you understand by a Blalock–Taussig shunt?

It is the anastomosis of the left subclavian artery to the left pulmonary artery with the intention to increase pulmonary blood flow.

Why is it less frequently seen in adults in the recent past?

With ready availability of cardiopulmonary bypass, such patients have total correction of their anomalies at an early age.

What do you know about the embryological development of Fallot's tetralogy?

It arises from the anterior displacement of the conal septum, which leads to unequal partitioning of the conus at the expense of the right ventricular infundibulum and results in the obstruction of the right ventricular outflow tract and failure to close the intraventricular foramen.

What is the treatment for Fallot's tetralogy?

- Total correction under the age of 1 year when there is no need for an outflow transannular patch. A second-stage total correction can be performed when the child is over the age of 2 years.
- Blalock–Taussig shunting is performed nowadays only if the anatomy is unfavourable for a total correction.
- Modified Blalock–Taussig shunting is the interposition of a tubular graft between the subclavian and pulmonary arteries.
- The Waterston shunt involves anastomosis of the back of the ascending aorta to the pulmonary artery. A Waterston shunt is performed when surgery is required under the age of 3 months because the subclavian artery is too small for a good Blalock–Taussig shunt.
- The Potts shunt involves anastomosis of the descending aorta to the back of the pulmonary artery.
- The Glenn operation involves anastomosis of the superior vena cava to the right pulmonary artery. The bidirectional Glenn procedure involves anastomosis of the superior vena cava to both pulmonary arteries.
- Pulmonary balloon valvuloplasty is sometimes used as an alternative for surgery.

What cardiac lesions favour an initial shunt?

- Anomalous coronary artery.
- Single pulmonary artery.
- Hypoplastic pulmonary arteries.
- Single pulmonary artery.

What is Fallot's triology?

ASD, pulmonary stenosis and right ventricular hypertrophy.

What is Fallot's pentalogy?

Fallot's tetralogy with associated ASD is known as Fallot's pentalogy.

What conditions are associated with Fallot's tetralogy?

- Right-sided aortic arch (in 30% of cases).
- Double aortic arch.

- Left-sided superior vena cava (in 10% of cases).
- Hypoplasia of the pulmonary arteries.
- ASD.

Mention the common congenital heart diseases.

VSD, ASD of the secundum type, patent ductus arteriosus and Fallot's tetralogy are the common congenital heart diseases, in order of frequency.

What are the CXR findings?

- Boot-shaped heart.
- Enlarged right ventricle.
- Decreased pulmonary vasculature.
- Right-sided aortic arch (in 30% of cases).

What do you know about the Taussig – Bing syndrome?

In this condition the aorta arises from the right ventricle; the pulmonary trunk overrides both ventricles at the site of an interventricular septal defect.

Etienne-Louis Arthur Fallot (1850–1911), Professor of Hygiene and Legal Medicine in Marseilles, published his *Contribution to the pathologic anatomy of morbus coeruleus cardiac cyanosis* in 1888. The tetralogy was first described by N Stensen, Professor of Anatomy in Copenhagen, in 1672.

Helen Brook Taussig (1898–1986) is the founder of American paediatric cardiology. She collaborated with Alfred Blalock (1899–1964), a vascular surgeon, in the development of palliative surgery for Fallot's tetralogy.

References

Blalock A & Taussig HB (1945) The surgical management of malformations of the heart in which there is pulmonic stenosis or patent ductus arteriosus. *JAMA* **128**: 189.

Case Records of the Massachusetts General Hospital (1985) Congestive heart failure and cyanosis 31 years after an operation for cyanotic congenital heart disease. *N Engl J Med* **313**: 171–178.

Fallot A (1888) Contribution à l'anatomie pathologique de la maladie bleue (cyanose cardiaque). *Marseille Médical* **25**: 418–420.

Higgins CB & Mulder DG (1972) Tetralogy of Fallot in the adult. *Am J Cardiol* **28**: 837.

Murphy JG, Gersh BJ, Mair DD et al (1993) Long-term outcome in patients undergoing surgical repair of tetralogy of Fallot. *N Engl J Med* **329**: 593–599.

Potts WJ, Smith S & Gibson S (1946) Anastomosis of the aorta to the pulmonary artery. *JAMA* **132**: 627.

Rosenthal A (1993) Adults with tetralogy of Fallot – repaired yes, cured no. *N Engl J Med* **329**: 655–656.

CASE 30   Absent Radial Pulse

Instruction

Examine this patient's pulses.

Salient features

- Left radial pulse is weaker than the right.

Proceed as follows:

- Examine all other pulses (including carotid, brachial, femoral, popliteal, posterior tibial and dorsalis pedis pulses).
- Tell the examiner that you would like to know about:
    Past history of insertion of an arterial line for blood gases or arterial pressure.
    Systemic symptoms in the past (Takayasu's arteritis).
    Past history of cardiac surgery (Blalock–Taussig shunt).
    Cervical rib.

Diagnosis

This patient has an absent radial pulse (lesion) which is due to a previous Blalock–Taussig shunt.

Questions

In which conditions may the pulse rate in one arm differ from that in the other?

Usually, slowing of the pulse on one side occurs distal to the aneurysmal sac. Thus, an aneurysm of the transverse or descending aortic arch causes a retardation of the left radial pulse. Also the artery feels smaller and is more easily compressed than usual. An aneurysm of the ascending aorta or common carotid artery may result in similar changes in the right radial pulse.

What are the causes of absent radial pulse?

- Aberrant radial artery or congenital anomaly (check the brachials and blood pressure).

- Tied off at surgery or previous surgical cut-down.
- Catheterization of the brachial artery with poor technique.
- Following a radial artery line for monitoring of blood gases or arterial pressure.
- Subclavian artery stenosis.
- Blalock–Taussig shunt on that side.
- Embolism into the radial artery (usually due to atrial fibrillation).
- Takayasu's arteritis (rare).

Advanced-level Questions

What do you know about Takayasu's arteritis?

It tends to affect young women and most of the cases have been from Japan. Prodromal systemic symptoms include fever, night sweats, anorexia, weight loss, malaise, fatigue, arthralgia and pleuritic pain. It predominantly involves the aorta and is of three types: Type I (Shimizu–Sano) which involves primarily the aortic arch and brachiocephalic vessels, Type II (Kimoto) which affects the thoracoabdominal aorta and particularly the renal arteries, and Type III (Inada) with features of Types I and III. Types I and III may be complicated by aortic regurgitation.

M. Takayasu (1860–1938), Japanese ophthalmologist.

CASE 31   Constrictive Pericarditis

Instruction

Examine this patient's cardiovascular system

Salient features

- The patient may appear cachectic.
- Pulse may be regular or irregularly irregular (one-third have atrial fibrillation).
- Prominent *x* and *y* descents in the JVP and the level of the jugular venous pulse may rise with inspiration (Kussmaul's sign).
- Apex beat is not palpable.
- Early diastolic pericardial knock along the left sternal border, which may be accentuated by inspiration.
- Lungs are clear but there may be pleural effusion.
- Markedly distended abdomen with hepatomegaly and ascites.
- Pitting leg oedema.

Diagnosis

This patient has constricitve pericarditis (lesion) due to radiation therapy for previous Hodgkin's disease (aetiology) and is now limited by dyspnoea and marked ascites (functional status).

Questions

Mention some causes of constrictive pericarditis?

● Tumour.
● Radiation therapy.
● Tuberculosis.
● Connective tissue disorders.

Advanced-level Questions

What is the mechanism for pericardial knock?

It is caused by the abrupt halting of rapid ventricular filling.

Mention the differential diagnosis of the early diastolic sound.

● Loud P_2 (see page 92).
● S_3 gallop (see page 34).
● Opening snap (mitral stenosis).
● Pericardial sound.
● Tumour plop (atrial myxoma).

What is Beck's triad?

The presence of low arterial blood pressure, high venous pressure and absent apex in cardiac tamponade is known as Beck's triad.

CS Beck (1894–1971), surgeon, Peter Bent Brigham Hospital in Boston.
W Broadbent (1868–1951), English physician who qualified from St Mary's Hospital Medical School, London. He described the Broadbent sign in constrictive pericarditis, which is an indrawing of the 11th and 12th left ribs with a narrowing and retraction of the intercostal space posteriorly; this occurs as a result of pericardial adhesions to the diaphragm.

CASE 32 Permanent Cardiac Pacemaker

Instruction

Examine this patient's cardiovascular system.

Salient features

- Dropped beats due to occasional ventricular ectopics.
- Infraclavicular scar indicating pacemaker insertion.

Proceed as follows:

- Palpate the infraclavicular area gently to confirm the presence of a pacemaker.
- Tell the examiner you would like to ask the patient about:
  Past history of syncope (Stokes–Adams attacks) and heart block.
  Dizziness (pacemaker syndrome).

Remember, electromagnetic interference during magnetic resonance imaging or lithotripsy may transiently cause malfunction of pacemakers.

Diagnosis

This patient has a permanent pacemaker (lesion) for previous heart block (aetiology) which is functioning adequately (functional status).

Questions

What are the indications for a permanent pacemaker?

- Symptomatic bradyarrhythmias.
- Asymptomatic Mobitz Type II atrioventricular block.
- Complete heart block.

Advanced-level Questions

What do you know about permanent pacemakers?

- They are connected to the heart by one or two electrodes and are powered by long-lasting (5–10 years) solid-state lithium batteries. Most pacemakers are designed to pace and sense the ventricles – called the VVI pacemakers because they pace the ventricle (V), sense the ventricle (V) and are inhibited (I) by the ventricular signal.

They are inserted under local anaesthesia and fluoroscopic guidance, subcutaneously under the pectoral muscles.

- In symptomatic sinus tachycardia, an atrial pacemaker may sometimes be implanted (AAI).
- In sick sinus syndrome, a dual-chamber pacemaker DDD (because it paces two or dual chambers, senses both (D) and reacts in two (D) ways, i.e. pacing in the same chamber is inhibited by spontaneous atrial and ventricular signals, and ventricular pacing is triggered by spontaneous atrial events) is implanted.
- Rate-responsive pacemakers measure activity, respiration, biochemical and electrical indicators, and change their pacing rate so that it is suitable for that level of exertion.

How soon after pacemaker insertion can a patient drive?

They may not drive until the pacemaker has been shown to be functioning correctly for at least 1 month after implantation. Patients must inform driving licensing authorities and the motor insurers.

What are the complications of pacemakers?

- Erosion through the skin due to mechanical factors.
- Infection.
- Lead displacement.
- Pacemaker malfunction.

What is the pacemaker syndrome?

It is seen in individuals with a single-chamber pacemaker who experience symptoms of low cardiac output (dizziness, etc.) when erect; it is attributed to the lack of atrial kick.

References

Nathan AW & Davis DW (1992) Is VVI pacing outmoded? *Br Heart J* **67**: 285–288.
Petch MC (1993) Who needs dual chamber pacing? *Br Med J* **307**: 215–216.
Travill CM & Sutton R (1992) Pacemaker syndrome: an iatrogenic condition. *Br Heart J* **68**: 163.

CASE 33 Pericardial Rub

Instruction

Listen to this patient's heart.

Salient features

- Scratching and grating sound heard best with the diaphragm.
- Early diastolic sound (pericardial knock).

Proceed as follows:

- Tell the examiner that you would like to take a history of:
  Precordial pain changing with posture (worse on lying down and relieved by sitting forward).
  Myocardial infarction.
  Viral infection (Coxsackie A and B viruses).
  Chronic renal failure.
  Trauma.
  Tuberculosis.
- Tell the examiner that you would like to do an ECG (see below).

Diagnosis

This patient has a pericardial rub (lesion) due to pericarditis secondary to uraemia (aetiology) and is not in pain (functional status).

Questions

What are the characteristic features of a pericardial friction rub?

It typically consists of three components: a presystolic rub (during atrial filling), a ventricular systolic rub (which is almost always present and usually the loudest component) and a diastolic rub which follows the second heart sound.

Advanced-level Questions

What are the characteristic electrocardiographic findings?

- ST elevation in most ECG leads with the concavity upwards.
- T-wave inversion occurs after the ST segment returns to baseline (unlike in acute myocardial infarction where the ST segment is concave downwards like a cat's back and there is some amount of T-wave inversion accompanying the ST elevation).

How common is pericardial rub in constrictive pericarditis?

It is not heard in constrictive pericarditis.

What is the treatment for acute pericarditis?

- Pain relief (codeine) and anti-inflammatory agents (non-steroidal anti-inflammatory drugs (NSAIDs) such as indomethacin).
- Treatment of the underlying cause.

What is Dressler's syndrome?

Dressler's syndrome is characterized by persistent **p**yrexia, **p**ericarditis and **p**leurisy. It was first described in 1956 when Dressler recognized that postmyocardial infarction chest pain is not due to coronary artery insufficiency. It usually occurs 2–3 weeks after myocardial infarction and is considered to be of autoimmune aetiology; it responds to NSAIDs.

W Dressler (1890–1969), US physician educated in Vienna. He worked at the Manimoides Hospital, Brooklyn, New York.

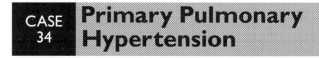

CASE 34 Primary Pulmonary Hypertension

Instruction

Listen to this patient's heart.

Salient features

- Young woman.
- Loud pulmonary second sound.
- Early diastolic murmur of pulmonary regurgitation best heard on inspiration (Graham-Steell murmur).

Proceed as follows:

- Tell the examiner that you would like to:
   Investigate for a tight or occult mitral stenosis.
   Examine the chest for chronic lung disease.
   Perform a ventilation–perfusion (V/Q) scan to exclude pulmonary emboli.
   Know whether the patient is on oral contraceptives, fenfluramine or aminorex.

Know whether the patient has habitually consumed plant products from *Crotalaria* species (particularly if from the Caribbean).

Diagnosis

This patient has pulmonary hypertension (lesion), and should be investigated for an underlying cause; she is in cardiac failure (functional status).

Questions

What are the symptoms of primary pulmonary hypertension?

Dyspnoea (60–89%), fatigue (19–73%), syncope, near syncope or dizziness (13–88%), oedema (3–37%) and palpitations (5–33%).

What are the signs of pulmonary hypertension?

- Large 'a' waves in JVP.
- Left parasternal heave.
- Loud or palpable P_2.
- Ejection click in the pulmonary area.
- Early diastolic murmur (Graham Steell murmur) due to pulmonary regurgitation.

Advanced-level Questions

How would you investigate such a patient?

- Chest radiograph: enlarged main pulmonary arteries with reduced peripheral branches, enlargement of the right ventricle.
- Pulmonary function testing, arterial blood-gas study.
- ECG: right ventricular and right atrial hypertrophy.
- V/Q scan to exclude pulmonary emboli.
- Echocardiography, right heart catheterization and pulmonary angiography.

What are the pathological features of primary pulmonary hypertension?

They are those of plexogenic pulmonary arteriopathy (which also occurs in post-tricuspid left-to-right atrial shunts such as VSD or PDA, and collagen vascular diseases), characterized by medial hypertrophy and concentric intimal fibrosis of the pulmonary arteries with complex plexiform lesions. Others have no plexiform lesions or concentric intimal fibrosis, but rather have recanalized thrombotic small pulmonary arteries which are said to be due to small thrombi or recurrent emboli. The least common histological pattern is veno-occlusive disease.

What is the prognosis in pulmonary hypertension?

The prognosis is poor with median survival of approximately 3 years from the time of diagnosis, with about one-third of patients surviving for 5 years. Death usually occurs suddenly, presumably from arrhythmias or right ventricular infarction.

What treatment is available for primary pulmonary hypertension?

- Oral anticoagulants (controversial).
- Calcium channel blockers: nifedipine, diltiazem.
- Intravenous epoprostenol (formerly prostacyclin or prostaglandin I_2), which is a potent short-acting vasodilator and inhibitor of platelet aggregation that is produced by the vascular endothelium.
- Heart–lung transplantation.

Graham Steell (1851–1942), assistant physician to the Manchester Royal Infirmary, described the murmur in a paper titled 'The murmur of high pressure in the pulmonary artery'.

References

Barst RJ, Rubin LJ, Long WA et al for the Primary Pulmonary Hypertension Study Group (1996) A comparison of continuous intravenous epoprostenol with conventional therapy for primary pulmonary hypertension. *N Engl J Med* **334**: 296–301.
Steell G (1888) The murmur of high pressure in the pulmonary artery. *Med Chron* (Manchester) **9**: 182–188.

CASE 35 Ebstein's Anomaly

Instruction

Listen to this patient's heart. He was told he had an innocent murmur during a school medical many years ago but now has a large globular heart on chest radiography.

Salient features

- Raised jugular venous pulse.

- Left parasternal heave.
- Pansystolic murmur which increases on inspiration.
- Hepatomegaly.

Proceed as follows:

- Tell the examiner that you would like to:
    Ascertain whether the patient has exertional cyanosis or dyspnoea.
    Exclude an atrial septal defect.
    Ask the patient about palpitations (paroxysmal supraventricular tachycardia).

Diagnosis

This patient has isolated tricuspid regurgitation (lesion) which is probably of congenital aetiology as there is no pulmonary hypertension. He has Ebstein's anomaly with cardiomegaly and cardiac failure (functional status).

Advanced-level Questions

What is the pathology in Ebstein's anomaly?

The tricuspid leaflets are abnormal and are displaced into the body of the right ventricle. The abnormally located tricuspid orifice produces a part of the right ventricle lying between the atrioventricular ring and the origin of the valve, which is continuous with the right atrial chamber. This proximal segment is known as the 'atrialized' portion of the right ventricle.

What are the mechanisms of cyanosis in these patients?

Right-to-left shunting at the atrial level, i.e. through a patent foramen ovale or atrial septal defect.

How would you investigate such a patient?

- CXR: large right atrium with oligaemic lung fields.
- ECG: RBBB (right bundle branch block), prolonged PR interval, P pulmonale (indicating right atrial enlargement), Type B Wolff–Parkinson–White syndrome (where the QRS complex is downward in lead V1).
- Echocardiography: diagnostic findings include the abnormal positional relation between the tricuspid valve and mitral valve with septal displacement of the septal tricuspid leaflet.
- Cardiac catheterization: in classical cases there is no place for this

investigation, which in the past has been associated with serious morbidity and mortality.

How are such patients treated?

- Tricupsid valve replacement plus closure of atrial septal defect.
- Tricuspid annuloplasty with plication of the atrialized portion of the right ventricle.

W Ebstein (1836–1912), German physician who also described the Armanni–Ebstein nephropathy (where there is glycogen vacuolation in the proximal convoluted tubules); L Armanni (1839–1903) was an Italian pathologist.

Reference

Celermajer DS, Bull C, Till JA et al (1994) Ebstein's anomaly: presentation and outcome from fetus to adults. *J Am Coll Cardiol* **23**: 170–176.

NEUROLOGY

EXAMINATION OF THE CRANIAL NERVES

First cranial nerve

- Ask the patient, 'Have you noticed any change in your sense of smell recently?' 'Can you differentiate between the odour of tea, coffee and bananas?'
- If the examiner requires you to test the sense of smell, use an odour that can be readily identified, such as soap or clove oil. If the patient has frequent nasal troubles, the value of this examination is limited.

Second cranial nerve

- First check visual acuity with a pocket Snellen's chart and finger counting.
- Make sure that the patient wears her spectacles should she use them, as one is not concerned with refractive errors.
- Check visual fields with a hat pin; your instructions to the patient should be clear and precise.
- Comment on the pupils (size, shape or inequality) and test their reaction to light (direct and indirect reaction) and to accommodation. The popular acronym PERRLA (**p**upils **e**qual, **r**ound and **r**eactive to **l**ight and **a**ccommodation) is a convenient description of normal pupillomotor function.
- Examine the fundus in a definite sequence: retina, retinal vessels, optic nerve and macula.

Third, fourth and sixth cranial nerves

- Test eye movements.

  Remember to ask the patient whether she sees a double image – this is the most sensitive sign of defective eye movement and may be present even when there is no apparent weakness of extraocular muscle or an abnormality of gaze.

  Saccadic movements are tested by asking the patient to look voluntarily to the right and left and up and down. Note whether these movements are carried out rapidly to the extremes of gaze.

Pursuit movements are examined by asking the patient to follow an object moved to the right and left and up and down. Note whether these movements are carried out smoothly without interruption.

- Remember to comment on nystagmus.

   Nystagmus is a repetitive drift of the eyeball away from the point of fixation, followed by a fast corrective movement towards it.

- Comment on ptosis if present (seen in third nerve palsy).

Fifth cranial nerve

- Test the masseters – 'Clench your teeth' – taking care to palpate the muscles.
- Test the pterygoids – 'Open your mouth' – and note the jaw deviates to the side of the lesion.
- Test corneal (not conjuctival) sensation by touching a wisp of cotton wool to the cornea while the patient looks upward and away from the examiner.
- Test facial sensation: keep in mind that this nerve supplies not only the face but also the anterior half of the scalp. Impairment of sensation limited to the face only is usually psychogenic in origin.
- Test jaw jerk: with the mouth half open, place your thumb over the patient's chin and lightly tap on the thumb. A mild jaw jerk or absent jerk is seen in normal individuals. In upper motor neuron lesions above the cervical cord, the jaw will manifest a marked jerk with this procedure.

Seventh cranial nerve

Remember that the facial nerve is a motor nerve.

- Test the lower half of the face:

   Ask the patient, 'Show me your teeth'.

   Note the nasiolabial fold, which often disappears in mild facial palsy.

- Test the upper half of the face:

   Ask the patient, 'Screw your eyes tightly shut and don't let me open them'.

   Have the patient wrinkle his or her forehead and note the movement of the muscles of the forehead.

Note. Taste may be lost on the anterior two-thirds of the tongue, but this is not usually tested.

Eighth cranial nerve

- Test by bringing a watch from beyond auditory acuity into the zone of hearing.
- Occlude each external auditory meatus with your finger and whisper short phrases, asking the patient to repeat them.
- Perform Rinne's and Weber's tests (use a tuning fork with a frequency of 256 or 512 cycles per second). Normally air conduction is better than bone conduction.
- Rinne's test: in obstructive deafness, bone conduction is better. In nerve deafness the normal relations are kept, i.e. air conduction is greater than bone conduction in the deaf ear.
- Weber's test: if the base of the tuning fork is placed on the middle of the forehead of a person with an obstructive deafness, he or she will hear it better in the deaf ear; with a nerve deafness, the fork will be heard better in the normal ear.

Ninth and tenth cranial nerves

- Ask the patient 'Open your mouth and say "aah"'; observe the soft palate with a torch (the soft palate is pulled to the normal side on saying 'aah').
- Tell the examiner that you would like to check gag reflex. An absence of gag reflex is significant only if it is unilateral.

Eleventh cranial nerves

- Ask the patient, 'Shrug your shoulders', and try to push them down simultaneously (this tests the trapezii muscles).
- Test the sternomastoids – by the patient's ability to resist lateral movement of the neck. Keep in mind that one rotates the head to the *right* by use of the *left* sternomastoid muscle.

Twelfth cranial nerve

- Ask the patient, 'Open your mouth'; comment on fasciculations of the tongue while in the mouth. Comment on wasting.
- Ask the patient, 'Stick your tongue out' (it deviates to the side of the lesion). Slight deviation of the tongue can be disregarded.

HA Rinne (1819–1868), German ear, nose and throat physician.
FE Weber-Liel (1832–1891), a German otologist.

NEUROLOGICAL EXAMINATION OF THE PATIENT'S UPPER LIMBS

1. *Introduce* yourself to the patient and ask him to take his top off so that both his arms are well exposed. If the patient is female, cover her breasts with suitable clothing so that she is decent.

2. *Comment on wasting, tremor* (see page 157), *fasciculations*.

3. *Assess tone*: 'Let your arms go loose and let me move them from you'.
   - Flex and extend wrists passively – cogwheel rigidity is elicited by this method.
   - Flex and extend at the elbows, pronate and supinate at the forearm – lead-pipe rigidity and clasp-knife spasticity is elicted by these methods.

4. *Test power*: 'I am going to test the strength of the muscles of your arms'.
   - Tell the patient, 'Hold your arms stretched out in front of you and then close your eyes'. Observe for drift, action tremor.
   - Shoulder abduction: 'Hold your arms outwards at your sides (like this) and keep them up; don't let me stop you'. Chief movers are the deltoids, C5. (**Note.** Supraspinatus is responsible for the initiation of abduction and for the first 60 degrees of this movement. However, this method of testing only assesses the power of the deltoids.)
   - Shoulder adduction: 'Push your arms in towards you and don't let me stop you'. Chief movers are the pectoral muscles, C6–8.
   - Elbow flexion: 'Bend your elbows and pull me towards you; don't let me stop you'. Chief mover is the biceps, C5.
   - Elbow extension: 'Straighten your elbows and push me away; don't let me stop you'. Chief mover is the triceps, C7.
   - Wrist extension: 'Clench your fist and cock your wrists up; don't let me stop you'. Chief mover is C7.
   - Wrist flexion: 'Now push the other way'. Chief mover is C7.
   - Finger abduction: 'Spread your fingers wide apart and don't let me push them together'. Chief movers are the dorsal interossei, T1 (ulnar nerve). **Note. D**orsal interossei **ab**duct: mnemonic, DAB.
   - Finger adduction: 'Hold this piece of paper between your fingers and don't let me snatch it away'. Chief movers are the palmar interossei, T1 (ulnar nerve). **Note. P**almar interossei **ad**duct: mnemonic, PAD.
   - Thumb abduction: 'Hold your palms facing the ceiling and now point your thumb towards the ceiling; don't let me stop you'. Chief mover is the abductor pollicis brevis, C8, T1 (median nerve).

- Flexion of fingers: 'Grip these two fingers of mine tightly and don't let them go'. Chief movers are the long and short flexors of the fingers, C8.

Note.
- The median nerve supplies the lateral two lumbricals, opponens pollicis, abductor pollicis brevis, flexor pollicis brevis: mnemonic, LOAF.
- The ulnar nerve supplies all other small muscles of the hand.
- The lumbricals are responsible for flexion at the metacarpophalangeal joint when the interphalangeal joints are in extension.
- Power is graded from 0 to 5:
  0, Absence of movement.
  1, Flicker of movement on voluntary contraction.
  2, Movement present when gravity is eliminated.
  3, Movement against gravity but not against resistance.
  4, Movement against resistance but not full strength.
  5, Normal power.

5. *Test deep tendon reflexes*:
   - Biceps jerk, C5, C6.
   - Triceps, C7.
   - Supinator, C5, C6.

Note.
- If the reflexes are absent, test after reinforcement – ask the patient to clench his or her teeth.
- *Inversion of the supinator reflex.* When the supinator jerk is elicited the normal response is a slight flexion of the fingers, contraction of the brachioradialis and flexion at the elbow joint. The jerk is said to be 'inverted' when finger flexion is the sole response, with contraction of the brachioradialis and elbow flexion being absent. There is associated absence of the biceps jerk and exaggeration of the triceps jerk.

  The inverted jerk indicates a lower motor neuron lesion at the fifth cervical level and an upper motor neuron lesion below this level. It could be due to cervical spondylosis, trauma to the cervical cord, spinal cord tumours at this level and syringomyelia.

6. *Finger reflexes*
   - Hoffman's sign:
   The examiner holds the patient's wrist in the horizontal pronated position with the fingers and wrists relaxed. Then the distal phalanx of the patient's middle finger is forcibly flexed. Normally no reflex occurs unless the patient is under emotional tension.

In upper motor neuron lesions, the patient's thumb undergoes a quick flexion–adduction–opposition movement while the other fingers move in flexion–adduction. This response is labelled as a 'positive' Hoffman's sign.

- Wartenberg's sign:
  The patient places his or her hand in partial supination resting on a table with the fingers slightly flexed. Then the examiner places his/her middle and index fingers on the volar surface of the patient's four fingers and taps his/her own fingers briskly with the tendon hammer. The response is one of flexion of the patient's four fingers and the distal phalanx of the thumb.
- Mayer's sign:
  With the patient's thumb abducted and the hand relaxed, the proximal phalanx of the middle finger is forcibly flexed towards the palm. Normally the thumb adducts. In upper motor neuron lesions the thumb usually remains in the position of abduction.

7. *Test co-ordination*
   - Finger–nose–finger test: 'Touch your nose with your index finger and now touch my finger'.
   - Rapid alternating movement of one hand over the other.

8. *Test sensation*
   - Light touch: use cottonwool and check each dermatome.
   - Pinprick: demonstrate first the sharp end and then the blunt end on the sternum; then check each dermatome for sharp or blunt sensation with the eyes closed.
   - Joint position sense: check in the distal interphalangeal joint of the thumb.
   - Vibration sense: use a tuning fork of 128 c.p.s. (although some authorities believe that a fork of 64 c.p.s. is more accurate). First test on the sternum so that the patient can recognize the vibration and then check over the fingers, moving proximally if the vibration sense is absent distally. Pallaesthesia is the ability to perceive the presence of vibration when an oscillating tuning fork is placed over certain bony prominences. Loss of vibratory perception is referred to as pallanaesthesia.

Remember:
- Joint sense and vibration sense are carried in the dorsal columns.
- Pain and temperature are carried in the lateral spinothalamic tracts.
- Light touch is carried in both the above tracts.

NEUROLOGICAL EXAMINATION OF THE PATIENT'S LOWER LIMBS

1. *Introduce* yourself and then ensure that the lower limbs are well exposed. It is important to ensure that the patient is decent – cover the genital area with a towel or any suitable clothing.

2. *Inspect for wasting, fasciculations* (tap the muscles of the leg and thigh to elicit fasciculations if not seen).

3. *Assess tone*
   - Ask the patient, 'Let your leg go loose and lax, and let me move it for you'; then passively flex and extend the leg at the knee and hip.
   - Roll the extended leg, feeling for resistance.
   - Put your hand behind the knee and pull it upwards, observing the foot to check whether or not it flops.
   - If there is spasticity or increased tone, then test for ankle clonus and patellar clonus.
   Patellar clonus: With the patient in the supine position, grasp the upper edge of the patella between the thumb and index finger and apply a quick constant pressure in a downward direction. Avoid prolonging this manoeuvre as it is often painful to the patient. In upper motor neuron lesions the patella may manifest a few jerks (unsustained clonus) or a constant jerking as long as the pressure is applied (sustained clonus).
   Ankle clonus: Ensure that the patient's knee is semi-flexed and the foot relaxed. The foot is suddenly pushed dorsally with moderate force and held there. In upper motor neuron lesions the posterior muscles of the leg will enter into a persistent contraction.

4. *Test power* (begin at the hips): 'I am going to test the strength of the muscles of your legs'.
   - Hip flexion: 'Lift your leg straight up and keep it there; don't let me stop you'. Chief mover is iliopsoas L1, L2.
   - Hip extension: 'Push your leg downwards into your bed and don't let me stop you'. Chief movers are glutei, L4, L5.
   - Hip adduction: 'Push your thigh inwards against my hand'. Chief movers are adductors of the thigh, L2–4.
   - Knee flexion: 'Bend your knee and pull your heel towards you; don't let me stop you'. Chief movers are the hamstrings, L5, S1.
   - Knee extension: 'Straighten your knee and don't let me stop you'. Chief movers are quadriceps, L3, L4.
   - Plantar flexion of the ankle: 'Push your foot downwards against my hand'. Chief mover is the gastrocnemius, S1.

- Dorsiflexion of the ankle: 'Move your foot up and don't let me stop you'. Chief movers are the tibialis anterior and long extensors, L4, L5.
- Inversion of the foot: 'Push your foot inwards against my hand'. Chief movers are tibialis anterior and posterior, L4.
- Eversion of the foot: 'Push your foot outwards against my hand'. Chief movers are the peronei, S1.
- Extension of the great toe: 'Pull your toe upwards and don't let me stop you'. Chief mover is the extensor hallucis longus, L5.

5. *Test the plantar response*: 'I am going to tickle the bottom of your foot'; use an orange stick to stimulate the outer portion of the sole and then across the ball to the base of the big toe. Always describe the response as either downgoing or upgoing. Normally the response is downgoing, i.e. all the toes flex towards the plantar surface. Upgoing plantars or the Babinski response is a feature of upper motor neuron lesions where the four small toes fan and turn towards the sole while the big toe extends dorsally. There is associated slight flexion of the hip and knee. The contraction of the tensor fasciae lata is referred to as the Brissaud's reflex and is a part of the spinal defence reflex mechanism. Other responses to plantar stimulation include: (a) quick avoidance response; (b) the grasp reflex; and (c) the support reaction. Remember that if the feet are cold (when outside the bedclothes for long) the response may be equivocal.

6. *Test deep tendon reflexes*
- Knee jerk, L4.
- Ankle jerk, S1. In the elderly, the plantar strike technique is said to be more reliable than the tendon-striking method for eliciting ankle jerks. The plantar strike technique of eliciting ankle jerks is as follows: the patient's legs are side by side and the foot is passively dorsiflexed; the reflex hammer strikes the examiner's own fingers, which are placed over the plantar surface.
- When the reflexes are absent, reinforce by asking the patient to pull outwards his or her clasped hands (Jendrassik manoeuvre). Do not tie your hands into a knot while testing the left ankle jerk from the patient's right-hand side. Avoid jabbing the patient while eliciting reflexes.

Note. By convention, deep tendon reflexes are graded as follows:
- 0   no response, abnormal.
- 1+   slight but definitely present response which may be normal or abnormal.
- 2+   brisk response, normal.

3+ very brisk response which may be normal or abnormal.

4+ a tap elicits clonus, abnormal.

Asymmetry of reflexes suggests abnormality.

7. *Test co-ordination*
   - Heel–shin test: Have the patient place the heel of one foot upon the knee of the opposite leg, and then move the heel downwards along the tibia. In a positive test, the patient has difficulty placing or holding the heel on the opposite knee or cannot keep the heel firmly on the tibia as the heel is moved downwards.

8. *Test sensation*
   Avoid testing in a given rhythm where the patient can expect to be stimulated at a given time. Always compare sensory responses in different areas of the same side of the body, as well as the two sides of the body.
   - Light touch.
   - Pinprick: test irregularly with the pin-point and pin-head, asking the patient whether the perceived sensation is sharp or blunt.
   - Joint position sense: hold the lateral aspect of the patient's big toe (not the dorsum of the toe) while eliciting this and move the toe gently up and down. The examiner's fingers should not rub against the skin of the adjoining toe during this test. Also, the joint should not be put in the extreme position of flexion during the test.
   - Vibration sense.

Note. When there is weakness of the limbs, tell the examiner that you would like to check sensation in the sacral area.

9. *Romberg's test*: 'Please stand up with your legs together and now close your eyes'. Take care to protect the patient if he or she sways or tends to fall. A positive test result is shown by pronounced swaying of the trunk. Sometimes functional cases will sway without having a true Romberg. This may be proved by diverting the attention of the patient by instituting the finger–nose test at the same time as Romberg is being tested. In functional cases the 'rombergism' will usually disappear.

10. *Check gait* and, if the heel–shin test is affected, then test tandem walking (asking the patient to walk along a straight line with one heel in front of the other foot). *Candidates frequently forget to check the gait when asked to examine the legs.*

Special manoeuvres in suspected upper motor neuron lesions

- Rossalimo's sign: The undersurface of the patient's toes are tapped with the examiner's fingers to produce abrupt extension (dorsiflexion) of the toes. In normal individuals there is no response, whereas in patients with upper motor neuron lesions all the toes respond with a quick plantar flexion.

In upper motor neuron lesions, the big toe will often dorsiflex (i.e. upgoing toe) when any of the following manoeuvres is conducted:

- Gordon reflex: on applying pressure to the muscle of the calf.
- Oppenheim sign: on applying heavy pressure with the thumb and index finger to the shin, stroking downwards from below the knee down to the ankle.
- Bing reflex: when the dorsum of the toe is pricked with a pin.
- Schaefer reflex: pinching the Achilles tendon enough to cause pain.
- Chaddock reflex: on stroking the lateral side of the foot, beginning below the malleolus and extending anteriorly along the dorsum of the foot to the base of the big toe.
- Gonda reflex: grasping the small toes between the fingers, slowly and forcibly flex the toe and then suddenly release the toe.

JJ Babinski (1857–1932), of Polish origin, graduated from the University of Paris with a thesis on multiple sclerosis. The Babinski response refers to upgoing plantars in upper motor neuron lesions. He described adiposogenitalis a year before Frolich.

References

Dohrmann GJ & Nowack WJ (1973) The upgoing great toe: optimal method of elicitation. *Lancet* **i**: 339–341.

Landau W (1971) Clinical definition of the extensor plantar reflex. *N Engl J Med* **285**: 1149–1150.

O'Keefe ST, Smith T, Valacio R, Jack CI, Playfer JR & Lye M (1994) A comparison of two techniques for ankle jerk assessment in elderly subjects. *Lancet* **344**: 1619–1620.

CASE 36 Bilateral Spastic Paralysis (Spastic Paraplegia)

Instruction

Carry out a neurological examination of this patient's lower limbs.

Salient features

- Increased tone in both lower limbs.
- Hyper-reflexia.
- Ankle clonus.
- Weakness in both lower limbs.

Proceed as follows:

- Check the sensory level and examine the spine.
- Tell the examiner that you would like to do the following:
    Ask about bladder symptoms and check sacral sensation.
    Ask about radicular pain.
    Ask whether the weakness was sudden or gradual.
    Examine the hands to rule out involvement of upper limbs.
    Check for cerebellar signs (multiple sclerosis, Friedreich's ataxia).
    Take a family history (hereditary spastic paraplegia).
    Take a history of birth anoxia (cerebral palsy).
- Try to localize the level of lesion using the following:
    Spasticity of the lower limb alone: lesion of thoracic cord (T2–L1).
    Irregular spasticity of lower limbs with flaccid weakness of scattered muscles of lower limbs: lesion of lumbosacral enlargement (L2–S2).
    Radicular pain – useful early in the disease, with time becomes diffuse and ceases to have localizing value.
    Superficial sensation – not good for localizing as the level of sensory loss may vary greatly in different individuals and in different types of lesions.

Diagnosis

This patient has bilateral spastic paraparesis (lesion) at L1 spinal level due to trauma (aetiology); it is complicated by bladder involvement (functional status).

Questions

What are the causes of spastic paraparesis?

Youth:
- Trauma.
- Multiple sclerosis.
- Friedreich's ataxia.

Adults:
- Multiple sclerosis.
- Trauma (motor vehicle or diving accident).
- Spinal cord tumour (meningioma, neuroma).
- Motor neuron disease.
- Syringomyelia.
- Subacute combined degeneration of the cord (associated peripheral neuropathy).
- Tabes dorsalis.
- Transverse myelitis.
- Familial spastic paraplegia

Elderly:
- Osteoarthritis of the cervical spine.
- Vitamin deficiency.
- Metastatic carcinoma.
- Anterior spinal artery thrombosis.
- Atherosclerosis of spinal cord vasculature.

Advanced-level Questions

What intracranial cause for spastic paraparesis do you know?

Parasagittal falx meningioma.

What do you know about transverse myelitic syndrome?

- Causes include: trauma, compression by bony changes or tumour, vascular disease.
- All the tracts of the spinal cord are involved.
- The chief clinical manifestation is spastic or flaccid paralysis.
- The lesion can be incomplete cord compression or total cord transection:

	Total cord transection	Incomplete cord compression
Paraplegia in flexion	+	+
Paralysis	Symmetrical	Asymmetrical
Flexor–withdrawal reflex	+ without return (withdrawal phase only)	Associated with return to original position
Other	Vasomotor and sphincter changes	Variable area of anaesthesia which is not consistent with motor loss

What do you know about paraplegia-in-flexion?

Paraplegia-in-flexion is seen in partial transection of the cord where the limbs are involuntarily flexed at the hips and knees because the extensors are more paralysed than the flexors. In complete transection of the spinal cord, the extrapyramidal tracts are also affected and hence no voluntary movement of the limb is possible, resulting in paraplegia-in-extension.

What investigations would you do?

- Magnetic resonance imaging (MRI) of the spine.
- Myelography.
- Computed tomography (CT) of the head.
- Check cerebrospinal fluid (CSF) for oligoclonal bands.
- Serum vitamin B_{12} levels.

Where is the lesion in patients with spastic weakness of one leg?

The lesion may be localized to the spinal cord or the brain. Progression to involve the arm does not help to differentiate between the spinal cord or the brain. Similarly, spread to the opposite leg does not necessarily indicate that the lesion is the spinal cord. Full investigation would include radiography of the spine and CT, but if the latter is normal then myelography may be required.

What do you know about hereditary spastic paraplegia?

This is an autosomal dominant condition, first described by Seeligmuller and Strumpell, in which spasticity is more striking than muscular weakness. The age of onset is variable and the condition has a relatively benign course. When the onset is in childhood, there may be shortening of the Achilles tendon, often requiring surgical lengthening. There is usually no sensory disturbance.

What do you know about tropical spastic paraplegia?

This is seen in Japan, the Caribbean and parts of western Africa and South America where women more often than men in their third and fourth decades have spastic paraparesis with neurogenic bladder. Viral infection due to human T-lymphotrophic virus 1 has been implicated as a cause of this disorder.

How do you localize the lesion to the 2nd and 3rd lumbar root level?

- Muscular weakness: hip flexors and quadriceps.
- Deep tendon reflexes affected: knee jerk.
- Radicular pain/paraesthesia: anterior aspect of thigh, groin and testicle.
- Superficial sensory deficit: anterior thigh.

How do you localize the lesion to the 4th lumbar root level?

- Muscular weakness: quadriceps, tibialis anterior and posterior.
- Deep tendon reflexes affected: knee jerk.
- Radicular pain/paraesthesia: anteromedial aspect of the leg.
- Superficial sensory deficit: anteromedial aspect of the leg.

How do you localize the lesion to the 5th lumbar root level?

- Muscular weakness: hamstrings, peroneus longus, extensors of all the toes.
- Deep tendon reflexes affected: none.
- Radicular pain/paraesthesia: buttock, posterolateral thigh, anterolateral leg, dorsum of foot.
- Superficial sensory deficit: dorsum of the foot and anterolateral aspect of the leg.

How do you localize the lesion to the 1st sacral root level?

- Muscular weakness: plantar flexors, extensor digitorum brevis, peroneus longus, hamstrings.
- Deep tendon reflexes affected: ankle jerk.
- Radicular pain/paraesthesia: buttock, back of thigh, calf and lateral border of the foot.
- Superficial sensory deficit: lateral border of the foot.

How do you localize the lesion to the lower sacral root level?

- Muscular weakness: none
- Deep tendon reflexes affected: none (but anal reflex impaired).
- Radicular pain/paraesthesia: buttock and back of thigh.
- Superficial sensory deficit: saddle and perianal areas.

What is the characteristic type of diplegia in cerebral palsy?

Diplegia associated with prematurity is a striking clinical entity – striking for the symmetry of neurological signs, for their distribution, for the relatively good intelligence of the patients, and for the comparative absence of seizures, the disability often being purely motor without sensory deficits.

What surgical treatment is available for the management of spastic diplegia in cerebral palsy?

Dorsal rhizotomy may be beneficial in selected patients.

What are the clinical features of spinal cord compression from epidural metastases?

The initial symptom is progressive axial pain, referred or radicular, which may last for days to months. Recumbency frequently aggravates the pain, unlike the pain of degenerative joint disease where it is relieved. Weakness, sensory loss and incontinence typically develop after the pain. Once a neurological deficit appears, it can evolve rapidly to paraplegia over a period of hours to days. In suspected cases MRI of the spine must be done by the next day. About 50% of cases in adults arise from breast, lung or prostate cancer. Compression usually occurs in the setting of disseminated disease. It is at the thoracic level in 70% of cases, lumbar in 20% and cervical in 10%, and occurs at mutliple, non-contiguous levels in less half of the cases. The tumour usually occupies the anterior or anterolateral spinal canal. CSF findings are non-specific in metastatic epidural compression. The cell count is usually normal, but protein levels may be raised because the flow of CSF is impeded. Lumbar puncture has been known to worsen the neurological deficit, presumably due to impaction of the cord.

References

Kuban KCK & Leviton A (1994) Cerebral palsy. *N Engl J Med* **330**: 188.
Park TS & Own JH (1992) Surgical management of spastic diplegia in cerebral palsy. *N Engl J Med* **326**: 745–749.
Rosenblum M (1989) Dissociation of AIDS-related vascular myelopathy and productive HIV-1 infection of the spinal cord. *Neurology* **39**: 892.
Young RR (1989) Treatment of spastic paraparesis. *N Engl J Med* **320**: 1553.

CASE 37 **Hemiplegia**

Instruction

Carry out a neurological examination of this patient.

Salient features

• Unilateral upper motor neuron seventh nerve palsy.

- The arm is held to the side, the elbow is flexed, and the fingers and wrist are flexed on to the chest.
- The leg is extended at both the hip and knee, while the foot is plantar flexed and inverted.
- Weakness of the upper and lower limbs on the same side with upper motor neuron signs – increased tone, hyperreflexia and upgoing plantar response.

> Hemiplegic weakness of the upper limbs affects the shoulder abductor, elbow extensors, wrist and finger extensors, and small hand muscles.
>
> Hemiplegic weakness of the lower limbs affects hip flexors, knee flexors and dorsiflexors and evertors of the foot.

- Do not forget sensory signs, in particular joint sensation which is important in rehabilitation.

Proceed as follows:

- Examine:
  For homonymous hemianopia and sensory inattention.
  For carotid bruits.
  For speech defects.
  The pulse for atrial fibrillation.
  The heart for murmurs.
- Tell the examiner that you would like to check the blood pressure and check the urine for sugar.

Diagnosis

This patient has had a stroke causing a right or left hemiplegia (lesion) which can be due either to a vascular event such as thrombosis, embolism or haemorrhage or to a neoplasm of the brain (aetiology). This patient is limited by hemiplegia and hemianopia (functional status).

Questions

What are the causes of hemiplegia?

Elderly:
- Vascular event (thrombosis, embolism or haemorrhage).
- Tumour.
- Subdural haematoma.
- Syphilis.

Youth:
- Multiple sclerosis.
- Tumour.
- Trauma.
- Embolism (look for underlying valvular heart disease, atrial fibrillation).
- Connective tissue disorder.
- Neurosyphilis.
- Intracranial infection: look for underlying acquired immune deficiency syndrome (AIDS), otitis media, cyanotic heart disease.

How would you manage such a patient?

- FBC, ESR.
- Urine sugar.
- ECG.
- Chest radiography.
- Echocardiography (looking for source of emboli), computed tomography (CT), carotid digital subtraction angiography (DSA) in selected patients.
- Physiotherapy, speech therapy and occupational therapy.
- Control of risk factors – stop smoking, hypertension, hyperlipidaemia, diabetes, stop oral contraceptives.

Advanced-level Questions

What are the measures used to determine the outcome after an acute stroke?

Some of the standard measures include:
- Barthel index is a reliable and valid measure of the ability to perform activities of daily living such as eating, bathing, walking and using the toilet.
- Modified Rankin Scale is a simplified overall assessment of function in which a score of 0 indicates the absence of symptoms and a score of 5 shows severe disability.
- Glasgow Outcome Scale is a global assessment of function in which a score of 1 indicates good recovery, a score of 2 moderate disability, a score of 3 severe disability, a score of 4 survival but in a vegetative state, and a score of 5 death.
- NIH Stroke Scale, a serial measure of neurological deficit, is a 42-point scale that quantifies neurological deficits in 11 categories. For example, a mild facial paralysis is given a score of 1 and complete right hemiplegia with aphasia, gaze deviation, visual field deficit, dysarthria and sensory loss is given a score of 25. Normal function without neurological deficit is scored as zero.

What is the role of thrombolysis in acute stroke?

Treatment with intravenous tissue plasminogen activator (tPA) when administered within 3 hours after onset of the ischaemic event (and in the absence of any sign of brain injury on CT) improves clinical outcome at 3 months. The CT scan in these patients must be examined very carefully for evidence of hemispheric brain ischaemia, which may increase the risk of deterioration with or without cerebral haemorrhage, after thrombolytic treatment.

How would you manage a patient with a transient ischaemic attack (TIA)?

- Advice to stop smoking.
- Aspirin.
- Duplex ultrasonography of the carotid vessels.
- Carotid artery DSA.

What do you understand by the term 'TIA'?

An acute loss of focal cerebral or ocular function with symptoms lasting less than 24 hours.

Why is it important to differentiate a carotid TIA from vertebrobasilar TIA?

Carotid TIAs may be amenable to surgery. Furthermore, a TIA in the anterior circulation is generally of more serious prognostic significance than a TIA in the posterior circulation.

What are the features of a carotid TIA?

Hemiparesis, aphasia or transient loss of vision in one eye only (amaurosis fugax).

What are the features of a vertebrobasilar TIA?

- Vertigo, dysphagia, ataxia and drop attacks (at least two of these should occur together).
- Bilateral or alternating weakness or sensory symptoms.
- Sudden bilateral blindness in patients aged over 40 years.

What are the clinical features that would interest you for the rehabilitation of a stroke?

- Independence in activities of daily living – bathing, dressing, toileting, transferring, continence and feeding.
- Independence in more complex activities such as meal preparation,

shopping, financial management, housekeeping, transportation, medication-taking and laundering.

What are the risk factors for stroke?

Hypertension, ischaemic heart disease, atrial fibrillation, peripheral vascular disease, diabetes, smoking, previous TIA, cervical bruit, hyperlipidaemia, raised haematocrit, oral contraceptive pill, cardiomyopathy.

Why is it important to treat TIAs?

Prospective studies have shown that within 5 years of a TIA:
>One out of six patients will have suffered a stroke.
>One out of four patients will have died (due either to stroke or heart disease).

What is the role of carotid endarterectomy in patients with a carotid TIA?

- For patients with severe stenosis (70–99%) the risks of surgery are significantly outweighed by the later benefits.
- For patients with mild stenosis (0–29% of cases) there is little 3-year risk of ipsilateral ischaemic stroke, even in the absence of surgery, so that any 3-year benefits of surgery are small and outweighed by its early risks.
- For patients with moderate stenosis (30–69% of cases) the balance of surgical risk and eventual benefit is still being evaluated.

What to you understand by the term 'RIND'?

Reversible ischaemic neurological disease, in which symptoms and signs reverse within 1 week but not within 24 hours.

What are lacunar infarcts?

Lacunar infarcts are seen in hypertensives and consist of small infarcts in the region of the internal capsule (causing partial hemiparesis or hemisensory impairment), pons (ataxia of cerebellar type, partial hemiparesis), basal ganglia or thalamus. They are often multiple. Lacunae are thought to be caused by occlusion of small branch arteries or by rupture of Charcot–Bouchard microaneurysms producing a small haematoma which resolves, leaving an area of infarction.

What are the deficits supplied by the anterior carotid artery?

The anterior carotid artery supplies the frontal lobes and the medial cerebral hemispheres with the exception of the visual cortex of the occipital lobes. Cortical areas supplied by this artery include the motor and sensory areas of the lower limbs, a 'micturition centre' and the supplementary motor cortex. Ischaemia in the territory of one anterior carotid artery produces weakness and mild sensory deficits in the opposite lower limb. Some patients with left anterior carotid artery ischaemia have a mild transient aphasia.

How do you classify stroke?

Bamford clinical classification of stroke

Total anterior circulation syndrome

- Unilateral motor deficit of face, arm and leg.
- Homonymous hemianopia.
- Higher cerebral dysfunction (e.g. aphasia, neglect).

Parietal anterior circulation syndrome

Any two of the following features:
- Unilateral motor and/or sensory deficit.
- Ipsilateral hemianopia or higher cerebral dysfunction.
- Higher cerebral dysfunction alone or isolated motor and/or sensory deficit restricted to one limb or the face.

Posterior circulation syndrome

One or more of the following features:
- Bilateral motor or sensory signs not secondary to brainstem compression by a large supratentorial lesion.
- Cerebellar signs, unless accompanied by ipsilateral motor deficit (see ataxic hemiparesis).
- Unequivocal diplopia with or without external ocular muscle palsy.
- Crossed signs, for example left facial and right limb weakness.
- Hemianopia alone or with any of the four items above.

Lacunar syndromes

Pure motor stroke
- Unilateral, pure motor deficit.
- Clearly involving two of three areas (face, arm and leg).
- With the whole of any limb being involved.

Pure sensory stroke
- Unilateral pure sensory symptoms (with or without signs).
- Involving at least two of three areas (face, arm and leg).
- With the whole of any limb being involved.

Ataxic hemiparesis
- Ipsilateral cerebellar and corticospinal tract signs.
- With or without dysarthria.
- In the absence of higher cerebral dysfunction or a visual field defect.

Sensorimotor stroke
- Pure motor and pure sensory stroke combined (i.e. unilateral motor or sensory signs and symptoms).
- In the absence of higher cerebral dysfunction or a visual field defect.

Charles Warlow, contemporary Professor of Neurosciences, Edinburgh.

References

Barnett HJM (1991) Beneficial effect of carotid endarterectomy in symptomatic patients with high-grade stenosis – North American Symptomatic Carotid Endarterectomy Trial Collaborators. *N Engl J Med* **325**: 445–453.

National Institute of Neurological Disorders and Stroke rtPA Stroke Study Group (1995) Tissue plasminogen activator for acute ischaemic stroke. *N Engl J Med* **333**: 1581–1587.

Warlow C (1991) European Carotid Surgery Trial; interim results for symptomatic patients with severe (70–99%) or patients with mild (0–29%) carotid stenosis. *Lancet* **337**: 1235.

CASE 38 **Ptosis and Horner's Syndrome**

Instruction

Look at this patient's face.

Salient features

Proceed as follows:

In the examination if you notice ptosis then you must answer the following questions:
- Is ptosis complete or incomplete?
- Is it unilateral or bilateral?

- Is the pupil constricted (Horner's syndrome) or dilated (third nerve palsy)?
- Are extraocular movements involved (third nerve palsy or myasthenia gravis)?
- Is the eyeball sunken or not (enophthalmos)?
- Is the light reflex intact (intact light reflex in Horner's syndrome)?

If the patient has Horner's syndrome then quickly proceed as follows:
- Examine the supraclavicular area:
  Percuss the supraclavicular area, looking for dullness of Pancoast's tumour.
  Look for scar of cervical sympathectomy (be prepared with indications for cervical sympathectomy).
  Look for enlarged lymph nodes.
- Examine the neck:
  For carotid and aortic aneurysms.
  For tracheal deviation (Pancoast's tumour).
- Examine the hands:
  For small muscle wasting.
  For pain sensation with a pin.
  For clubbing.
  (These should help in making a diagnosis of syringomyelia or Pancoast's tumour.)
- Tell the examiner that you would like to ask the patient whether or not there is absence of sweating on one side of the face.
- If there is no clue so far about the cause, tell the examiner that you would like to examine for nystagmus, cerebellar signs, cranial nerves and pale optic discs, and pyramidal signs to ascertain brainstem vascular disease or demyelination.

Diagnosis

This patient has Horner's syndrome (lesion) associated with dullness in the supraclavicular area indicating a Pancoast's tumour (aetiology).

Questions

What causes Horner's syndrome?

The syndrome is due to the involvement of the sympathetic pathway. It starts in the sympathetic nucleus and travels through the brainstem and spinal cord to the level of C8/T1/T2 to the sympathetic chain, stellate ganglion and carotid sympathetic plexus.

What are the features of Horner's syndrome?

It is characterized by:
- Miosis (resulting from paralysis of the dilator of the pupil).
- Partial ptosis or pseudo-ptosis (due to paralysis of the upper tarsal muscle).
- Enophthalmos (due to paralysis of the muscle of Müller).
- Often, slight elevation of the lower lid (because of paralysis of lower tarsal muscles).

What additional feature would you see in congenital Horner's syndrome?

There would be heterochromia of the iris, i.e. the iris remains grey-blue.

How would you determine the level of lesion using only history?

The level of the lesion is determined by the distribution of the loss of sweating:
- Central lesion – sweating over the entire half of the head, arm and upper trunk is lost.
- Lesions of the neck:
   Proximal to the superior cervical ganglion – diminished sweating on the face.
   Distal to the superior cervical ganglion – sweating is not affected.

Advanced-level Questions

How would you differentiate whether the lesion is above the superior ganglion (peripheral) or below the superior cervical ganglion (central)?

Test	Above	Below
Sweating	Such lesions may not affect sweating at all as the main outflow to the facial blood vessels is below the superior cervical ganglion	Such lesions affect sweating over the entire, head, neck, and arm upper trunk. Lesions in the lower neck affect sweating over the entire face
Cocaine 4% in both eyes	Dilates the normal pupil No effect on the affected side	Dilates both pupils
Adrenaline 1:1000 in both eyes	Dilates affected eye No effect on normal side	No effect on both sides

Note. In peripheral lesions there is depletion of amine oxidase due to postganglionic denervation. As a result this sensitizes the pupil to 1:1000 adrenaline, whereas it has no effect on the normal pupil or in central lesions (where the presence of the enzyme rapidly destroys the adrenaline).

Mention one cause of intermittent Horner's syndrome.

Migraine.

What are the causes of ptosis?

- Unilateral:
    Third nerve palsy.
    Horner's syndrome.
    Myasthenia gravis.
    Congenital or idiopathic.
- Bilateral:
    Myasthenia gravis.
    Dystrophia myotonica.
    Ocular myopathy or oculopharyngeal dystrophy.
    Mitochondrial dystrophy.
    Tabes dorsalis.
    Congenital.
    Bilateral Horner's syndrome (as in syringomyelia).

If the patient has Pancoast's tumour, what is the most likely underlying pathology?

Squamous cell carcinoma.

JF Horner (1831–1886), Professor of Ophthalmology in Zurich, conceded that Claude Bernard had recognized the syndrome before him.
Henry K Pancoast (1875–1939) was the first Professor of Radiology in the USA at the University of Pennsylvania.

Reference

Giles CL & Henderson JW (1958) Horner's syndrome: an analysis of 216 cases. *Am J Ophthalmol* **46**: 289–296.

CASE 39 Argyll Robertson Pupil

Instruction

Examine this patient's eyes.

Salient features

- The pupils are small and irregular.
- Light reflex is absent.
- Accommodation reflex is intact.
- There may be depigmentation of the iris.

Proceed as follows:

- Tell the examiner that you would like to do the following:
    Examine for vibration and position sense.
    Test for Romberg's sign and deep tendon reflexes (decreased).
    Ask the patient about lancinating pains.
    Check syphilitic serology.
    Check urine sugar.
- Remember that these pupils show little response to atropine, physostigmine or methacholine.

Diagnosis

This patient has Argyll Robertson pupil (lesion) and you would like to investigate for underlying neurosyphilis or leutic infection (aetiology).

Questions

What are the causes of Argyll Robertson pupil?

- Neurosyphilis – tabes dorsalis.
- Diabetes mellitus and other conditions with autonomic neuropathy.
- Pinealoma.
- Brainstem encephalitis.
- Multiple sclerosis.
- Lyme disease.
- Sarcoidosis.
- Syringobulbia.
- Tumours of the posterior portion of the third ventricle.

Advanced-level Questions

What do you know about the nerve pathways of the light reflex?

- The afferent is through the optic nerve and the efferent limb is through the third cranial nerve. The relevant optic nerve fibres responsible for the light reaction leave those responsible for the perception of light to terminate in the pretectal region of the midbrain, from whence a further relay passes to the Edinger–Westphal nucleus.
- Disturbances of the pupillary right reflex occur when there is involvement of the following:
  Superior colliculus.
  Decussation of Meynert.
  Edinger–Westphal nucleus (supplies the constrictor muscles of the iris).

Where is the lesion in Argyll Robertson pupil?

Damage to the pretectal region of the midbrain is believed to be responsible for the Argyll Robertson pupil of neurosyphilis.

Which muscle in the eye is responsible for the accommodation reflex?

Paralysis of accommodation occurs when the ciliary muscle is involved.

Mention a few causes of a small pupil.

- Senile miosis.
- Pilocarpine drops in the treatment of glaucoma.

What is 'reversed' Argyll Robertson pupil?

The pupils react to light but not to accommodation – seen in parkinsonism caused by encephalitis lethargica.

What do you understand by the term anisocoria?

Anisocoria is gross inequality of the pupils. Causes include:
- About 20% of normal individuals.
- Third nerve palsy.
- Iritis.
- Blind or amblyopia in one eye (pupil larger in the affected eye).
- Cerebrovascular accidents.

- Severe head trauma.
- Hemianopia due to optic tract involvement.

Note. Eccentric pupil occurs when the pupil is not in the centre of the iris. It may result from trauma or iritis and need not be pathognomonic of neurological disease.

Douglas MCL Argyll Robertson (1837–1909) of Edinburgh described these pupils in 1869 with neurosyphilis. His studies on the effects of the extracts of the Calabar bean (*Physostigma venenosum*) on the pupil were widely acclaimed. He was the President of the Royal College of Surgeons of Edinburgh.

References

Dacso CC & Bortz DL (1989) Significance of the Argyll Robertson pupil in clinical medicine. *Am J Med* **86**: 199.

Loewnfeld IE (1969) The Argyll Robertson pupil, 1869–1969, a critical survey of the literature. *Surv Ophthalmol* **14**: 199–299.

Lowenstein O (1956) The Argyll Robertson pupillary syndrome: mechanism and localisation. *Am J Ophthalmol* **42**: 105.

Poole CJM (1984) Argyll Robertson pupils due to neurosarcoidosis: evidence for site of lesion. *Br Med J* **289**: 356.

Robertson DA (1869) Four cases of spinal myosis; with remarks on the action of light on the pupil. *Edinb Med J* **15**: 487.

CASE 40   Holmes–Adie Syndrome

Instruction

Examine this patient's eyes.

Salient features

- The patient is usually a young woman.
- The pupil is large, regular or circular.
- The pupil will react sluggishly or fail to react to light. However, if a strong and persistent stimulus is used it can be shown that the pupil contracts excessively to a very small size and when the stimulus is removed it returns to its former size gradually – this is known as the 'myotonic' pupil.

Proceed as follows:

- Tell the examiner that you would like to check the ankle jerks and you expect them to be absent.

Diagnosis

This woman has a sluggishly reacting pupil with absent ankle jerks (lesion) due to Holmes–Adie Syndrome (aetiology) and is a benign disorder (functional status).

Questions

What is the significance of this condition?

It is benign and must not be mistaken for Argyll Robertson pupil.

What are the causes of a dilated pupil?

- Mydriatic eye drops.
- Third nerve lesion.
- Holmes–Adie syndrome.
- Lens implant, iridectomy.
- Deep coma, death.

What are the causes of a small pupil?

- Old age.
- Pilocarpine eye drops.
- Horner's syndrome.
- Argyll Robertson pupil.
- Pontine lesion.
- Narcotics.

Advanced-level Questions

What do you know about the factors that control the size of the pupil?

The sphincter muscle of the pupil (causing miosis) is supplied by the cholinergic parasympathetic nerves, whereas the dilator of the pupil (causing mydriasis) is supplied by noradrenergic sympathetic fibres. The parasympathetic fibres arise from the Edinger–Westphal nucleus. They travel by the IIIrd cranial nerve to the ciliary ganglion. Postganglionic fibres arise from the ciliary ganglion and are distributed by the ciliary nerve.

Where is the lesion in Adie's tonic pupil?

It is due to damage to the parasympathetic fibres from within the ciliary ganglion.

What is the difference between Adie's tonic pupil and Holmes–Adie syndrome?

Adie's tonic pupil with absent deep tendon jerks is called Holmes–Adie syndrome.

How does the Holmes–Adie pupil react to weak pilocarpine (0.125%) or 2.5% methacholine?

It usually constricts, indicating a supersensitivity to acetylcholine secondary to parasympathetic denervation resulting from degeneration of postganglionic neurons and neurons in the ciliary ganglion. There is no effect on a normal pupil.

Which conditions may accompany this syndrome?

Dysautonomias such as:

- Ross's syndrome (segmental loss of sweating).
- Cardiac arrhythmias.

Sir Gordon M Holmes (1876–1965) and WJ Adie (1886–1935) were London neurologists who described the condition independently in 1931. Saenger and Strasburger indepedently described the syndrome in 1902; it was first recorded in English literature by Markus in 1905.

References

Adie WJ (1932a) Tonic pupils and absent tendon reflexes: a benign disorder sui generis. Its complete and incomplete forms. *Brain* **55**: 98.

Adie W (1932b) Complete and incomplete forms of the benign disorder characterised by tonic pupils and absent tendon reflexes. *Br J Ophthalmol* **16**: 449.

Holmes G (1931) Partial iridoplegia associated with symptoms of other disease of the nervous system. *Trans Ophthalmol Soc UK* **41**: 209.

CASE 41   Homonymous Hemianopia

Instruction

Examine this patient's eyes.
Examine this patient's visual fields.

Salient features

- Homonymous hemianopia.

Proceed as follows:

- Check the visual acuity; examine the fundus.
- Tell the examiner that you would like to do a full neurological examination to look for an underlying cause:
  Stroke.
  Intracranial tumour.

Diagnosis

This patient has a homonymous hemianopia (lesion) for which I would like to determine the aetiology, such as a stroke or tumour.

Advanced-level Questions

Where is the lesion?

The lesion is in the optic tract and beyond (visual acuity is intact when the macula is spared):

Site of lesion	Type of homonymous hemianopia
Optic tract and first part of radiations	Incongruous
Optic radiations	Generally congruous
Temporal lobe	Superior quadrantic defect in each eye
Posterior parietal lobe	Inferior quadrantic defect in each eye

What further investigations would you do?

- Formal field testing: perimetry is particularly important if the patient holds a driver's licence.
- CT head scan.

CASE 42   Bitemporal Hemianopia

Instruction

Examine this patient's eyes.
Examine this patient's visual fields.

Salient features

- Bitemporal hemianopia which is due to a median lesion of the optic chiasma.

Proceed as follows:

- Examine the hands and face for acromegaly.
- Tell the examiner that you would like to look for signs of hypopituitarism (see page 402). The probable causes are as follows:
  Pituitary tumour.
  Craniopharyngioma.
  Suprasellar meningioma.
  Aneurysms.
  Metastases.
  Glioma.

Diagnosis

This patient has bitemporal hemianopia (lesion) and I would like to investigate for a median mass lesion compressing the optic chiasma.

Questions

How would you investigate this patient?

- Formal field testing – perimetry.
- Skull radiography (calcification of craniopharyngioma and size of the pituitary fossa which is best seen in the lateral skull radiograph).
- CT head scan.

Instruction

Examine this patient's visual fields.

Salient features

- Central scotoma.

Proceed as follows:

- Tell the examiner that you would like to examine the fundus.
- Remember that the optic discs may be:
  Pale (optic atrophy).
  Normal (retrobulbar neuritis).
  Swollen and pink (papillitis).

Diagnosis

This patient has a central scotoma (lesion) due to optic atrophy (aetiology).

Mention a few underlying causes for central scotoma.

- Demyelinating disorders (multiple sclerosis).
- Optic nerve compression by tumour, aneurysm.
- Glaucoma.
- Toxins – methanol, tobacco, lead, arsenical poisoning.
- Ischaemia – including central retinal artery occlusion due to thromboembolism, temporal arteritis, syphilis, idiopathic acute ischaemic neuropathy.
- Hereditary disorders – Friedreich's ataxia, Leber's optic atrophy.
- Paget's disease.
- Vitamin B_{12} deficiency.
- Secondary to retinitis pigmentosa.

CASE 44 Tunnel Vision

Instruction

Examine this patient's eyes..
Examine this patient's visual fields.

Salient features

- Intact central vision with constriction of the peripheral fields.

Proceed as follows:

- Examine for the following:
    Optic atrophy (primary and secondary).
    Retinitis pigmentosa (see page 606).
    Choroidoretinitis (see page 609).
    Glaucoma.

Diagnosis

This patient has tunnel vision (lesion) due to retinitis pigmentosa (aetiology).

What are the other causes of tunnel vision?

- Hysteria.
- Slight contraction of field occurs when there is a significant refractive error.

Note. Before making a diagnosis of hysteria, contraction of the visual fields due to extreme fatigue, poor attention, inadequate vision, diminished visual acuity or delayed reaction time must be excluded.

How would you differentiate hysteria from an organic cause of tubular vision?

In organic causes the field of vision widens progressively as the test objects are held further away from the eye, but in the hysterical person this widening is not seen and the entire width of the field is as great at 1 foot from the eye as it is at 5, 10 or 15 feet.

CASE 45 Parkinson's Disease

Instruction

Examine this patient.

Salient features

- Usually florid cases are seen in the examination and the striking abnormalities are:
  An expressionless or 'mask-like' face (fixed stare, infrequent blinking and ironed-out wrinkles).
  Drooling of saliva.
  Resting or pill-rolling movement (most common in the distal extremities).

Proceed as follows:

- Comment on the expressionless face, pill-rolling movement and drooling of saliva so that the examiner knows that you have observed these abnormalities. Elicit bradykinesia by asking the patient to touch her thumb with each finger in turn.
- Examine the tone, in particular at the wrist for cog-wheel rigidity.
- Proceed to do the glabellar tap (tap the forehead just above the bridge of

the nose repeatedly: in normal subjects the blinking will stop whereas the patient with Parkinson's disease continues to blink – referred to as Myerson's sign. It must be remembered that this sign is unreliable.)

- Ask the patient to walk, and comment on the paucity of movement including the absence of arm swing and festinating gait (the patient walks with a stooped posture as if trying to catch up with her centre of gravity). The feet may scrape the floor in taking steps so the patient trips easily (be prepared to prevent the patient from falling when examining the gait).

- Tell the examiner that you would like to:
  Ask the patient a few questions with a view to assessing her speech.
  Assess handwriting (tremulous and small, micrographia).
  Elicit a drug history, particularly regarding neuroleptics.

- Tell the examiner that you would like to look for:
  Postural hypotension (Shy–Drager syndrome, L-dopa treatment).
  Impaired vertical gaze (Steele–Richardson–Olzewski syndrome).
  Seborrhoea.

Note. The diagnosis of Parkinson's disease is entirely clinical but the results of certain investigations may help in recognizing alternative causes for parkinsonism.

Diagnosis

This patient has features of Parkinson's disease (lesion) which is due to long-standing use of phenothiazines (aetiology). The patient is severely disabled by the bradykinesia (functional status).

Questions

What comprises Parkinson's disease?

- Upper body dyskinesia must be present – it is a symptom complex containing many of the following features:
  Slowness of movement (bradykinesia).
  Poverty of movement (mask-like facies, diminished arm swing).
  Difficulty in initiating movement.
  Diminished amplitude of repetitive alternative movement.
  Inordinate difficulty in accomplishing some simultaneous or sequential motor acts.

- Rigidity is usually but not always present:
  Leadpipe rigidity where the increase in tone is equal in flexors and extensors of all four limbs but slightly more in flexors resulting in a part flexed 'simian' posture.

Cog-wheel rigidity is due to superimposed or underlying tremor.
- Postural instability is usually a late feature.
- Tremor – absent in about one-third of patients with Parkinson's disease
  at presentation and throughout its course in some.
  Resting, 3–5 Hz pill, pronation and supination rolling tremor of the
  upper limb.
  Tremor is intermittent (can usually be brought about by getting the
  subject to count backwards with the eyes closed and hands
  dangling over the armrests of the seat).
  The tremor is intensified by emotion or stress and disappears during
  sleep.
  The legs, head and jaw may shake as well. Jaw tremor is rare but is
  most distressing where the teeth may pound together until they
  become unbearably painful.

Advanced-level Questions

What are the pathological changes in Parkinson's disease?

The most typical pathological hallmarks of Parkinson's disease are:
- Neuronal loss with depigmentation of the substantia nigra.
- Lewy bodies, which are eosinophilic cytoplasmic inclusions in neurons
  consisting of aggregates of normal filaments.
  The following associations have been made with clinical features and
pathological changes:

Clinical deficit	Pathology
Motor symptoms	Degeneration of dopaminergic nigrostriatal pathway
Cognitive defects	Degeneration of dopaminergic mesocortical and mesolimbic pathways
Autonomic dysfunction	Dopamine depletion in the hypothalamus
'Freezing phenomenon'	Degeneration of the noradrenergic locus ceruleus
Dementia	Degeneration of the cholinergic nucleus

What is the mental status of patients with Parkinson's disease?

- In the initial stages, intellect and senses are usually preserved. Many
  patients have some intellectual deterioration – a slowness of thought
  and of memory retrieval (bradyphrenia), and subtle personality
  changes.
- Global dementia may develop in one-fifth of patients.
- Depression occurs in one-third of patients.
- Acute confusion can be precipitated by drug therapy.

Note. Parkinson's disease must be kept in mind in elderly patients presenting with a history of frequent falls.

What are the causes of Parkinson's disease?

- True parkinsonism:
    Idiopathic (due to degeneration of the substantia nigra) – also known as Parkinson's disease.
    Drug induced (chlorpromazine, metaclopramide, prochlorperazine).
    Anoxic brain damage such as cardiac arrest, exposure to manganese and carbon monoxide.
    Post-encephalitic – as a result of encephalitis lethargica or von Economo's disease.
    1-Methyl-4-phenyl-1,2,3,6-tetrahydropyridine toxicity – seen in drug abusers.
    Multiple system atrophy.
    Progressive supranuclear atrophy.
- Pseudoparkinsonism:
    Essential tremor.
    Atherosclerotic (vascular) pseudoparkinsonism (mention that in the past atherosclerosis was thought to be a cause of Parkinson's disease but this is no longer accepted as a cause).

What is the difference between rigidity, spasticity and gegenhalten?

- Rigidity indicates increased tone affecting opposing muscle groups equally and is present throughout the range of passive movement. When smooth it is called 'lead-pipe' rigidity and when intermittent is termed 'cog-wheel' rigidity. It is common in extrapyramidal syndromes, Wilson's disease, Creutzfeld–Jakob disease.
- Spasticity of the clasp knife type is characterized by increased tone which is maximal at the beginning of movement and suddenly decreases as passive movement is continued. It occurs chiefly in the flexors of the upper limb and extensors of the lower limb (anti-gravity muscles).
- Gegenhalten, or paratonia, is where the increased muscle tone varies, and becomes worse the more the patient tries to relax.

What do you understand by the 'wheelchair sign' in Parkinson's disease?

Patients with advanced disease and 'on-off' motor fluctuations require a wheelchair when 'off' and when 'on' are seen to walk about (sometimes pushing the chair!). These patients are rarely permanently wheelchair-bound; in contrast, those who never leave their wheelchair usually do not have Parkinson's disease.

What is the role of protein diets in patients who have episodes of sudden and substantial loss of mobility?

High protein diets should be avoided in these patients, because a large influx of dietary amino acids can interfere with the transport of L-dopa into the brain.

How is the severity of Parkinson's disease graded?

Hoehn–Yahr staging grades Parkinson's disease into five stages:

Newly diagnosed disease	Stage I
Moderately severe disease	Stages II and III
Advanced disease	Stages IV and V

How would you manage a patient with Parkinson's disease?

1. Symptomatic therapy:
- When tremor is the main problem – anticholinergic drugs such as trihexyphenidyl, benztropine.
- When bradykinesia is the main problem – L-dopa with a decarboxylase inhibitor such as carbidopa or benserazide. Second-line drugs include amantidine and synthetic dopamine agonists (bromocriptine, pergolide).
2. Protective therapy:
- Selegiline (deprenyl), a monoamine oxidase B inhibitor, is said to retard the progression of early Parkinson's disease. It is not clear whether the beneficial effect of selegiline derives from a symptomatic benefit (i.e. by increasing dopaminergic transmission) or by decreasing the rate of neuronal death. There is no beneficial effect of tocopherol (a component of vitamin E that traps free radicals) in this condition. Recent evidence suggests that selegiline may increase mortality.

In which condition is L-dopa absolutely contraindicated?

Melanoma.

What do you know about 'drug holidays' in levodopa therapy?

Drug holidays (i.e. discontinuation of therapy) was previously claimed to enhance the efficacy of treatment when it was resumed; is now known to be dangerous (deaths have occurred) and of doubtful value.

What do you know about dopamine receptors?

At least four types of receptor have been reported: D_1 and D_2 are the two major families of dopamine receptors. For neurotransmission to occur, a complex consisting of a dopamine receptor and G protein (guanine nucleotide-binding protein) must be formed. This complex then usually couples to the enzyme adenylate cyclase which controls the formation of the second messenger, cyclic AMP. Alteration of the second messenger leads to a cascade of events that ultimately determines the transfer of information between nerve cells. The D_{2A} receptor is involved in the therapeutic response elicited by dopaminergic agonists in parkinsonism, although the mechanism is not clear at a physiological level. The role of the D_1 family is unclear – whether the activation of these receptors leads to useful effects (i.e. reduction of parkinsonian deficits), undesireable effects (e.g. dyskinesia), or both. Bromocriptine, pergolide and lisuride all stimulate D_2 receptors, whereas bromocriptine and lisuride are D_1 receptor antagonists and pergolide is a D_1 receptor agonist.

Mention some newer drugs used in the treatment of Parkinson's disease.

• Dopamine antagonists: cabergoline, ropinirole, terguride, talipexole.
• Inhibitors of catechol *O*-methyltransferase: Ro 40-7592, nitecapone (OR 462).
• Inhibitors of glutamate receptors: CPP (3-(2-carboxy-piprazin-4-yl)propyl-1-phosphonate), lamotrigine.
• GM-1 ganglioside – when monkeys were treated with this drug from cow's brain their motor function was returned to normal.

What is the role of fetal tissue in Parkinson's disease?

Parkinson's disease is characterized by loss of midbrain dopamine neurons that innervate the caudate and putamen. Patients tend to have a reduced response to levodopa after 5–20 years of therapy, with 'on–off' fluctuations consisting of dyskinesia alternating with immobility. Animal experiments have suggested that fetal dopaminergic neurons can survive transplantation and restore neurological function. Trials are underway to determine whether fetal grafts can improve motor function in patients with Parkinson's disease. Fetal ventral mesencephalic tissue is implanted in the patient's postcommissural putamen.

What is the role of thalamotomy in Parkinson's disease?

Thalamotomy used to be the main treatment until 1950, but with the introduction of levodopa it became less popular. However, there has been a revival of stereotactic surgery prompted by the failure of levodopa in four main aspects: in severe tremor, levodopa-induced dyskinesia, advanced Parkinson's disease and akinetic–rigid syndromes. Four types of stereotactic surgery are practised:

- Thalamotomy for intractable tremor where a radiofrequency lesion is placed in the venterointermediate nucleus (VIM) of the thalamus. It is unsuitable for bilateral tremor as bilateral thalamotomy tends to cause impairment of speech.
- Thalamic stimulation with a fine electrode in the VIM nucleus and a pacemaker inserted under the skin on the chest. This relieves tremor and can be performed bilaterally. Neither procedure improves akinesia, the most disabling aspect of Parkinson's disease.
- Posteroventral pallidotomy – improves akinesia, rigidity and levodopa-induced dyskinesia but is less effective for tremor.

Note. Patients with dementia and hallucinations tolerate all surgical procedures poorly and any benefit in patients with rapidly progressive parkinsonism is likely to be short lived.

What are Parkinson plus syndromes?

Some patients have other neurological deficits in addition to Parkinson's disease. Examples of these so-called Parkinson plus syndromes are:
- Steele–Richardson–Olszewski disease (akinesia, axial rigidity of the neck, bradyphrenia, supranuclear palsy).
- Multiple system atrophy.
  Olivopontocerebellar degeneration.
  Strionigral degeneration.
  Progressive autonomic failure (Shy–Drager syndrome).
- Basal ganglia calcification.

What is tardive dyskinesia?

Tardive dyskinesia is seen in patients taking neuroleptics. Its manifestations are orofacial dyskinesia such as smacking, chewing lip movements, discrete dystonia or choreiform movements and – rarely – rocking movements. Withdrawal of the offending drug will improve these symptoms over a period of 3–4 years, except in a small minority of patients.

Mention some heredodegenerative parkinsonian disorders.

- Hallervorden–Spatz disease: autosomal recessive; patients also have dementia, dystonia, choreoathetosis, retinitis pigmentosa. There is increased iron deposition and increased cysteine in the globus pallidus.
- Fahr's disease or familial basal ganglia calcification: patients also have chorea, dementia and palilalia.
- Olivopontocerebellar and spinocerebellar degenerations: autosomal dominant, associated cerebellar ataxia and retinitis pigmentosa.

James Parkinson (1755–1824) first reported six cases of this syndrome in 1817 (at the age of 62 years).

JC Steele, JC Richardson and J Olszewski were all US neurologists.

K von Economo (1876–1931), an Australian neurologist, also wrote on Wilson's disease.

CD Marsden, contemporary Professor of Neurology, National Hospital, Queen's Square, London; his chief interest is Parkinson's disease and movement disorders.

References

Calne DB (1993) Treatment of Parkinson's disease. *N Engl J Med* **329**: 1021.

Cotzias GC, Van Woert MH & Schiffer IM (1967) Aromatic amino acids and modification of Parkinson's disease. *N Engl J Med* **276**: 374–379.

Kordower JH, Freeman TB, Snow BJ et al (1995) Neuropathological evidence of graft survival and striatal reinnervation after the transplantation of fetal mesencephalic tissue in patients with Parkinson's disease. *N Engl J Med* **332**: 1118–1124.

Parkinson Study Group (1993) Effect of tocopherol and deprenyl (selegiline) on the progression of disability in early Parkinson's disease. *N Engl J Med* **328**: 176–183.

Quinn N (1995) Parkinsonism – recognition and differential diagnosis. *Br Med J* **310**: 447–452.

CASE 46 Cerebellar Syndrome

Instruction

Examine this patient, who presented with a history of falling to one side. Demonstrate the cerebellar signs.

Salient features

Proceed as follows:

- Tell the examiner you would like to ask the patient a few questions to assess his speech.
- Ask the patient to keep his arms outstretched; then give them a small push downward and look for rebound phenomenon.
- Examine for rapid alternating movements with the hand.
- Do the finger–nose test: look for past-pointing and intention tremor.
- Do the heel–shin test.
- Examine the gait, in particular tandem walking. If ataxia is not marked, the patient's gait may be tested with eyes closed; he often progresses to the side of the lesion.

- Tell the examiner that you would like to examine the fundus for optic atrophy as demyelination is the commonest cause of cerebellar signs.

Diagnosis

This patient has a cerebellar syndrome with optic atrophy (lesion) due to multiple sclerosis (aetiology) and is markedly ataxic (functional status).

Questions

How may cerebellar signs manifest?

- Disorders of movement:
    Nystagmus.
    Scanning dysarthria.
    Lack of finger–nose co-ordination (past-pointing) – dysmetria.
    Rebound phenomenon – inability to arrest strong contraction on sudden removal of resistance. This is known as Holmes' rebound phenomenon.
    Intention tremor.
    Dysdiadochokinesia – impairment of rapid alternating movements (clumsy).
    Dyssynergia – movements involving more than one joint are broken into parts.
- Hypotonia.
- Absent reflexes or pendular reflexes.
- Lack of co-ordination of gait – patient tends to fall towards the side of the lesion.

Note.
1. The classical clinical triad of cerebellar disease is: Ataxia, Atonia, Asthenia.
2. The cerebellum is not primarily a motor organ. It is developed phylogenetically from a primary vestibular area and is involved in modulation of motor activity. It receives afferents from the vestibular nuclei, spinal cord and cerebral cortex via the pontine nuclei.

What are the causes of cerebellar syndrome?

- Demyelination (multiple sclerosis).
- Brainstem vascular lesion.
- Phenytoin toxicity.
- Alcoholic cerebellar degeneration (there is atrophy of the anterior vermis of the cerebellum).

- Space-occupying lesion in the posterior fossa including cerebellopontine angle tumour.
- Hypothyroidism (a reversible cause).
- Paraneoplastic manifestation of bronochogenic carcinoma.
- Friedreich's ataxia and other hereditary ataxias.
- Congenital malformations at the level of the foramen magnum.

Advanced-level Questions

How are cerebellar signs localized?

- Gait ataxia (inability to do tandem walking): anterior lobe (palaeocerebellum).
- Truncal ataxia (drunken gait, titubation): flocculonodular or posterior lobe (archicerebellum).
- Limb ataxia, especially upper limbs and hypotonia: lateral lobes (neocerebellum).

What is the difference between sensory ataxia and cerebellar ataxia?

	Cerebellar ataxia	Sensory ataxia
Site of lesion	Cerebellum	Posterior column or peripheral nerves
Deep tendon reflexes	Unchanged or pendular	Lost or diminished
Deep sensation	Normal	Decreased or lost
Sphincter disturbances	None	Decreased when posterior column involved, causing overflow incontinence

If you were allowed to do one investigation, which one would you choose in a patient with a suspected cerebellar lesion?

Magnetic resonance imaging (MRI).

Sir Gordon M Holmes (1876–1965), consultant neurologist, National Hospital for Nervous Diseases, Queen Square, London, whose observations on wartime gunshot wounds allowed him to study cerebellar disease. He was the editor of the journal *Brain*.

References

Gilman S (1986) Cerebellum and motor dysfunction. In: Asbury AK, McKhann GM, McDonald WI, eds. *Diseases of the Nervous System*, pp. 401–422. Philadelphia: WB Saunders.

Holmes G (1922) The Croonian lectures on the clinical symptoms of cerebellar disease and their interpretation. *Lancet* **i**: 1177, 1231.

Holmes G (1922) The Croonian lectures on the clinical symptoms of cerebellar disease and their interpretation. *Lancet* **ii**: 59, 111.

Holmes G (1939) The cerebellum of man. *Brain* **62**: 1–30.

CASE 47 Jerky Nystagmus

Instruction

Examine this patient's eyes.
Test the patient's eye movements.

Salient features

- Horizontal nystagmus with fast components to right or left side (when eliciting nystagmus take care to keep your finger at least 2 feet away from the patient and avoid going laterally beyond the extent of binocular vision).

Proceed as follows:

- Look for other cerebellar signs (see page 137).
- Tell the examiner that you would like to do the following:
  Examine the fundus for optic atrophy (multiple sclerosis).
  Take a history of vertigo (vestibular nystagmus).

Note. Remember that if the patient has vertical nystagmus in addition to horizontal nystagmus it is more likely to be vestibular nystagmus or brainstem disease.

Diagnosis

This patient has a jerky nystagmus with optic atrophy (lesion) due to multiple sclerosis (aetiology). I would like to examine her neurological system to evaluate the disability (functional status).

Questions

What do you understand by the term 'nystagmus'?

Nystagmus is a series of involuntary, rhythmic oscillations of one or both eyes. It may be horizontal, vertical or rotatory.

Advanced-level Questions

What is pendular nystagmus?

In pendular nystagmus, the oscillations are equal in speed and amplitude in both directions of movement. It may be seen on central gaze when the vision is poor, as in severe refractive error or macular disease.

What do you understand by the term 'jerky' nystagmus?

Jerky or phasic nystagmus is a condition in which eye movement in one direction is faster than that in the other. This is usually seen in the horizontal plane and is brought out by lateral gaze to one or both sides. It is seen with lesions of the cerebellum, vestibular apparatus or their connections in the brainstem.

What is dissociated nystagmus?

Dissociated or ataxic nystagmus is irregular nystagmus in the abducting eye. It is bilateral in multiple sclerosis, brainstem tumour or Wernicke's encephalopathy. It is unilateral in vascular disease of the brainstem. It is due to a lesion in the medial longitudinal fasciculus (which links the sixth nerve nucleus on one side to the medial rectus portion of the third nerve on the other).

Where is the lesion in vestibular nystagmus?

It may be in one of two locations:
- Peripheral (labyrinth or vestibular nerve), as in labyrinthitis, Ménière's syndrome, acoustic neuroma, otitis media, head injury.
- Central (affecting vestibular nuclei), as in stroke, multiple sclerosis, tumours, alcoholism.

What do you know about 'downbeat' and 'upbeat' nystagmus?

Downbeat nystagmus is associated with brainstem lesions, meningoencephalitis and hypomagnesaemia. Upbeat nystagmus is caused by lesions of the anterior vermis of the cerebellum.

K Wernicke (1848–1904) graduated from Poland; although aware that a toxic factor was important in the aetiology, he did not realize that this syndrome was due to a nutritional deficiency.

P Ménière (1799–1862), French ear, nose and throat specialist.

CASE 48 Speech

Instruction

Ask this patient some questions.

Salient features

Proceed as follows:

- Ask the patient simple questions regarding personal details such as name, age, occupation, address and handedness (remember that over 90% of left-handed people have a dominant left hemisphere).
- Test the following:
  Comprehension
  > Put your tongue out.
  > Shut your eyes.
  > Touch your nose.
  > Smile.
  > Two-step commands, such as touch your left ear with your right hand.

  Orientation
  > Time–date.
  > Place.

  Name familiar objects
  > Pen.
  > Coin.
  > Watch.

  Articulation
  > Ask the patient to repeat the following:
  >> British constitution.
  >> West Register Street.
  >> Baby hippopotamus.
  >> Biblical criticism.
  >> Artillery.

  Abbreviated mental test
  > Address to recall: 42 West Street.
  > Age.
  > Date of birth.
  > Time.
  > Year.
  > Recognition of two persons such as doctor and nurse.
  > Name of this place.

Name of the monarch or prime minister.
Year of World War I or World War II.
Count backwards from 20 to 1.
Serially subtract 7 from 200.
- Tell the examiner that you would like to check the 'primitive' reflexes:
  Snout reflex: brought about by tapping the upper lip slightly. There is
      puckering or protrusion of the lips with percussion. The
      muscles around the mouth and the base of the nose contract.
  Palmomental reflex: occurs when a disagreeable stimulus is drawn
      from the thenar eminence at the wrist to the base of the thumb.
      There is ipsilateral contraction of the orbicularis oris and
      mentalis muscles. The corner of the mouth elevates slightly
      and the skin over the chin wrinkles.
  Sucking reflex: elicited by tapping or lightly touching the lips with a
      tongue blade or the examiner's finger. Sucking movements of
      the lips occur when they are stroked or touched.

Note. The above three reflexes are normal in infants, may be present
in normal individuals and are said to be present in a larger number of
patients with neurological disease. They are most often seen in those
with diffuse cerebral conditions that affect the frontal lobes and
pyramidal tracts. The occurrence of more than one reflex is more
suggestive of disease than normality.
  Grasp reflex: obtained when the examiner's hand is gently inserted
      into the palm of the patient's hand (when the patient is
      distracted, usually by engaging him in conversation). With a
      positive response the patient grasps the examiner's hand and
      continues to grasp it as it is moved. The presence of the grasp
      reflex indicates disease of the supplementary motor area of the
      frontal cortex.
  Jaw jerk (see page 98).

Diagnosis

This patient has expressive dysphasia (lesion) due to a stroke (aetiology)
and is unable to express himself (functional status).

Questions

What do you understand by the term 'dysphasia'?

Dysphasia is a disorder of the content of speech which usually follows a
lesion of the dominant cortex:
- When the *speech defect* is expressive dysphasia or nominal dysphasia
    or motor dysphasia, the *site of the lesion in the cortex* is the posterior
    inferior part of the dominant frontal lobe, i.e. *Broca's area*.

- When the *speech defect* is sensory dysphasia or receptive dysphasia the *site of the lesion* is the superior temporal lobe or *Wernicke's area*.

What do you understand by the term 'dysarthria'?

Dysarthria is an inability to articulate properly due to local lesions in the mouth or disorders of speech muscles or their connections. There is no disorder of the content of speech. The causes of dysarthria are:
- Stutter.
- Paralysis of cranial nerves – Bell's palsy, 9th, 10th and 11th nerves.
- Cerebellar disease – staccato, scanning speech.
- Parkinson's speech – slow, quiet, slurred, monotonous.
- Pseudobulbar palsy – monotonous, high-pitched 'hot potato' speech.
- Progressive bulbar palsy – nasal.

Advanced-level Questions

What are the components of speech?

- Phonation: abnormality is called dysphonia.
- Articulation: abnormality is called dysarthria.
- Language: abnormality is called dysphasia.

What are the other dominant hemisphere functions?

- Right–left orientation.
- Finger identification.
- Calculation.

What are the non-dominant hemisphere functions?

- Drawing ability.
- Topographic ability.
- Construction.
- Dressing.
- Facial recognition.
- Awareness of body and space.
- Motor persistence.

What are the parietal lobe signs?

- Loss of accurate localization of touch, position, joint sense and temperature appreciation.
- Loss of two-point discrimination.

- Astereognosis.
- Dysgraphaesthesia.
- Sensory inattention.
- Attention hemianopia, homonymous hemianopia, or lower quadrantic hemianopia.

What do you understand by the term agnosia?

Agnosia is a failure to recognize objects despite the fact that the sensory pathways for sight, sound or touch are intact. This is tested by asking the patient to feel, name and describe the use of certain objects.

What are the different types of agnosia?

Different types of agnosia include:
- Tactile agnosia and astereognosis: where the patient is unable to recognize objects placed in his hands despite the fact that the sensory system of the hands and fingers is intact and there is adequate motor function to allow him to examine the object. The lesion is in the parietal lobe.
- Prosopagnosia: inability to recognize a familiar face. The lesion is in the parieto-occipital lobe.
- Visual agnosia: inability to recognize objects despite the fact that the main visual pathways to the occipital cortex are preserved. The lesion is in the parieto-occipital lobe.
- Anosognosia: the lack of awareness or realization that the limbs are paralysed, weak or have impaired sensation. The lesion is usually in the non-dominant parietal lobe.

What you understand by the term apraxia?

Apraxia is the inability to perform purposeful volitional movements in the absence of motor weakness, sensory deficits or severe inco-ordination. Usually the defect is in the dominant parietal lobe, with disruption of connections to the motor cortex and to the opposite hemisphere.

What are the different types of apraxia?

Different types of apraxia include:
- Dressing apraxias: patient is unable to put on his clothes correctly.
- Gait apraxia: difficulty in walking, although patients may show intact leg movements when examined in bed.
- Ideomotor apraxia: patients are unable to perform movements on command, although they may do this automatically, e.g. lick their lips.

- Ideational apraxias: difficulty in carrying out a complex series of movements, e.g. to take a match from a box to light a cigarette.
- Constructional apraxia: patient has difficulty in arranging patterns on blocks or copying designs.

What do you know about dyslexia?

Reading difficulties, including dyslexia, occur as a part of a continuum that also includes normal reading ability. It is not an all-or-none phenomenon but, like hypertension, occurs in degrees. It has been defined as a disorder that is manifested by difficulty in learning to read despite conventional instruction, adequate intelligence and sociocultural opportunity.

Sir Charles Sherrington (1857–1952), Oxford University, and Lord Edgar Douglas Adrian (1889–1977), Cambridge University, were awarded the Nobel Prize in 1932 for their discoveries regarding the functions of neurons.

References

de Noordhout AM & Delwaide PJ (1988) The palmomental reflex in Parkinson's disease. *Arch Neurol* **45**: 425–427.
Damasio AR (1992) Aphasia. *N Engl J Med* **326**: 531–539.

CASE 49   Expressive Dysphasia

Instruction

Ask this patient a few questions.

Salient features

- Patient has difficulty in finding the appropriate words, comprehension is intact and repetition may or may not be intact.

Proceed as follows:

- Tell the examinter that you would like to carry out a neurological examination of the patient for a right-sided stroke.

Diagnosis

This patient has expressive dysphasia (lesion) due to a right-sided stroke (aetiology).

Questions

Where is the lesion?

In Broca's area, which is located in the posterior portion of the third left frontal gyrus. It is the motor association cortex for face, tongue, lips and palate. It contains the motor patterns necessary to produce speech.

How would you manage this patient?

• CT head scan to localize the affected area.
• Aspirin.
• Referral to the speech therapist.
• General rehabilitation of a patient with stroke.

Pierre Paul Broca (1824–1880) was Professor of Surgery in Paris. His notable achievements were in anthropology and his suggestion of cerebral localization of speech was first made at a French Anthropological Society meeting in 1861. He is reported to have described muscular dystrophy (before Duchenne), venous spread of cancer (before Rokitansky) and rickets as a nutritional disorder (before Virchow).

References

Damasio AR (1992) Medical progress: aphasia. *N Engl J Med* **326**: 531–539.
Geshwind N (1971) Aphasia. *N Engl J Med* **284**: 654.

CASE 50 Cerebellar Dysarthria

Instruction

Ask this patient a few questions.

Salient features

• The speech may be scanning (enunciation is difficult, words are produced slowly and in a measured fashion) or staccato (in bursts). Scanning speech is more common in multiple sclerosis, whereas staccato speech is more common in Friedreich's ataxia.
• Articulation is uneven, words are slurred and variations in pitch and loudness occur.

Proceed as follows:

- Tell the examiner that you would like to carry out a neurological examination of the patient for cerebellar signs.

See *Cerebellar syndrome* (page 136) for discussion.

Diagnosis

This patient has scanning speech (lesion) due to cerebellar involvement secondary to chronic alcohol abuse (aetiology).

Questions

What do you understand by the term 'dysarthria'?

Dysarthria is impaired articulation of speech. It may result from lesions of muscles, myoneural junctions or motor neurons of lips, tongue, palate and pharynx. Common causes include mechanical defects such as ill-fitting dentures or cleft palate. Dysarthria may also result from impaired hearing which begins in early childhood.

Advanced-level Questions

How would you test the different structures responsible for articulation?

- Lips: ask the patient to say, 'me, me, me'.
- Tongue: ask the patient to say, 'la, la, la'.
- Pharynx: ask the patient to say, 'kuh, gut'.
- Palate, larynx and expiratory muscles: ask the patient to say, 'ah'. In palatal paralysis the patient's speech is worse when the head is bent forwards.

Articulation can also be tested by asking the patient to repeat the following:
- British constitution.
- Hippopotamus.
- Methodist Episcopal.
- Constantinople is the capital of Turkey.

CASE 51 Third Cranial Nerve Palsy

Instruction

Examine this patient's eyes.

Salient features

- Unilateral ptosis (from paralysis of the levator palpebrae superioris).
- Dilated pupil reacting slowly or incompletely to light (paralysis of the constrictor of the pupil).
- Paralysis of accommodation (from involvement of ciliary muscle).
- Squint and diplopia resulting from weakness of muscles supplied by the third cranial nerve (superior, inferior, medial recti and inferior oblique). The eye will be in the position of abduction, i.e. down and out (if the fourth and sixth nerves are intact).
- Diplopia may not be obvious until the affected eyelid is elevated manually.

Proceed as follows:

- Exclude associated fourth cranial nerve lesion (supplies the superior oblique) by tilting the head of the patient to the same side – the affected eye will intort if the fourth cranial nerve is intact. Remember superior oblique intorts the eye (SIN). Inferior oblique externally rotates the eye.
- Tell the examiner that you would like to check:
  The urine for sugar (diabetes mellitus).
  The blood pressure (hypertension).

Note. Vascular lesions (such as those associated with diabetes and arteritis) which infarct the third nerve may produce a complete oculomotor palsy with pupillary sparing. The pupillomotor fibres are around the periphery of the third nerve. Compression of the mass or aneurysm often involves the pupil.

Diagnosis

This patient has a R/L third nerve palsy (lesion) due to diabetes mellitus (aetiology).

Questions

What are the common causes of a third nerve palsy?

- Hypertension and diabetes are the most common causes of pupil-sparing third nerve palsy. (**Note.** The presence of pain is not a good discriminating feature between diabetes and aneurysm, as pain is present in both.) Diabetic third nerve palsy usually recovers within 3 months.
- Multiple sclerosis.
- Aneurysms of posterior communicating artery (painful ophthalmoplegia).
- Trauma.
- Tumours, collagen, vascular disorder, syphilis.
- Ophthalmoplegic migraine.
- Encephalitis.
- Parasellar neoplasms.
- Meningioma at the wing of sphenoid.
- Basal meningitis.
- Carcinoma at the base of the skull.

How would you investigate such a patient?

- Test blood pressure and urine for sugar.
- ESR to exclude temporal arteritis (in the elderly).
- Edrophonium test to exclude myasthenia if the pupil is not involved.
- Thyroid function tests and orbital ultrasonography to exclude thyroid disease.
- CT scan of the head.
- Arteriography, especially when the pupil is involved and there is severe pain.

Advanced-level Questions

When would you suspect a lesion of the third nerve nucleus?

In the following instances:
- Unilateral third nerve palsy with contralateral superior rectus palsy and bilateral partial ptosis.
- Bilateral third nerve palsy (with or without internal ophthalmoplegia associated with spared levator function).

What do you know about the muscles of extraocular movement?

Each eye is moved by three pairs of muscles and the precise action of these muscles depends on the position of the eye; the actions are as follows:
- Medial and lateral recti (first pair of muscles): adduct and abduct the eye respectively.
- Superior and inferior recti: elevate and depress the abducted eye.

- Superior and inferior obliques: depress and elevate the adducted eye.

Note. Superior and inferior recti act in the **ab**ducted position (mnemonic RAB).

Do you know of any eponymous syndromes in which the third cranial nerve is involved?

- Weber's syndrome: ipsilateral third nerve palsy with contralateral hemiplegia. The lesion is in the midbrain.
- Benedikt's syndrome: ipsilateral third nerve palsy with contralateral involuntary movements such as tremor, chorea and athetosis. It is due to a lesion of the red nucleus in the midbrain.
- Claude's syndrome: ipsilateral oculomotor paresis with contralateral ataxia and tremor. It is due to a lesion of the third nerve and red nucleus.
- Nothnagel's syndrome: unilateral oculomotor paralysis combined with ipsilateral cerebellar ataxia.

M Benedikt (1835–1920), an Austrian physician, described this syndrome in 1889.
Sir HD Weber (1823–1918) qualified in Bonn and worked at Guy's Hospital, London.
Henri Claude (1869–1945), a French psychiatrist.
Carl Wilhelm Nothnagel (1841–1905), an Austrian physician.

Reference

Adaur KK (1982) Current concepts in neurology: diagnosis and management of facial paralysis. *N Engl J Med* **307**: 348–351.

CASE 52 Sixth Cranial Nerve Palsy

Instruction

Examine this patient's eyes.

Salient features

- The eye is deviated medially and there is failure of lateral movement.
- The diplopia is maximal when looking towards the affected side. The two images are parallel and separated in the horizontal plane. The outer image comes from the affected eye and disappears when the eye is covered.

Proceed as follows:

- Tell the examiner that you would like to check the following:
  Blood pressure and urine sugar.
  Hearing and corneal sensation (early signs of acoustic neuroma).

Diagnosis

This patient has a sixth nerve palsy (lesion) due to diabetes mellitus (aetiology) and is having severe diplopia (functional status).

Questions

What are the causes of sixth nerve palsy?

- Hypertension.
- Diabetes.
- Raised intracranial pressure (false localizing signs).
- Multiple sclerosis.
- Basal meningitis.
- Encephalitis.
- Acoustic neuroma, nasopharyngeal carcinoma.

Advanced-level Questions

Where is the nucleus of the sixth nerve located?

In the pons. (**Note.** The nuclei of the first four cranial nerves are situated above the pons and those of the last four cranial nerves are situated below the pons.)

What are the structures in close proximity to the sixth nerve nucleus and fascicles?

These include:
- Facial and trigeminal nerves.
- Corticospinal tract.
- Median longitudinal fasciculus.
- Parapontine reticular formation.
  A combination of clinical findings pointing to the involvement of these structures indicates the presence of an intrapontine lesion.

What you know about the peripheral course of the abducens nerve?

It is a lengthy one from the brainstem and base of the skull, through the petrous tip and cavernous sinus, to the superior orbital fissure and orbit. Lesions at any of these sites may affect the nerve.

Have you heard of Gradenigo's syndrome?

Inflammation of the tip of the temporal bone may involve the fifth and sixth cranial nerves as well as the greater superficial petrosal nerve, resulting in unilateral paralysis of the lateral rectus nerve, pain in the distribution of the trigeminal nerve (particularly its first division) and excessive lacrimation.

Do you know any eponymous syndromes where the pons is infarcted and consequently the sixth cranial nerve is involved?

- Raymond's syndrome: ipsilateral sixth nerve paralysis and contralateral paresis of the extremities.
- Millard–Gubler syndrome, in which there is ipsilateral sixth and seventh nerve palsy with contralateral hemiplegia.
- Foville's syndrome has all the features of Millard–Gubler paralysis with lateral conjugate gaze palsy.

Mention other syndromes with sixth nerve involvement.

- Duane's syndrome: widening of the palpebral fissure on abduction and narrowing on adduction.
- Gerhardt's syndrome: bilateral abducens palsy.
- Möbius syndrome: paralysis of extraocular muscles, especially abducens, with paresis of facial muscles.

What do you know about Tolosa–Hunt syndrome?

It is a syndrome characterized by unilateral recurrent pain in the retro-orbital region with palsy of the extraocular muscles resulting from involvement of the third, fourth, fifth and sixth cranial nerves. It has been attributed to inflammation of the cavernous sinus.

C Gradenigo (1859–1926), an Italian otolaryngologist, described this syndrome in 1904.
E Tolosa, a Spanish neurosurgeon.
WE Hunt, an American neurosurgeon.
ALJ Millard (1830–1915), a French physician.
AM Gubler (1821–1915), Professor of Therapeutics in France.
ALF Foville (1799–1878), Professor of Physiology at Rouen, described his syndrome in 1848.

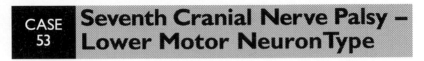

CASE 53 Seventh Cranial Nerve Palsy – Lower Motor Neuron Type

Instruction

Look at this patient's face.
Examine the cranial nerves.

Salient features

- Weakness of muscles of one half of the face – patient is unable to screw her eyes tightly shut or move the angle of the mouth on the affected side.
- Loss of facial expression.
- Widened palpebral fissure.

Proceed as follows:

- Look for the following when the patient is unaware of being observed:
  Flatter nasolabial folds on the affected side.
  Mouth on the affected side droops and participates manifestly less while talking.
  The eyelid on the affected side closes just after the opposite eyelid.
- Look at the external auditory meatus for herpes zoster (Ramsay Hunt syndrome).
- Look for parotid gland enlargement.
- Tell the examiner that you would like to do the following:
  Examine for taste (loss of taste with the involvement of chorda tympani).
  Check for hearing (for hyperacusis resulting from involvement of the nerve to stapedius muscle).
  Examine tympanic membrane for otitis media.
  Test the urine for sugar (diabetes).

Diagnosis

The patient has lower motor neuron seventh cranial nerve palsy (lesion) which is idiopathic (aetiology). She is distressed because the condition causes severe disfigurement while talking (functional status).

Questions

How would you differentiate between upper and lower motor neuron palsy?

In lower motor neuron palsy the whole half of the face on the affected side is involved. In upper motor neuron palsy the upper half of the face (the forehead) is spared.

Advanced-level Questions

What are the causes of bilateral facial nerve palsy?

- Guillain–Barré syndrome (see page 251).
- Sarcoidosis in the form of uveoparotid fever (Heerfordt's disease).
- Melkersson–Rosenthal syndrome, which is a triad of facial palsy, recurrent facial oedema and plication of the tongue.

Note. Myasthenia may mimic bilateral facial nerve palsy.

What are causes of unilateral facial nerve palsy?

Lower motor neuron (all the muscles of one half of the face are affected):
- Bell's palsy (idiopathic). Recent studies using a polymerase chain reaction have implicated herpes simplex viral infection in Bell's palsy.
- Herpes zoster.
- Cerebellopontine angle tumours.
- Parotid tumours.
- Old polio.
- Otitis media.
- Skull fracture.

Upper motor neuron (forehead spared):
- Stroke (hemiplegia).

Is the facial nerve a motor nerve or a sensory nerve?

The facial nerve is predominantly a motor nerve and supplies all muscles concerned with facial expression and the stapedius muscle. Uncommonly, it may have a sensory component which is small – the nervus intermedius of Wrisberg. It conveys taste sensation from the anterior two-thirds of the tongue and, probably, cutaneous impulses from the anterior wall of the external auditory canal.

What do you know of nervus intermedius?

Nervus intermedius or pars intermedia of Wrisberg is the sensory or the parasympathetic root of the facial nerve, and is lateral and inferior to the motor root. Inside the internal auditory meatus it lies between the motor root and the eighth cranial nerve. The sensory cells are located in the geniculate ganglion (at the bend of the facial nerve in the facial canal) and their nerve fibres enter the pons with the motor root. The geniculate ganglion is continued distally as the chorda tympani, which carries taste and preganglionic parasympathetic fibres. This nerve consists of contributions from three areas:

- Superior salivary nucleus (in the pons) supplies secretory fibres to the glands.
- Gustatory or solitary nucleus (in the medulla) receives taste fibres via the chorda tympani.
- Dorsal part of the trigeminal nerve receives cutaneous sensation from the external auditory meatus and the skin behind the ear (distributed with the facial nerve proper).

How would you manage Bell's palsy?

- Physiotherapy: massage, electrical stimulation, splint to prevent drooping of the lower part of the face.
- Protection of the eye during sleep.
- A short course of dexamethasone 2 mg three times a day for 5 days and tapered over the next 5 days (should be given within 48 hours of onset).

What are the branches of the facial nerve?

- Greater superficial petrosal nerve (supplies lacrimal, nasal and palatine glands).
- Nerve to stapedius muscle.
- Chorda tympani (supplies taste to anterior two-thirds of tongue, submaxillary and sublingual glands).
- Motor branches (exit from the stylomastoid foramen).

How would you localize facial nerve palsy?

- Involvement of the nuclei in the pons – associated ipsilateral sixth nerve palsy.
- Cerebellopontine angle lesion – associated fifth and eighth nerve involvement.
- Lesion in the bony canal – loss of taste (carried by the lingual nerve) and hyperacusis (due to involvement of the nerve to stapedius).

Mention reflexes involving the facial nerve.

- Corneal reflex (see page 250).

- Palmomental reflex (see page 142).
- Suck reflex.
- Snout reflex (see page 142).
- Orbicularis oculi reflex or glabellar reflex (see page 129).
- Palpebral–oculogyric reflex.
- Orbicularis oris reflex.

Mention a few examples of facial synkinesis.

Facial synkinesis means that attempts to move one group of facial muscles result in contraction of associated muscles. It may be seen during anomalous regeneration of facial nerve. For example:

- If fibres originally connected with muscles of the face later innervate the lacrimal gland, anomalous secretion of tears (crocodile tears) may occur while eating.
- If fibres originally connected with the orbicularis oculi innervate the orbicularis oris, closure of the eyelids causes retraction of the mouth.
- Opening of the jaw may cause closure of the eyelids on the corresponding side (jaw-winking).

Have you heard of Möbius' syndrome?

Congenital facial diplegia, congenital oculofacial paralysis and infantile nuclear aplasia. It consists of congenital bilateral facial palsy associated with third and sixth nerve palsies.

What is the relationship between diabetes and Bell's palsy?

Diabetes is said to be an important cause in about 10% of cases of Bell's palsy. In one study Bell's palsy was associated with abnormal glucose tolerance in two-thirds of patients.

Sir Charles Bell (1774–1842) was Professor of Surgery in Edinburgh and a founder member of the Middlesex Hospital in London. He discovered that the anterior and posterior spinal nerve roots were motor and sensory respectively.
James Ramsay Hunt (1874–1937), Professor of Neurology in New York.
PJ Möbius (1853–1907), a German neurologist.

References

Adour KK, Bell DN & Wingerd J (1974) Bell's palsy: dilemma of diabetes mellitus. *Arch Otolaryngol.* **99**: 114.
Korczyn AD (1971) Bell's palsy and diabetes mellitus. *Lancet* **i**: 108.
Melkersson E (1928) Case of recurrent facial paralysis with angioneurotic oedema. *Hygiea* (Stockholm) **90**: 737–741.

Rosenthal C (1931) Klinisch-erbbiologischer Beitrag zur Konistitutionspathologie; Gemeinsames Auftreten von (rezidivierender familiärer) Facialislähmung, angioneurotischem Gesichtsödem and Lingua plicata in Arthritismus-Familien. *Z Neurol Psychiatr* **131**: 475–501.

CASE 54 Tremors

Instruction

Look at this patient's hands.
Demonstrate tremors.

Salient features

Patient 1

- Coarse resting tremor which is slow (4–6 per second).
- Adduction–abduction of the thumb with flexion–extension of fingers (pill-rolling movement).
- The tremor is halted by purposive movements of the hands. The upper limb tremor often increases as the patient walks.

Proceed as follows:

- Tell the examiner that you would like to do the following:
  Look for cog-wheel rigidity.
  Comment on mask-like facies.
  Check gait for festinant gait.
  Ask the patient's relatives whether sleep relieves the tremor and whether emotion makes it worse.

Diagnosis

This patient with resting tremor and mask-like facies (lesion) has Parkinson's disease (aetiology) and is severely disabled by the tremor (functional status).

Patient 2

- There is a 10-second physiological tremor which is brought on when the arms are outstretched. It can be amplified by laying a sheet of paper on the hands.

Proceed as follows:

- Tell the examiner that you would like to do the following:
    Check for thyrotoxicosis.
    Take a history for alcoholism.
    Take a drug history (salbutamol, terbutaline, lithium).
    Occupational history to mercury ('hatters' shakes').
    Know whether tremor runs in the family and is relieved by alcohol
        (benign essential tremor).

Diagnosis

This patient has fine tremor with an enlarged thyroid gland (lesion), which
could be due to hyperthyroidism (aetiology).

Patient 3

- The patient does not have a resting tremor or a tremor with outstretched
    hands.

Proceed as follows:

- Check the past-pointing – the intention tremor of cerebellar disease.
- Tell the examiner that you would like to check for other cerebellar signs
    (see page 136).

Diagnosis

This patient has an intention tremor (lesion) due to cerebellar syndrome
(aetiology).

Patient 4

- Unsteadiness when standing still; by contrast patient has little or no
    difficulty while walking, which relieves the symptoms
- Fine rippling of the muscles of the legs may be seen or felt when the
    patient attempts to stand still; after a short interval the patient
    becomes increasingly unsteady and is forced to take a step to regain
    balance.

Diagnosis

This patient has primary orthostatic tremor (lesion).

Questions

What are the tremors?

Involuntary movements that result from alternating contraction and relaxation of groups of muscles, producing rhythmic oscillations about a joint or a group of joints.

How would you classify tremors?

- Resting tremor, as in Parkinson's disease.
- Postural tremor (brought on when the arms are outstretched) due to the following:
    Exaggerated physiological tremor, caused by anxiety, thyrotoxicosis, alcohol, drugs.
    Brain damage seen in Wilson's disease, syphilis.
- Intention tremor (aggravated by voluntary movements) in cerebellar disease.

Mention a few involuntary movements.

- Chorea.
- Athetosis.
- Hemiballismus
- Fasciculation
- Torticollis.
- Clonus.

Advanced-level Questions

What do you know about the investigation and management of primary orthostatic tremor?

In primary orthostatic tremor:
- EMG shows rhythmic activation of lower limb muscles at a frequency of 4–18 Hz.
- Positron emission tomography shows increased activity in the cerebellum.
- Treatment is supportive and patient is often relieved to know the diagnosis, especially when a psychiatric cause has been suspected previously.

Mercury poisoning was known as 'hatter's shakes' because workers involved in the manufacture of felt hats were exposed to mercury.

Reference

Fahn S (1972) Differential diagnosis of tremors. *Med Clin North Am* **56**: 1363–1375.

CASE 55 Peripheral Neuropathy

Instruction

Examine this patient's legs.
Carry out a neurological examination of this patient's legs.

Salient features

● Bilateral symmetrical sensory loss for all modalities with or without motor weakness.

Proceed as follows:

● Look for evidence of the following:
  Diabetes mellitus (diabetic chart, insulin injection sites, insulin pump).
  Alcoholic liver diease (palmar erythema, spider naevi, tender liver).
  Drug history.
  Rheumatoid arthritis.
  Uraemia.
  Malignancy.
  (Mnemonic: DAD,RUM)
● Palpate for thickened nerves and look for Charcot's joints.
● Tell the examiner that you would like to do the following:
  Look for anaemia and jaundice (vitamin B_{12} deficiency).
  Check urine for sugar.
  Take a history of alcohol consumption and a drug history.

Diagnosis

This patient has symmetrical, bilateral sensory loss for touch and pain (lesion) due to diabetes mellitus (aetiology).

Questions

Mention a few causes of thickened nerves.

● Amyloidosis.
● Charcot–Marie–Tooth disease.
● Leprosy.
● Refsum's disease (retinitis pigmentosa, deafness and cerebellar damage).
● Déjérine–Sottas disease (hypertrophic peripheral neuropathy).

What are the causes of motor neuropathy?

- Guillain–Barré syndrome.
- Peroneal muscular atrophy.
- Lead toxicity.
- Porphyria.
- Dapsone toxicity.
- Organophosphorous poisoning.

What are the causes of mononeuritis multiplex?

- **W**egener's granulomatosis.
- **A**myloidosis.
- **R**heumatoid arthritis.
- **D**iabetes mellitus.
- **S**LE.

- **P**olyarteritis nodosa.
- **L**eprosy
- **C**arcinomatosis, **C**hurg–Strauss syndrome.
      (Mnemonic: WARDS, PLC).

Mention a few causes of predominantly sensory neuropathy.

- Diabetes mellitus.
- Alcoholism.
- Deficiency of vitamins B_{12} and B_1.
- Chronic renal failure.
- Leprosy.

What are the types of neuropathy described in diabetes mellitus?

- Symmetrical, mainly sensory, polyneuropathy.
- Asymmetrical, mainly motor, polyneuropathy (diabetic amyotrophy).
- Mononeuropathy.
- Autonomic neuropathy.

What drugs are used for painful peripheral neuropathy of diabetes?

Tricyclic antidepressants, phenytoin, carbamazepine and topical capsaicin.

Advanced-level Questions

What are the other effects of alcohol on the central nervous system?

- Wernicke's encephalopathy (ophthalmoplegia, nystagmus, confusion and neuropathy).
- Korsakoff's psychosis (recent memory loss and confabulation).
- Cerebellar degeneration.
- Marchiafava–Bignami disease (symmetrical demyelination of corpus callosum).
- Central pontine myelinolysis.
- Amblyopia.
- Epilepsy.
- Myopathy and rhabdomyolysis.

K Wernicke (1848–1904) worked in Poland.
SS Korasakoff (1853–1900), a Russian neuropsychiatrist.
J Churg (b. 1910) qualified in Poland and was Professor of Pathology in New York.
L Strauss, a pathologist in New York.

References

Harati Y (1987) Diabetic peripheral neuropathies. *Ann Intern Med* **107**: 546.
Garland H (1955) Diabetic amyotrophy. *Br Med J* **2**: 1287.

CASE 56

Charcot–Marie–Tooth Disease (Peroneal Muscular Atrophy)

Instruction

Examine this patient's legs.

Salient features

- Wasting of muscles of calves and thighs which stops abruptly, usually in the lower third of the thigh, and is described as 'stork' or 'spindle' legs, 'fat bottle' calves and 'inverted champagne bottles'.
- Pes cavus, clawing of toes, contractures of the Achilles tendon.
- Weakness of dorsiflexion.
- Absent ankle jerks, plantars are downgoing or equivocal.
- Mild sensory impairment or no sensory loss. Some patients have decreased responses to pain in the stocking distribution.

Proceed as follows:

- Feel for lateral popliteal nerve thickening (seen in some cases only).
- Look at the hands for small muscle wasting and clawing.
- Tell the examiner that you would like to:

Know whether there is a family history of disease.
Look for enlarged greater auricular nerves.
Examine the spine for scoliosis.
Examine the gait (high-steppage gait of foot-drop).

Note. There are two distinctive clinical features of this disease:
1. The muscular atrophy begins in the distal portions of the affected muscles in the lower and upper limbs, unlike the global atrophy of motor neuron disease or muscular dystrophy. The atrophy then creeps upwards, involving all muscles.
2. Second, the degree of disability is minimal in spite of marked deformity.

Diagnosis

This patient has 'inverted champagne bottle' legs with sensory neuropathy (lesion) which is due to hereditary Charcot–Marie–Tooth disease (aetiology). She has severe foot-drop and requires calipers (functional status).

Advanced-level Questions

What is the mode of inheritance?

Both autosomal dominant and recessive inheritances are seen in different families. The responsible gene is usually located on the short arm of chromosome 17 and less often shows linkage to chromosomes 1 or X. In hereditary motor sensory neuropathy (HMSN) type I with dominant inheritance, the locus is on the long arm of chromosome 1.

What are the three recognized forms?

- HMSN type I – a demyelinating neuropathy (marked slowing of conduction in motor nerves; absent deep tendon reflexes).
- HMSN type II – an axonal neuropathy (little or no slowing of nerve conduction; normal deep tendon reflexes).
- Distal spinal muscular atrophy.

What other uncommon features may these patients have?

Optic atrophy, retinitis pigmentosa, spastic paraparesis.

In which other conditions is pes cavus is seen?

Friedreich's ataxia.

What is the natural history of the disease?

The disease usually arrests in middle life.

How does the forme fruste of the disease manifest?

The forme fruste may be seen in family members of patients with Charcot–Marie–Tooth disease and manifests as pes cavus and absent ankle jerks.

Mention other hereditary neuropathies.

- Roussy–Lévy syndrome (where features of progressive muscular atrophy may be combined with tremor and ataxia).
- Hereditary amyloidosis.
- Refsum's disease (phytanic acid accumulates in the central and peripheral nervous systems).
- Fabry's disease (where there is a deficiency of α-galactosidase).
- Tangier disease.
- Bassen–Kornzweig disease (abetalipoproteinaemia, absence of low density lipoproteins and vitamin E deficiency).
- Metachromatic leukodystrophy (where galactosyl sulphatide accumulates in the central and peripheral nervous systems).

Mention a few conditions that Charcot is credited to have described for the first time.

- Ankle clonus.
- Tabes dorsalis and Charcot's joints.
- Multiple sclerosis.
- Peroneal muscular atrophy.
- Multiple cerebral aneurysms, called Charcot–Bouchard aneurysms.
- Hysteria.

The syndrome was originally described by JM Charcot (1825–1923) and P Marie (1853–1940) in 1886 at the Saltpêtrière in Paris, and independently by HH Tooth at St Bartholomew's Hospital and the National Hospital for Nervous Diseases, Queen Square, London, at the same time. P Marie was a world-famed neurologist. He published extensively on aphasia. He succeeded Charcot's lineage of Raymond, Brissaud and Dejerine at the Saltpêtrière in 1918.

References

Hallam PJ, Harding AE, Bercano J, Barker DF & Malcolm S (1992) Duplication of the part of chromosome 17 is commonly associated with hereditary motor and sensory neuropathy type I (Charcot–Marie–Tooth disease type 1). *Ann Neurol* **31**: 570.

Roa BB, Garcia C, Suter U et al (1993) Charcot–Marie–Tooth type 1A: association with a spontaenous mutation in the PMP22 gene. *N Engl J Med* **329**: 96–101.

CASE 57 Dystrophia Myotonica

Instruction

Look at this patient's face.
Examine this patient's cranial nerves.

Salient features

- While shaking hands with the patient, note the myotonia.
- Frontal baldness. (**Note.** The patient may be wearing a wig and it is important to mention that he is wearing one.)
- Ptosis (bilateral or unilateral) with a *smooth* forehead.
- Cataracts or evidence of surgery for cataracts.
- Difficulty in opening the eyes after firm closure.
- Expressionless face ('hatchet face') with wasting of temporalis, masseters and *sternomastoids*.

Proceed as follows:

- Test:
  Sternomastoids.
  Distal muscles of the upper limbs, wasting, percussion myotonia over thenar muscles and weakness.
  Deep tendon jerks (depressed).
- Tell the examiner that you would like to do the following:
  Ask the patient whether or not he has dysphagia (oesophageal involvement).
  Check the urine for sugar (diabetes mellitus).
  Test higher intellectual function (low IQ).
  Examine for gynaecomastia and testicular atrophy.

Diagnosis

This patient has frontal balding, myotonia, cataracts and wasting of the sternomastoids (lesion) due to dystrophia myotonica (aetiology). He has dysphagia and severe muscular weakness (functional status).

What is the inheritance of this condition?

Autosomal dominant; the gene is located on chromosome 19q13.3. The condition usually presents in the third and fourth decades. The disease tends to be worse in successive generations (known as anticipation). As a result the grandparent may merely have cataracts while the grandchild develops a severe progressive form of the disease. Positional cloning has helped to identify the myotonic dystrophy gene and localized a dynamic mutation with an increase in the number of trinucleotide repeats (AGC repeat). The repeat size typically increases from generation to generation, providing a molecular basis for the clinical phenomenon of anticipation.

What are the other features of this condition?

- Cardiomyopathy and cardiac conduction defects.
- Respiratory infection (low serum immunoglobulin G levels).
- Somnolence.
- External ophthalmoplegia (occasionally).

What do you understand by myotonia?

It is continued contraction of the muscle after voluntary contraction ceases, followed by impaired relaxation.

What therapeutic modalities are available?

Procainamide or phenytoin have been used in *disabling* myotonia. No treatment has altered the course of progressive weakness.

What other forms of myotonia do you know?

Myotonia congenita or Oppenheim's disease, an autosomal dominant condition which presents at birth with feeding difficulties. The myotonia improves with age and there is no dystrophy. Although this is considered to be a myopathy, changes have been reported in the motor nuclei of the spinal cord and motor cortex.

In which myopathies is distal weakness prominent?

- Myotonic dystrophy.
- Welander's distal myopathy.

If this patient requires major surgery, what fact would you keep in mind?

Patients with dystrophia myotonica tend to do poorly after the administration of general anaesthetic (due to impaired cardiorespiratory malfunction) and will require intensive postoperative observation.

Mention some causes of bilateral ptosis?

- Myasthenia gravis.
- Congenital muscular dystrophies.
- Ocular myopathy.
- Syphilis.

What is the pathognomonic pattern of cataract in dystrophia myotonica?

Stellate cataract.

The patient's sister is worried about risks to her offspring. What tests would you do?

- Clinical examination.
- Electromyography (EMG).
- Slit-lamp examination for cataracts.

Is prenatal diagnosis available?

Yes – in some families. The myotonic dystrophy gene is linked to the ABH secretor gene. However, not all families are informative.

What is the characteristic EMG finding?

Waxing and waning of the potentials, known as the dive-bomber effect.

How would you manage such patients?

- Foot drop is controlled by calipers or molded-foot orthoses.
- Myotonia when disabling may respond to phenytoin (avoid quinidine and procainamide as they can worsen cardiac conduction).
- Advanced heart block with or without syncope should be considered for pacemaker insertion.

Délége in 1890 first described the association of myotonia with muscular atrophy. Batten and Gibb, and Steinert, in 1909 independently described the clinical features of symptom complex. Curschmann in 1912 emphasized the dystrophic symptoms and applied the term 'dystrophia myotonica'.

References

Batten FE (1909) The myopathies or muscular dystrophies: critical review. *Q J Med* **3**: 313.

Batten FE & Gibb HP (1909) Myotonia atrophica. *Brain* **32**: 187.

Fu-YH, Pizzuti A, Fenwick RG Jr et al (1992) An unstable triplet repeat in a gene related to myotonic muscular dystrophy. *Science* **255**: 1256–1258.

Harley HG, Brook JD, Rundle SA et al (1992) Expansion of an unstable DNA region and phenotypic variation in myotonic dystrophy. *Nature* **355**: 545–546.

Harper PS (1989) *Myotonic Dystrophy*, 2nd edn. London: Saunders.

Mahadevan M, Tilfidis C, Sabourin L et al (1992) Myotonic dystrophy mutation: an unstable CTG repeat in the 3′ untranslated region of gene. *Science* **255**: 1253–1255.

Ptacek LJ, Johnson KJ & Griggs RC (1993) Genetics and physiology of the myotonic muscle disorders. *N Engl J Med* **328**: 482.

Shelbourne P, Davis J, Buxton, T, Anvret M, Biennow E & Bondivelle M (1993) Direct diagnosis of myotonic dystrophy with a disease-specific DNA marker. *N Engl J Med* **328**: 471.

Steinert H (1909) Myopathogische Bietrage; I. Ueber das klinische und antomische Bild des Muskelschwunds der Myotoniker. *Dtsch Z Nervenheilk* **37**: 58.

CASE 58 Proximal Myopathy

Instruction

Perform a neurological examination of this patient's arms or legs.

Salient features

- Weakness of proximal muscles.
- Patient has difficulty in standing from the sitting position (getting up from chairs, getting off the commode) or difficulty in combing her hair – elicit this history.

Proceed as follows:

- Check the gait, looking for waddling gait (see page 178).
- Look for an underlying cause:
  Diabetic amyotrophy (asymmetrical, usually in the lower limbs in non-insulin-dependent diabetes mellitus).
  Cushing's syndrome (characteristic facies, history of steroid ingestion; see page 392).
  Thyrotoxicosis (look for eye signs, goitre, rapid pulse, tremor).
  Polymyositis (heliotropic rash, tender muscles).

Drug history (alcohol, steroids, chloroquine).
Carcinomatous neuropathy.
Osteomalacia (bone pain).
Hereditary muscular dystrophy.

Diagnosis

This patient has weakness of the proximal muscles of the lower limbs (lesion) due to Cushing's syndrome (aetiology) and is severely limited by the weakness (functional status).

Questions

What is Gowers' sign?

In severe proximal myopathy of the lower limbs, the patient on rising from the floor uses her hands to climb up herself. It has been classically described in Duchenne muscular dystrophy.

What do you know about diabetic amyotrophy?

It is an asymmetrical motor polyneuropathy which presents with asymmetrical weakness and wasting of the proximal muscles of the lower limbs and sometimes upper limbs, diminished or absent knee jerk and sensory loss in the thigh. It is usually accompanied by severe pain in the thigh, often awakening the patient at night. The prognosis is good and most patients recover over months or years with diabetic control.

Advanced-level Questions

What is the difference between type 1 and type 2 muscle fibres?

- Type 1 muscle fibres are high in myoglobin and oxidative enzymes and have many mitochondria. They perform tonic contraction and are involved in weight-bearing and movements requiring sustained force. Chloroquine causes vacuolation of myocytes, predominantly type 1 fibres.
- Type 2 muscle fibres are rich in glycolytic enzymes; they perform rapid phasic contractions and are involved in sudden movements and in purposeful motion. In steroid myopathy the muscle fibre atrophy predominantly affects these fibres.

Sir WR Gowers (1845–1915), Professor of Medicine at University College Hospital, London, invented a haemoglobinometer, personally illustrated an atlas of ophthalmology, wrote a book on spinal cord diseases and a manual on the nervous system. He also founded a society of medical stenographers.

Reference

Kumamoto T, Araki S, Watanabes S, Ikebe N & Fukuhara N (1989) Experimental
    chloroquine myopathy: morphological and biochemical studies. *Eur Neurol*
    29: 202.

CASE 59 — Deformity of a Lower Limb

Instruction

Examine the lower limbs of this patient who has had this abnormality since childhood.

Salient features

- Wasting and deformity of one lower limb (or both with one side being more affected than the other).
- Fasciculations.
- Normal tone in both lower limbs.

Proceed as follows:

- Check the sensory system (L5 and/or S1 sensory loss in spina bifida).
- Examine the spine:
    Kyphoscoliosis (seen in poliomyelitis, indicating involvement of trunk muscles).
    Tuft of hair in the lower lumbosacral spine (closed spina bifida).
- Comment on bony deformity in the affected leg.
- **Note.** Always check the gait and test for Romberg's sign.
- Tell the examiner that you would like to ask the patient about the following:
    History of trauma to the spine and/or leg.
    Bladder and bowel symptoms.

Diagnosis

This patient has unilateral wasting and deformity of the R/L leg (lesion) due to poliomyelitis in childhood (aetiology) and wears calipers on that leg (functional status).

Questions

What is the differential diagnosis?

- Old poliomyelitis.
- Spina bifida.

What are the causes of lower motor neuron signs in the legs?

- Peripheral neuropathy.
- Prolapsed intervertebral disc.
- Diabetic amyotrophy.
- Poliomyelitis.
- Cauda equina lesions.
- Motor neuron disease.

Advanced-level Questions

What is the cause of polio?

Polio is due to a picornavirus of the genus Enterovirus; there are three antigenic types – type I (Brunhilde), type II (Lansing) and type III (Leon).

Is the muscular involvement of polio in childhood progressive?

Usually paralytic polio remains stable after the initial attack. However, in some patients new muscle weakness and atrophy involving previously affected muscles or even unaffected muscles occurs and this deterioration can occur as long as 30 years after the first attack – known as post-poliomyelitis muscular atrophy (PPMA). The progression of this involvement is slow and is said to be distinct from motor neuron disease. It is not entirely clear why only some patients are affected but it has been reported that it is more likely to occur in those with widespread paralysis and poor immune status.

Is poliomyelitis preventable?

Yes, three types of poliovaccine are available (each containing all three strains of the virus):
- Oral polio vaccine of Sabin consists of live attenuated virus.
- Killed or inactivated vaccine of Salk.
- Enhanced potency vaccine of van Wezel.

With which vaccine is paralytic poliomyelitis associated?

Vaccine-associated paralytic poliomyelitis (VAPP) is associated with oral polio vaccine, particularly in immunodeficient individuals. Such individuals and their household contacts should be given inactivated vaccine.

What do you know about 'provocation poliomyelitis'?

Provocation poliomyelitis is caused by the administration of intramuscular injections during the incubation period of wild-type poliovirus or shortly after exposure to oral poliovaccine (either as a vaccine recipient or through contact with a recent recipient).

What do you understand by the term spina bifida?

Spina bifida means an incomplete closure of the bony vertebral canal and is commonly associated with a similar anomaly of the spinal cord. The commonest site is the lumbosacral region but the cervical spine can be involved. It may associated with hydrocephalus.

What are the features of closed spina bifida?

- Cutaneous: lumbosacral lipoma, hypertrichosis, sinus or dimple above the sacrum, naevus or scarring.
- Unilateral shortening of one leg and foot with a deficiency of the muscles below the knee. There may be calcaneovalgus or equinovarus deformity. Sensory loss in the 5th lumbar and 1st sacral dermatome is common.
- Neuropathic bladder, enuresis.
- Bony changes on X-ray: sacral dysgenesis, scoliosis, laminar fusion of vertebral body, pedicle erosion and bony spurs.

Is the neurological deficit in closed spina bifida progressive?

This issue is contentious as much of the deficit is fixed antenatally and any progression is a result of growth and posture. However, in some patients the late appearance of bladder dysfunction indicates that the neurological deficit is progressive in these individuals.

Mention some teratogenic factors responsible for neural canal defects.

- Maternal diabetes and sacral dysgenesis.
- Sodium valproate in pregnancy and neural tube defects.

Mention some prenatal screening tests for spina bifida.

- Amniotic α-fetoprotein levels.
- Amniotic acetylcholinesterase estimation.
- High-resolution diagnostic ultrasonography.

MH Romberg (1795–1873), German neurologist and Professor of Medicine in Berlin.

The 1952 Nobel Prize was jointly awarded to John F Enders (1897–1985), Thomas H Weller (1915–) both of Children's Medical Center and Harvard Medical School, Boston, and Frederick C Robbins (1916–) of Western Reserve University, Cleveland, Ohio, for their discovery of the ability of poliomyelitis viruses to grow in cultures of various types of tissue.

References

Beale AJ (1990) Polio vaccines. Time for a change in immunization policy? *Lancet* **335**: 839.

Cashman NR, Maselli R, Wollman RL et al (1987) Late denervation in patients with antecedent paralytic poliomyelitis. *N Engl J Med* **317**: 7.

Dalakas MC, Elder G, Hallett M et al (1986). A long-term follow-up study of patients with post-poliomyelitis neuromuscular symptoms. *N Engl J Med* **314**: 959.

Howard RS, Wiles CM & Spencer GT (1988) The late sequel of poliomyelitis. *Q J Med* **66**: 219.

Stanley OH & Chambers TL (1982) Sodium valproate and neural tube defects. *Lancet* **ii**: 1282.

Strebel PM, Ion-Nedelcu N, Baughman AL, Sutter RW & Cochi SL (1995) Intramuscular injections within 30 days of immunization with oral poliovaccine – a risk factor for vaccine-associated paralytic poliomyelitis. *N Engl J Med* **332**: 500–506.

CASE 60 Multiple Sclerosis

Instruction

Examine this patient's eyes (*patient 1*).

Salient features

- Optic atrophy.
- Nystagmus.
- Internuclear ophthalmoplegia.

Proceed as follows:

- Tell the examiner that you would like to look for features of cerebellar syndrome and do a full neurological examination.

Instruction

Examine this patient's legs (*patient 2*).

Salient features

- Spastic paraparesis (increased tone, upgoing plantars, weakness, brisk reflexes and ankle or patellar clonus).
- Impaired co-ordination on heel–shin test (if there is marked weakness, this test may be unreliable).

Proceed as follows:

- Check abdominal reflexes (absent or diminished in over 80% of cases).
- Tell the examiner that you would like to do the following:
    Take a history of incontinence of bladder, impotence or constipation (Steinberg's triad).
    Look for optic atrophy and cerebellar signs.

In such patients remember that spinal cord compression should be ruled out before making a diagnosis of multiple sclerosis.

Some examiners may consider it insensitive to use the term 'multiple sclerosis' in front of the patient and may prefer that the candidate uses the term 'demyelinating disorder' instead.

Diagnosis

This patient has optic atrophy and spastic paraparesis (lesion) due to multiple sclerosis, and is wheelchair bound (functional status).

Questions

What investigations would you consider?

- Spinal radiography, including both cervical and thoracic regions.
- Lumbar puncture: total protein concentration may be raised (in 60% of cases), with an increase in the level of immunoglobulin G (in 40%) and oligoclonal bands (in 80%) on electrophoresis.
- Visual evoked potentials: despite normal visual function there may be prolonged latency in cortical response to a pattern stimulus. This indicates a delay in conduction in the visual pathways.
- MRI scan of the brain: about 50% of patients with early multiple sclerosis in the spinal cord show abnormal areas in the periventricular white matter.
- Serum vitamin B_{12} – to exclude subacute degeneration of the spinal cord.

Mention a few causes of bilateral pyramidal lesions affecting the lower limbs?

- Cord compression.
- Multiple sclerosis.
- Cervical spondylosis.
- Transverse myelitis.
- Motor neuron disease.
- Vitamin B_{12} deficiency.
- Cerebrovascular disease.

Advanced-level Questions

What are the main ways in which multiple sclerosis can present?

- Optic neuritis (in 40% of cases) resulting in partial loss of vision.
- Weakness of one or more limbs.
- Tingling in the extremities due to posterior column involvement.
- Diplopia.
- Nystagmus, cerebellar ataxia.
- Vertigo.

What is the natural history of multiple sclerosis?

The course of the disease is extremely variable. The onset may be acute, subacute or insidious. The course may be rapidly downhill, or may spontaneously remit for periods lasting from days to years before a second exacerbation.

What is Lhermitte's sign?

A tingling or electric shock-like sensation which radiates to the arms, down the back or into the legs on flexion of the patient's neck. It has also been called the barber's chair sign. It indicates disease near the dorsal column nuclei of the higher cervical cord. Causes include multiple sclerosis, cervical stenosis, subacute combined degeneration of the cord.

What is Uhthoff's symptom?

The exacerbation of symptoms of multiple sclerosis during a hot bath.

Do you know of any criteria for diagnosis of multiple sclerosis?

Poser's criteria: a history of two episodes of neurological deficit and objective clinical signs of lesions at more than one site within the central nervous system establishes the diagnosis of definite multiple sclerosis. In the presence of only one clinical sign the demonstration of an additional lesion by laboratory tests – such as evoked potentials, MRI, CT or urological studies – also fulfils the criteria.

A diagnosis of probable multiple sclerosis is defined as either two attacks with clinical evidence of one lesion or one attack with clinical evidence of two lesions.

Which conditions may be considered forme fruste of multiple sclerosis?

● Optic neuritis.
● Single episode of transverse myelitis with optic neuritis.

What is the role of steroids in acute optic neuritis and the development of multiple sclerosis?

In acute optic neuritis treatment with a 3-day course of high-dose intravenous methylprednisolone (followed by a short course of prednisone) reduces the rate of development of multiple sclerosis over a 2-year period.

Does pregnancy affect the clinical features of multiple sclerosis?

Pregnancy itself may have a mildly protective effect but there is an increased risk of relapse during the puerperium; overall, the effect on the course of the disease is probably negligible.

What is the role of exercise in the treatment of such patients?

Patients should be encouraged to keep active during remission and to avoid excessive physical exercise during relapses.

What is the role of MRI in multiple sclerosis?

MRI can identify up to 80% of patients with multiple sclerosis. T_2-weighted images show hyperintense focal periventricular lesions. Although periventricular white matter lesions are typical of multiple sclerosis, they are not pathognomonic. Small infarcts, disseminated metastases, moya-moya disease and inflammatory diseases can produce a similar picture. High-resolution MRI may provide useful prognostic information in patients who present with an acute clinically isolated syndrome suggestive of multiple sclerosis. On 5-year follow-up over half the patients who had asymptomatic white matter lesions at presentation had developed clinically definite multiple sclerosis, compared with 3% of patients with normal results at presentation. The disease progressed rapidly if the scan showed four or more lesions at presentation, and a greater number of lesions also correlated with development of moderate or severe disability.

Mention some other demyelinating disorders.

- Devic's disease: myelitis with optic neuritis. There has been debate as to whether this is a form of multiple sclerosis or a monophasic illness.
- Leukodystrophies.
- Tuberous sclerosis (patchy demyelination; see page 587).
- Schilder's disease (diffuse cerebral sclerosis; may present with cortical blindness when the occipital cortex is involved).

Is there any treatment for multiple sclerosis?

Recent evidence suggests that the two forms of interferon β (i.e. 1b and 1a) may delay, though not yet abolish, the progress of irrecoverable neurological deficit.

JL Lhermitte (1877–1959), a French neurologist and neuropsychiatrist, wrote exclusively on spinal injuries, myoclonus, internuclear ophthalmoplegia and chorea.

References

Beck RW, Cleary PA, Anderson MM Jr et al (1993) The Optic Neuritis Study Group. *N Engl J Med* **326**: 581–588.

Beck RW, Cleary PA, Trobe JD et al (1993) The effect of corticosteroids for acute optic neuritis on the subsequent development of multiple sclerosis. The Optic Neuritis Study Group. *N Engl J Med* **329**: 1764–1769.

IFNB Multiple Sclerosis Study Group (1993) Interferon β-1b is effective in relapsing–remitting multiple sclerosis. *Neurology* **43**: 655–667.

McDonald WI (1995) New treatments for multiple sclerosis. *Br Med J* **310**: 345–346.

Morrissey SP, Miller DH, Kendall BE et al (1993) The significance of brain magnetic resonance imaging abnormalities at presentation with clinically isolated syndromes suggestive of multiple sclerosis. *N Engl J Med* **116**: 135–146.

CASE 61   Abnormal Gait

Instruction

Look at this patient while he walks.
Test this patient's gait.

Salient features

1. *Cerebellar gait*: the patient has a broad-based gait, reeling and lurching to one side.

Proceed as follows:

- Tell the examiner that you would like to examine the patient for other cerebellar signs (see page 137).

2. *Parkinsonian gait*: the steps are small and shuffling, and the patient walks in a haste (festinates). The entire body stoops forwards, knees bent, head hunched forward, and the feet must hurry to keep up with it as if trying to catch up with the centre of gravity. There is associated loss of arm swing and mask-like facies.

Proceed as follows:

- Tell the examiner that you would like to look for other signs of Parkinson's disease (page 129).

3. *Hemiplegic gait*: the gait is slow, spastic and shuffling. With each step the pelvis is tilted upward on the involved side to aid in lifting the foot off the ground, and the entire affected limb is circumducted, rotated in a semicircle at the pelvis. The upper limb is flexed, adducted and does not swing, and the lower limb is extended.

4. *Sensory ataxia:* the feet stamp, the movement of the legs bearing no relation to the position of the legs in space since proprioception is impaired or absent. The patient has to look down at the ground to compensate for the loss of proprioception. The patient walks on a wide base; the feet are lifted too high off the ground and are brought down too vigorously.

Proceed as follows:

- Check for Romberg's sign, vibration and position sense.
- Sensory ataxic gait may be due to the following:

Tabes dorsalis.
Subacute combined degeneration of the cord.
- Tell the examiner that you would like to look for Argyll Robertson pupils and anaemia.

5. *High steppage gait* is usually unilateral and results from foot drop. The patient has to lift the foot high in order to avoid dragging the forefoot.
- It may be due to the following:
   Lateral popliteal nerve palsy.
   Poliomyelitis.
   Charcot–Marie–Tooth disease.
   Lead or arsenic poisoning.

6. *Scissor gait* is seen in spastic paraplegia. The adductor spasm may be so severe as to lead to the legs crossing in front of one another. Short steps with the front of the feet clinging to the ground result in a wearing out of the toes of shoes.

Proceed as follows:

- Tell the examiner that the underlying aetiology would probably be cord compression, multiple sclerosis or cerebral palsy.

7. *Waddling gait*: the legs are held wide apart and the patient shifts weight from one side to the other as he walks. Comment on the lumbar lordosis. It is seen in advanced pregnancy and proximal weakness (Cushing's syndrome, osteomalacia, thyrotoxicosis, polymyositis, diabetes, hereditary muscular dystrophies).

Advanced-level Questions

What do you understand by the term astasia abasia?

This is seen in psychogenic disturbances in which the patient is unable to walk or cannot stand. The patient falls far to the side on walking but usually regains balance before hitting the ground. The legs may be thrown out wildly or the patient may kneel with each step.

What do you understand by the term marche à petits pas?

This is to describe a gait in which the movement is slow and the patient walks with very short, shuffling and irregular steps with loss of associated movements. It is seen in normal-pressure hydrocephalus. This gait bears some resemblance to that seen in Parkinson's disease.

CASE 62 Wasting of the Small Muscles of the Hand

Instruction

Examine this patient's hands.
Ask the patient whether her hands are painful.

Salient features

- Wasting of thenar and hypothenar eminences and dorsal interossei.

Proceed as follows:

- Look for deformity and swelling.
- Look for fasciculations.
- Check sensation over the hand, especially index and little fingers.
- Test grip and pincer movements.
- Test for median and ulnar nerve compression.
- Ask the patient to unbutton clothes or to write.
- Palpate for cervical ribs and compare radial pulses.
- Look for Horner's syndrome.
- Examine the neck and test neck movements.

Diagnosis

This patient has bilateral wasted hands (lesions) due to cervical myelopathy (aetiology) and is unable to button her clothes (functional status).

Remember that the causes of bilateral wasted hands are as follows:
- Rheumatoid arthritis.
- Old age.
- Cervical spondylosis.
- Bilateral cervical ribs.
- Motor neuron disease.
- Syringomyelia.
- Charcot–Marie–Tooth disease.
- Guillain–Barré syndrome.
- Bilateral median and ulnar nerve lesions.

If the wasting is see in only one hand then in addition to the above causes consider the following:
- Brachial plexus trauma.
- Pancoast's tumour.

- Cervical cord lesions.
- Malignant infiltration of the brachial plexus.

Questions

In unilateral wasting what is the level of the lesion?

C8, T1. These muscles are predominantly supplied by the ulnar nerve (the median nerve supplies the thenar eminence), the inner cord of the brachial plexus, the T1 spinal root and the anterior horn cells. Thus lesions of these structures may all produce wasting of the small muscles of the hand:
  (a) Lesions of the radial, median and ulnar nerves (trauma).
  (b) Brachial plexus (trauma, cervical lymph nodes, cervical ribs, tumour of superior sulcus of lung).
  (c) Anterior root (cervical spondylosis).
  (d) Anterior horn cell (motor neuron disease, tumours of spinal cord, syringomyelia, poliomyelitis).

CASE 63 Dermatomyositis

Instruction

Examine this patient.

Salient features

Skin
- Heliotrope rash or purplish-blue rash around the eyes, back of the hands, dilated capillary loops at the base of fingernails, erythema of knuckles accompanied by a raised violaceous scaly eruption (Gottron's sign). The erythema spares the phalanges (unlike that of systemic lupus erythematosus in which the phalanges are involved and the knuckles are spared).
- The erythematous rash may be present on the neck and upper chest (often in the shape of a V), shoulders (shawl sign), elbows, knees and malleoli.
- The cuticles may be irregular, thickened and distorted, and the lateral and palmar areas of the fingers become rough and cracked with irregular 'dirty' horizontal lines, resembling those in a mechanic's hands.

Muscles
- Proximal muscle weakness and tenderness of muscles.
- Weakness of neck flexors in two-thirds of cases.

Proceed as follows:

- Tell the examiner that you would like to take a history of the following:
  Dysphagia.
  Dysphonia.
- Ask the patient whether the red rash is made worse by exposure to sunlight.
- If the patient is more than 40 years old, tell the examiner that you would like to look for an underlying neoplasm.

Diagnosis

This patient has Gottron's papules and proximal muscle weakness (lesion) due to dermatomyositis (aetiology).

Questions

What investigations would you like to do?

- Estimation of serum creatine phosphokinase (CPK) levels (mirrors disease activity).
- EMG.
- Muscle biopsy.

In which other conditions is there proximal muscle weakness with high serum creatine kinase levels?

It may be caused by drugs such as lovastatin, chloroquine and colchicine, especially in patients on chronic haemodialysis. (Remember that steroids cause proximal muscle weakness with normal serum creatine kinase levels.)

How would you treat such patients?

- Most patients respond to steroids; prednisolone is the first-line drug for the empirical treatment of polymyositis and dermatomyositis.
- Resistant cases may benefit from methotrexate, azathioprine and high-dose intravenous immunoglobulin.
- Those with an underlying neoplasm may remit after treatment of the tumour.

Advanced-level Questions

What are the EMG findings in an affected muscle?

Spontaneous fibrillation, salvos of repetitive potentials, and short duration of polyphasic potentials of low amplitude.

What features will a muscle biopsy show?

Necrosis and phagocytosis of muscle fibres, and interstitial and perivascular infiltration of inflammatory cells.

How would you classify polymyositis – dermatomyositis?

The classification of Bohan et al (1977) is as follows:
Group I: primary idiopathic polymyositis.
Group II: primary idiopathic dermatomyositis.
Group III: dermatomyositis (or polymyositis) associated with neoplasia.
Group IV: childhood dermatomyositis (or polymyositis) associated with vasculitis.
Group V: polymyositis (or dermatomyositis) with associated collagen vascular disease.

Mention a few disorders associated with myositis.

Sarcoid myositis, focal nodular myositis, infectious polymyositis (Lyme disease, toxoplasma), inclusion body myositis, eosinophilic myositis.

What do you understand by the term overlap syndrome?

Overlap syndrome indicates that characteristics of two different disorders are common to both. Dermatomyositis overlaps with systemic sclerosis and mixed connective tissue disease. Specific signs of systemic sclerosis and mixed connective tissue disease, such as sclerotic thickening of the dermis, contractures, oesophageal hypomotility, microangiopathy and calcium deposits, are present in dermatomyositis. Patients with the overlap syndrome of dermatomyositis and systemic sclerosis may have a specific antinuclear autoantibody anti-PM/Scl, directed against a nucleolar protein complex.

Heinrich Adolf Gottron (1890–1974), a German dermatologist.

References

Bohan A, Peter JB, Bowman R et al (1977) A computer assisted analysis of 153 patients with polymyositis and dermatomyositis. *Medicine* **56**: 255.

Dalakas MC (1993) Medical progress: polymyositis, dermatomyositis, and inclusion body myositis. *N Engl J Med* **325**: 1487.

Dalakas MC, Illa I, Dambrosia JM et al (1993) Controlled trial of high-dose intravenous immune globulin infusions as treatment for dermatomyositis. *N Engl J Med* **329**: 1993–2000.

Lakhanpal S, Bunch TW, Ilstrup DM et al (1986) Polymyositis–dermatomyositis and malignant lesions. Does an association exist? *Mayo Clin Proc* **61**: 645.

CASE 64 — Facioscapulohumeral Dystrophy (Landouzy–Déjérine Syndrome)

Instruction

Perform a neurological examination of this patient's cranial nerves and upper limbs.

Salient features

In the face:
- Prominent ptosis.
- Difficulty in closing the eyes.
- Marked facial weakness, resulting in a dull expressionless face with lips open and slack, and inability to whistle or puff the cheeks.
- Speech is impaired owing to difficulty in articulation of labial consonants.

In the neck:
- Wasted sternomastoids and marked weakness of neck muscles.

Shoulder girdle:
- Winging of the scapula.
- Lower pectorals and lower trapezii severely affected.
- Weakness of triceps and biceps.
- True hypertrophy of deltoids to compensate for other muscles.
- Absent biceps and triceps jerk.

Uncommon features: congenital absence of pectoralis, biceps or brachioradialis; tibialis anterior may be the only muscle involved outside the shoulder girdle.

Diagnosis

This patient has weakness of the muscles of the face, neck and shoulder girdle (lesion) due to inherited facioscapulohumeral dystrophy (aetiology).

Questions

What is the mode of inheritance?

Autosomal dominant; both sexes are equally affected. The gene has been recently localized to the long arm of chromosome 4.

Are higher mental functions affected in this condition?

The IQ is normal in such patients.

What is the life span in such a patient?

Normal.

What is the age of onset of this disorder?

Between 10 and 40 years.

Are levels of muscle enzymes raised in this condition?

No; the enzyme levels remain normal.

LTJ Landouzy (1845–1917), Professor of Therapeutics in Paris; although remembered for the description of the syndrome which bears his name, his major research interest was tuberculosis.
JJ Déjérine (1849–1917), a French neurologist, was a pioneer in the localization of function in the brain. This syndrome was described in 1885.

Reference

Wijmenga C, Hewitt JE, Sandakuijl LA et al (1992) Chromosome 4q DNA rearrangement associated with facioscapulohumeral muscular dystrophy. *Nature Genet* **2**: 26.

CASE 65   Limb Girdle Dystrophy

Instruction

Perform a neurological examination of this patient's upper and lower limbs.

Salient features

Upper limbs:
- Biceps and brachioradialis are involved late; wrist extensors are first involved when it extends to the wrist.
- Deltoids may show pseudohypertrophy and are spared until late.

Lower limbs:
- In the early stages of the disease, hip flexors and glutei are weak.

- There is early wasting of medial quadriceps and tibialis anterior.
- Lateral quadriceps and calves may show hypertrophy.

Note. The face is never affected.

Diagnosis

This patient has weakness of the proximal muscles of the arms and legs (lesion) due to limb girdle dystrophy (aetiology).

Advanced-level Questions

What is the mode of inheritance?

Autosomal recessive, males and females equally affected.

What is the age of onset?

Between 10 and 30 years, causing disability 10–20 years after onset.

How is the intelligence affected?

It is unaffected and IQ is normal.

Is the life span affected?

No.

What happens to the serum enzymes?

Levels of serum enzymes are slightly affected or normal.

John Walton, Professor of Neurology at Oxford and Newcastle, was made a peer following his retirement and carries the title of Lord Walton of Detchant. His chief interest was muscular diseases.

Sir Roger Bannister, Master of Pembroke College at Oxford, worked at the National Hospital for Nervous Diseases, Queen Square, and St Mary's Hospital, London, and his main interest was chronic autonomic failure. He was the first person to run the 4-minute mile.

CASE 66 Myasthenia Gravis

Instruction

This patient complains of drooping of the eyelids in the evenings; examine this patient.

Salient features

- The patient may have obvious ptosis.
- Remember that *fatiguability* is the hallmark of myasthenia gravis.

Proceed as follows:

- Check for worsening of ptosis on sustained upward gaze.
- Check extraocular movements for diplopia and variable squint.
- Comment on snarling face when the patient attempts to smile.
- Weakness without loss of reflexes, or alteration of sensation or co-ordination. The weakness may be generalized; it may affect the limb muscles, often proximal in distribution, as well as the diaphragm and neck extensors.
- Tell the examiner that you would like to know whether or not the weakness is more marked in the evening.
- Tell the examiner that myasthenia is associated with thyrotoxicosis, diabetes mellitus, rheumatoid arthritis, SLE and thymoma.

Diagnosis

This patient has diplopia at the end of each day with ptosis; the weakness is marked on repeated exertion of the muscle (lesion) and is due to myasthenia gravis (aetiology).

Questions

At what age is myasthenia common?

The incidence has two age peaks, with one peak in the second and third decades affecting mostly women and a peak in the sixth and seventh decades affecting mostly men.

What groups of muscles are commonly involved?

Muscles affected are as follows, in order of likelihood: extraocular, bulbar, neck, limb girdle, distal limbs and trunk.

What investigations would you like to do in this patient?

- Edrophonium (Tensilon) test.
- Vital capacity.
- Imaging of the mediastinum: chest radiography, CT or MRI of the chest.
- Acetylcholine receptor antibodies (present in more than 80% of cases).
- Plasma thyroxine (to rule out an associated thyroid disorder).
- Antistriated muscle antibody (seen in association with thymoma).
- Test for systemic lupus erythematosus: antinuclear antibody, rheumatoid factor, antithyroid antibodies.
- Tuberculin test if immunosuppressive therapy is contemplated.
- EMG (abnormalities include a decremental response to tetanic train stimulation at 5–10 Hz, and evidence of neuromuscular blockade is seen on single-fibre EMG in the form of jitter and blocking of motor action potentials).

What is the differential diagnosis?

- Botulism.
- Eaton–Lambert syndrome.

What are the treatment modalities available?

- Symptomatic treatment entails adminstration of an anticholinesterase drug, e.g. pyridostigmine given up to five times per day.
- Definitive treatment entails immunosuppression, e.g. steroids, azathioprine, cylosporin, plasmapheresis, thymectomy.

Mention a drug that can cause myasthenia.

D-Penicillamine therapy given for rheumatoid arthritis.

Why may a 'gin and tonic' exacerbate myasthenia?

The quinine in tonic water causes muscle weakness.

If this patient develops an infection, which group of antibiotics would you avoid?

Aminoglycosides.

Mention a few exacerbating features.

Fatigue, exercise, infection, emotion, change of climate, pregnancy, magnesium enemas, drugs (aminoglycosides, propranolol, morphine, barbiturates, procainamide, quinidine).

Advanced-level Questions

How is the myasthenia graded?

Osserman grading is used:
Grade I: involves focal disease (e.g. restricted to ocular muscles).
Grade II: generalized disease that is mild (grade IIa) or moderate (IIb).
Grade III: severe generalized disease.
Grade IV: crisis with life-threatening respiratory impairment.

What do you know about Eaton–Lambert syndrome?

Eaton–Lambert syndrome is a myasthenic disorder associated with malignancy. The pelvic girdle and thighs are almost invariably involved. EMG is diagnostic. In the rested muscle there is marked depression of neuromuscular transmission after a single submaximal stimulus and marked facilitation of response during repetitive stimulation at rates greater than 10 per second.

What is myasthenic crisis?

Exacerbation of myasthenia. The need for artificial ventilation occurs in about 10% of patients with myasthenia. Those with bulbar and respiratory involvement are prone to respiratory infection. The crisis can be precipitated by respiratory infection and surgery. Such patients should be closely monitored for pulmonary function. Those with artificial ventilation are not given cholinergics as this avoids stimulation of pulmonary secretions and uncertainties about overdosage.

How does a cholinergic crisis manifest?

Excessive salivation, confusion, lacrimation, miosis, pallor and collapse. It is important to avoid edrophonium in such patients.

Mention a few associated disorders.

Thyroid disorders (thyrotoxicosis, hypothyroidism), rheumatoid arthritis, diabetes mellitus, dermatomyositis, pernicious anaemia, SLE, Sjögren's disease, sarcoidosis, pemphigus.

What is the role of thymectomy in such patients?

In the case of thymoma, thymectomy is necessary to prevent tumour spread, although most thymomas are benign. In the absence of a tumour, thymectomy has been found to be beneficial in 85% of patients and 35% go into drug-free remission. The improvement is noticed 1–10 years after surgery. The role of thymectomy in ocular myasthenia, in adults over 55 years of age and in children, is still under debate.

How is myasthenia graded clinically?

- Osserman's grading of severity:
    Grade I: ocular myasthenia.
    Grade IIA: mild generalized myasthenia with slow progression; no crises; drug responsive.
    Grade IIB: moderate generalized myasthenia; severe skeletal and bulbar involvement, but no crises; drug response is less satisfactory.
    Grade III: acute fulminating myasthenia: rapid progression of severe symptoms of respiratory crises and poor drug response; high incidence of thymoma; high mortality rate.
    Grade IV: late severe myasthenia; same as grade III but takes 2 years to progress from Class I to II; crises; high mortality rate.

- Newsom-Davies clinical subgroups include:
    1. Patients with thymoma, equal sex incidence, peak age of onset 30–50 years, no HLA association and poor response to thymectomy.
    2. Young onset (< 40 years), typically female, thymic medullary germinal centres present, strong association with HLA-B8 and -DR3, and usually a good response to thymectomy.
    3. Older onset (> 40 years), more common in males, thymic involution, an association with HLA-B7 and -DR9, and doubtful response to thymectomy.

LM Eaton (1905–1958), Professor of Neurology at the Mayo Clinic, Rochester, Minnesota.
EH Lambert (b. 1915), Professor of Physiology, University of Minnesota.
Sir Samuel Wilks (1824–1911), physician, Guy's Hospital, London. Myasthenia gravis was known as Wilks' syndrome.
Myasthenia gravis was first described by the physiologist Thomas Willis in 1672 and by Erb in 1878. It was also known as Hoppe–Goldflam disease after HH Hoppe (1867–1919), a US neurologist, and SV Goldflam (1852–1932), a Polish neurologist. John Newsom-Davies, FRS, contemporary Professor of Clinical Neurology, Oxford.
Alastair Composton, PhD, FRCP, contemporary Professor of Neurology, Cambridge.

References

Drachman DB (1994) Myasthenia gravis. *N Engl J Med* **330**: 1797–1810.

Fambrough DM, Drachman DB & Satyamurti S (1973) Neuromuscular junction in myasthenia gravis: decreased acetylcholine receptors. *Science* **182**: 293–295.

Lambert EH & Eaton LM (1957) Electromyography and electric stimulation of nerves in diseases of the motor unit. *JAMA* **163**: 1117.

O'Neill JH, Murray NM & Newsom-Davies J (1988) The Eaton–Lambert syndrome. *Brain* **111**: 577 (a review of 50 cases).

Osserman KE (1958) *Myasthenia Gravis*. New York: Grune and Stratton.

Vincent A & Newsom-Davies J (1985) Acetylcholine receptor antibody as a diagnostic test for myasthenia gravis: results in 153 validated cases and 2967 diagnostic assays. *J Neurol Neurosurg Psychiatry* **48**: 1246–1252.

Willis T (1672) *De Anima Brutorum*. Oxford: Theatro Sheldoniano.

CASE 67 **Thomsen's Disease (Myotonia Congenita)**

Instruction

Look at this patient.

Salient features

- Diffuse muscle hypertrophy.
- Myotonia – may be apparent while shaking hands with the person.

Proceed as follows:

- Tell the examiner that you would like to do the following:

  Ask the patient whether or not there is any seasonal variation in symptoms – myotonia is worse in winter due to the cold.

  Take a family history (inheritance is usually autosomal dominant; gene on long arm of chromosome 7).

Diagnosis

This patient has diffuse muscular hypertrophy with myotonia (lesion) due to Thomsen's disease (aetiology).

Advanced-level Questions

How is the disease recognized in infancy?

Myotonia is present from birth and may be recognized by the child's peculiar cry. Also noticed in early infancy are difficulty in feeding and inability to reopen the eyes while having the face washed.

When does muscle hypertrophy manifest?

It is usually apparent in the second decade.

What is the cause of muscle hypertrophy?

It is due to almost continual involuntary isometric exercise.

What is the life expectancy in such patients?

These patients have a normal life expectancy.

What drugs would you use to ameliorate the myotonia?

Procainamide, quinidine.

In which other conditions is myotonia seen?

- Myotonia dystrophica.
- Paramyotonia congenita (episodic myotonia after exposure to the cold).
- Following the administration of drugs such as clofibrate.

AJT Thomsen (1815–1896) was a Danish physician who described this condition in his family and himself in 1876.

CASE 68 Friedreich's Ataxia

Instruction

Perform a neurological examination of this patient's legs.

Salient features

- Pes cavus.
- Pyramidal weakness in legs.
- Cerebellar signs, ataxia being a constant sign.
- Impaired vibration and joint sense.
- Romberg's sign positive.
- Distal muscle wasting (in 50% of cases), especially in the hands.

Proceed as follows:

- Tell the examiner that you would like to do the following investigations:
  Check for nystagmus (present in 25% of the cases), scanning speech, intention tremor.
  Examine the heart for hypertrophic cardiomyopathy.
  Check the eyes for optic atrophy (present in 30% of cases).
  Check the spine for kyphoscoliosis.
  Check the urine for sugar (10% of patients have diabetes).
  Check IQ, looking for intellectual deterioration.

Diagnosis

This patient has kyphoscoliosis, pes cavus and a combination of pyramidal, cerebellar and sensory deficits (lesions) in the lower limbs due to Friedreich's ataxia (aetiology); he is severely disabled by his deformity.

Advanced-level Questions

What is the mode of inheritance?

Autosomal recessive or, rarely, sex linked.

What is the age of onset?

Between 6 and 18 years of age.

Why are the deep tendon reflexes absent even though plantars are upgoing?

This is due to a combination of pyramidal weakness with peripheral neuropathy.

In which other conditions is there a mixture of cerebellar, pyramidal and dorsal column signs?

Multiple sclerosis.

Mention a few conditions with absent knee jerks and upgoing plantars.

- Peripheral neuropathy in a stroke patient.
- Motor neuron disease.
- Conus medullaris – cauda equina lesion.
- Tabes dorsalis.
- Subacute combined degeneration of the spinal cord.

What is the forme fruste of this condition?

Pes cavus or hammer toes, without any other signs, are seen in family members of such patients.

On which chromosome is the gene for this disorder localized?

Chromosome 9.

What are the clinical criteria for diagnosis of Friedreich's ataxia?

Harding's criteria:
- Essential criteria are onset before the age of 25 years, ataxia of limbs and gait, absent knee and ankle jerks, extensor plantars, autosomal recessive inheritance, motor conduction velocity greater than 40 m s^{-1}, small or absent sensory nerve action potentials, dysarthria within 5 years of onset.
- Additional criteria (present in two-thirds) are scoliosis, pyramidal weakness of lower limbs, absent upper limb reflexes, loss of vibration and joint position sense in the legs, abnormal ECG, pes cavus.
- Other features (present in less than 50% of cases) are nystagmus, optic atrophy, deafness, distal muscle wasting and diabetes.

What is the prognosis of Friedreich's ataxia?

Friedreich's ataxia usually progresses slowly and few patients live for more than 20 years after the onset of symptoms. Occasionally it may appear to be arrested, and abortive cases may be encountered in apparently healthy relatives of affected patients.

What are the pathological changes in Friedreich's ataxia?

- Marked loss of cells in the posterior root ganglia.
- Degeneration of peripheral sensory fibres.
- Involvement of the posterior and lateral columns of the cord.

Name a few syndromes with spinocerebellar degeneration.

- Roussy–Lévy disease: hereditary spinocerebellar degeneration with atrophy of lower limb muscles and loss of deep tendon reflexes.
- Refsum's disease (see page 607).
- Bassen–Kornzweig syndrome (see page 607): caused by cellular deficiency of vitamin E (α-tocopherol) resulting from a defect in the α-tocopherol-transfer protein and abetalipoproteinaemia associated with a defect of very low density lipoproteins.

- Olivopontocerebellar degeneration: first described in 1882; autosomal dominant inheritance and has been mapped to HLA loci on the short arm of chromosome 6; a highly polymorphic CAG repeat sequence has been found in this region. The CAG repeat sequence is longer than normal and unstable in affected patients.
- Machado–Joseph disease: dominant inheritance, first described in families of Portuguese origin. Clinical features include progressive ataxia, ophthalmoparesis, spasticity, dystonia, amyotrophy and parkinsonism. This disorder has been linked to chromosome 14 and is caused by the expansion of unstable CAG repeat sequences.
- Dentatorubral pallidoluysian atrophy is similar to Machado–Joseph disease but maps on the short arm of chromosome 12. The abnormally expanded CAG repeat sequences identified in the gene for olivopontocerebellar degeneration, Machado–Joseph disease and dentatorubral pallidoluysian atrophy each result in the expression of a specific ataxin.

Nikolaus Friedreich (1825–1882), Professor of Pathology and neurologist in Heidelberg, described this condition, in a series of papers from 1861 to 1876.
Anita Harding (1953–1995) Professor of Neurology at the National Hospital, Queen Square, London, died at the age of 42 years from colonic cancer.
G Roussy (1874–1948), a French neuropathologist.
G Lévy (b. 1881), a French neurologist.
Sigvald Refsum (1907–1991), a Norwegian neurologist, was successively Professor of Neurology at Bergen University and at the National Hospital in Oslo.

References

Harding AE (1981) Friedreich's ataxia: a clinical and genetic study of 90 families with an analysis of early diagnostic criteria and intrafamilial clustering of clinical features. *Brain* **104**: 589.
Lord Walton of Detchant (1991) S Refsum (obituary). *Br Med J* **303**: 919.
Rosenberg RN (1995) Spinocerebellar ataxias and ataxins. *N Engl J Med* **333**: 1351–1353.

CASE 69 Motor Neuron Disease

Instruction

Examine this patient's cranial nerves.
Examine this patient's upper limbs.
Examine this patient's lower limbs.

Salient features

- Fasciculations, absent reflexes and weakness in the upper limbs.
- Spasticity, exaggerated reflexes and upgoing plantars in lower limbs.
- Sluggish palatal movements, absent gag reflex, brisk jaw jerk.

A combination of the above signs may be seen.

Diagnosis

This patient has a combination of upper and lower motor neuron signs (lesions) due to motor neuron disease (aetiology), although I would like to exclude cervical cord compression. The patient is wheelchair bound as a result of the disease (functional status).

Questions

What important cause should be ruled out before making a firm diagnosis of motor neuron disease?

Cord compression may produce a similar clinical picture and hence it is important to do an MRI scan of the spine and/or a myelogram to exclude it.

Advanced-level Questions

What are the characterisitic features of this disease?

- It rarely begins before the age of 40 years.
- Presence of upper and lower motor neuron involvement of a single spinal segment, and motor dysfunction involving at least two limbs or one limb and bulbar muscles.
- Sensory symptoms or signs are not seen.
- Ocular movements are not affected.
- There are never cerebellar or extrapyramidal signs.
- Sphincters are involved late, if at all.
- Remission is unknown and the disease is fatal within 5–7 years (due to bronchopneumonia).

What are the clinical patterns of motor neuron disease?

- Bulbar: bulbar or pseudobulbar palsy (25% of cases).
- Amyotrophic lateral sclerosis (50% of cases): flaccid arms and spastic legs.
- Progressive muscular atrophy (25% of cases): a lesion in the anterior horn cells affecting distal muscles. Characteristically there is retention of deep tendon reflexes in the presence of severe muscular atrophy.

- Primary lateral sclerosis (rare): signs progress from an upper motor neuron to a lower motor neuron type.

Others affect lower motor neurons and include:

- Werdnig–Hoffman's disease: presents in the neonatal period as a 'floppy infant' and known as infantile progressive spinal muscular atrophy.
- X-linked spinal muscular atrophy: the patient has associated testicular atrophy resulting in oligospermia and gynaecomastia. It is associated with the amplification of a trinucleotide repeat in the coding sequence of the androgen receptor gene; the severity of the disease is directly related to the number of repeats present.
- Spinal muscular atrophy linked to locus on the large arm of chromosome 5.

What are the other types of motor neuron disease?

- Madras motor neuron disease, common in southern India, where the onset is early (before the age of 30), with asymmetrical limb weakness and wasting, bulbar and facial involvement occurs along with sensorineural deafness. The course is more benign than the disorder observed in Europe and America.
- Amyotrophic lateral sclerosis associated with a parkinsonism–dementia complex in Guam. It also tends to have an earlier onset and a more protracted course than the sporadic cases seen in Europe and America.

What is the pathology of motor neuron disease?

The clinical manifestations are a result of degeneration of Betz cells, pyramidal tracts, cranial nerve nuclei and anterior horn cells. Both upper and lower motor neurons may be involved, but sensory involvement is not seen.

What is the explanation of fasciculation?

It is due to spontaneous firing of large motor units formed by branching fibres of surviving axons that are striving to innervate muscle fibres that have lost their nerve supply.

What are the cerebrospinal fluid (CSF) changes in the disease?

- The CSF is usually normal (the protein level may be slightly raised).

What do you know about the heredity of amyotrophic lateral sclerosis?

Most cases are sporadic. Five to ten per cent of cases are familial, and familial amyotrophic lateral sclerosis is linked to a gene on the long arm of chromosome 21. This genetic locus appears to be the copper–zinc-binding superoxide dismutase gene, with various missense mutations identified in different families.

Is there any treatment for motor neuron disease?

No treatment has been shown to influence the course of the disease. Riluzole, a glutamate antagonist, is being used in bulbar palsy. Patients often require treatment for painful muscle cramps, constant drooling, severe fatiguability, sleep problems, incipient contractures, subluxation of the shoulder joint, dysphagia and neuralgia – all of which can be ameliorated. Patients often have extreme lability of emotion, particularly in the early stages of amyotrophic lateral sclerosis. In order to alleviate distress before or during respiratory failure, which is usually the terminal event, narcotic drugs should not be withheld.

What is the rationale for using riluzole?

The suggestion that accumulation of toxic levels of glutamate at synapses may cause neuronal death through a calcium-dependent pathway. Riluzole has been shown to be useful in patients with disease of bulbar onset but not in those with disease of spinal onset.

Is there any test to monitor the rate of disease progression?

Antibodies to L-type voltage-gated calcium channels are present in the serum of patients with sporadic amyotrophic lateral sclerosis, and antibody titres correlate with the rate of disease progression.

What is the role of magnetic cortical stimulation in amyotrophic lateral sclerosis?

Magnetic cortical stimlation uses time-varying magnetic fields to induce electrical currents within the brain painlessly. It is said to activate cortical motor neurons trans-synaptically through thalamocortical and corticocortical afferents, and allows detection of degeneration of cortical Betz cells. In patients with amyotrophic lateral sclerosis the sensitivity of this technique to detect upper motor neuron involvement in those with clinical signs is high, but the sensitivity of the technique in those without clinical signs is unknown.

Is there any animal model for amyotrophic lateral sclerosis?

Transgenic mouse model possessing mutations in the gene encoding the cytosolic form of the enzyme copper–zinc superoxide dismutase.

Lou Gehrig, the American baseball player, died from amyotrophic lateral sclerosis 50 years ago.
Charcot gave a detailed clinical and pathological description of amyotrophic lateral sclerosis in 1865.
Professor Stephen Hawking, the Cambridge theoretical physicist, is the most famous sufferer of motor neuron disease. It claimed the lives of the actor David Niven, the football manager Don Revie and the wartime pilot Sir Leonard Cheshire, VC.

References

Bensimon G, Lacomblez L, Meninger V & ALS/Riluzole Study Group (1994) A controlled trial of riluzole in amyotrophic lateral sclerosis. *N Engl J Med* **330**: 585–591.

Gajdusek DC (1982) Foci of motor neuron disease in high incidence in isolated populations of East Asia and the western Pacific. In: Rowland LP (ed.) *Human Motor Neuron Diseases*, pp. 363. New York: Raven Press.

Mitsumoto H, Hanson MR & Chad DA (1988) Amyotrophic lateral sclerosis. Recent advances in pathogenesis and therapeutic trials. *Arch Neurol* **45**: 189.

O'Brien T, Kelly M & Saunders C (1992) Motor neuron disease: a hospice perspective. *Br Med J* **304**: 471–473.

Rosen DR, Siddique T, Patterson D et al (1993) Mutations in Cu/Zn superoxide dismutase gene are associated with familial amyotrophic lateral sclerosis. *Nature* **362**: 59.

Siddique T, Figlewicz DA, Periak-Vance MA et al (1991) Linkage of a gene causing familial amyotrophic lateral sclerosis to chromosome 21 and evidence of genetic locus heterogeneity. *N Engl J Med* **324**: 1381.

Smith RG, Hamilton S, Hofmann F et al (1992) Serum antibodies to L-type calcium channels in patients with amyotrophic lateral sclerosis. *N Engl J Med* **327**: 1721–1728.

Spencer PS, Nunn PB, Hugon T et al (1987) Guam amyotrophic lateral sclerosis–parkinsonism–dementia linked to a plant excitant neurotoxin. *Science* **237**: 517.

Srinivas K, Jagannathan K & Valmikinathan K (1984) The spectrum of motor neuron disease in Madras. In: Rose FC (ed.) *Research Progress in Motor Neuron Disease*, pp. 142. London: Pitman.

CASE 70 Neurofibromatosis

Instruction

Examine this patient.

Salient features

- Multiple neurofibroma and café-au-lait spots.

Proceed as follows:

- The axilla for freckles.
- Visual acuity and fundus for optic glioma.
- Hearing and corneal sensation for acoustic neuroma.
- The iris for Lisch nodules (often apparent only by slit-lamp examination) – present on over 90% of patients.
- The spine for kyphoscoliosis.
- Tell the examiner that you would like to check the blood pressure (for renal artery stenosis or phaeochromocytoma).

Remember the triad for neurofibromatosis – neurofibroma, café-au-lait spots and Lisch nodules – allows identification of virtually all patients with neurofibromatosis type 1.

Diagnosis

This patient has multiple café-au-lait spots and neurofibromas (lesion) due to von Recklinghausen's disease (aetiology) which are cosmetically disfiguring (functional status).

Advanced-level Questions

What are criteria for neurofibromatosis type I (von Recklinghausen's disease)?

Neurofibromatosis type 1 may be diagnosed when two or more of the following are present:
- Six or more café-au-lait spots, the greatest diameter of which is more than 5 mm in prepubertal patients and more than 15 mm in postpubertal patients.
- Two or more neurofibromas or one plexiform neurofibroma. Plexiform neurofibroma is considered by some to be a defining lesion of neurofibroma type 1.
- Freckling in the axilla or inguinal region (Crowe's sign).
- Optic glioma.

- Two or more Lisch nodules (iris hamartoma).
- A distinctive osseous lesion such as sphenoid dysplasia or thinning of long bone cortex with or without pseudoarthroses.
- A parent, sibling or child with neurofibromatosis according to the above criteria.

What are the criteria for neurofibromatosis type 2?

- Bilateral eighth nerve palsy confirmed by CT or MRI.
- A parent, sibling or child with neurofibromatosis type 2 and either unilateral eighth nerve mass or any two of the following: neurofibroma, meningioma, glioma, schwannoma or juvenile posterior subcapsular lenticular opacity.

What is the significance of the Lisch nodules?

Lisch nodules are melanocytic hamartomas that appear as well-defined, dome-shaped elevations projecting from the surface of the iris and are clear to yellow and brown. They are an important tool in establishing the diagnosis of neurofibromatosis type 1 and in providing accurate genetic screening.

What is the histology of the skin tumours?

The peripheral nerve tumours are of two types:
- Schwannomas: arise in cranial and spinal nerve roots and also in peripheral nerve trunks.
- Neurofibromas: composed of a proliferation of all elements of the peripheral nerve including neuritis, Schwann cells and fibroblasts. In sensory nerve twigs they appear as subcutaneous nodules, while in peripheral nerve trunks they may appear as a fusiform enlargement or a plexiform neurofibroma.

Is a biopsy of the neurofibromas required to make a diagnosis?

No, as the diagnosis is usually evident on clinical grounds.

What are the associated abnormalities of neurofibroma?

- Lung cysts.
- Retinal hamartomas.
- Skeletal lesions: rib notching and other erosive bony defects, intraosseous cystic lesions, subperiosteal bony cysts, dysplasia of the skull, bowed legs and pseudoarthrosis of the tibia.

- Intellectual disability.
- Aqueductal stenosis.
- Epilepsy.
- Sarcomatous change.

What do you know about the inheritance of these two disorders?

Both are autosomal dominant syndromes, type 1 being carried on chromosome 17q11.2 and type 2 on chromosome 22. The gene for neurofibromatosis type 1 encodes a protein called neurofibromin which downregulates the function of the p21 ras oncoprotein. The gene for type 2 neurofibromatosis is also a tumour suppressor gene which encodes a protein that links integral membrane proteins of the cytoskeleton. How this protein is involved in tumorigenesis is not clear. Family members at risk for type 2 neurofibromatosis should be screened regularly with hearing tests and brainstem auditory evoked responses.

How would you manage these patients?

- Most are asymptomatic and require no treatment.
- Large plexiform neurofibromas should be usually left alone.
- Small neurofibromas can be removed if painful.
- Optic gliomas are treated with radiation.

Friedreich Daniel von Recklinghausen (1833–1910) was Professor of Pathology successively at Könisberg, Wüurzburg and Strasbourg. He also described another disease, arthritis deformans neoplastica, to which his name is attached.

The elephant man, John Merrick, is commonly believed to have suffered from neurofibromatosis, but according to *Science* (1994; **264**: 188) a rare condition Proteus syndrome is the more likely diagnosis.

Professor Lisch first described the association of the Lisch nodule with neurofibromatosis in 1937. These nodules were first described by Waardenburg in 1918 but he did not appreciate the association with neurofibromatosis.

References

Barker D, Wright E, Nquyen K et al (1987) Gene for von Recklinghausen's neurofibromatosis is in the pericentric region of chromosome 17. *Science* **236**: 110.

Gutmann DH & Collins FS (1993) The neurofibromatosis type 1 gene and its protein product, neurofibromin. *Neuron* **10**: 335.

Lisch K (1937) Ueber Beteiligung der Augen, insbesondere das Vorkommen von Irisnötchen bei der Neurofibromatose (Recklinghausen). *Z Augenheilkd* **93**: 137–143.

Lubs ME, Bauer MS, Formas ME & Djokic B (1991) Lisch nodules in neurofibromatosis type 1. *N Engl J Med* **324**: 1264.

Martuza RL & Eldridge R (1988) Neurofibromatosis 2. *N Engl J Med* **318**: 685.

Riccardi VM (1991) Neurofibromatosis: past, present and future. *N Engl J Med* **324**: 1283.

Rouleau GA, Merel P, Lutchman M et al (1993) Alteration in a new gene encoding a putative membrane-organising protein causes neurofibromatosis type 2. *Nature* **363**: 515.

CASE 71 Syringomyelia

Instruction

Examine this patient's arms.

Salient features

- Wasting and weakness of the small muscles of the hands and forearm (if fasciculation is seen, then the other diagnosis that comes to mind at this stage is motor neuron disease).
- Tone and deep tendon reflexes are diminished.
- Loss of pain and temperature sensation with intact vibration, light touch and joint position sense – this deficit is the underlying cause for any burns present.
- There may be Charcot's joints of the shoulder and elbow.

Proceed as follows:

- Examine vibration sense over the fingers, lower end of radius, elbow and clavicles (note that vibration sense is impaired only at a later stage).
- Look for Horner's syndrome.
- Examine the neck posteriorly for scar of previous surgery.
- Ask whether you may examine the following:
    The lower limbs for pyramidal signs.
    The face for loss of temperature and pain sensation (starting from the outer part of the face and progressing forward, looking for the 'onion-skin pattern' of sensory loss due to a lesion in the spinal nucleus of the fifth cranial nerve which extends from the pons down to the upper cervical cord).
    For lower cranial nerve palsy.
    For nystagmus and ataxia (due to involvement of the medial longitudinal bundle from C5 upwards).
    For kyphoscoliosis (due to paravertebral muscle involvement).

- Tell the examiner that you would like to take a history of painless trauma or burns with cigarettes, hot water.

Diagnosis

This patient has dissociated sensory loss (lesion) due to syringomyelia (aetiology), and has had severe painless trauma or burns (functional status).

Questions

How common is syringomyelia?

It is a rare disorder affecting both sexes equally; the usual age of onset is the fourth or fifth decade.

How do you explain the clinical features?

- At the level of the syrinx:
    Anterior horn cell involvement causing a lower motor neuron lesion.
    Involvement of the central decussating fibres of the spinothalamic tract producing dissociated sensory loss and late development of neuropathic arthropathy and other trophic changes.
- Below the level of the syrinx:
    Involvement of pyramidal corticospinal tracts resulting in spastic paraparesis (sphincter function is usually well preserved).
- Involvement of cervical sympathetics:
    Horner's syndrome (miosis, enophthalmos, ptosis).

Advanced-level Questions

What is la main succulente?

In some patients with syringomyelia the hands have an ugly appearance as a result of trophic and vasomotor disturbances; these commonly result in cold, cyanosed and swollen fingers and palms.

What are the other causes of dissociated sensory loss?

- Anterior spinal artery occlusion (affecting the dorsal horn and lateral spinothalamic tract).
- Diabetic small-fibre polyneuropathy.
- Hereditary amyloidotic polyneuropathy.
- Leprosy (the latter three conditions affect small peripheral nerve axons).

What investigations would you do?

MRI scan. In the past, myelography was performed to confirm the diagnosis but was associated with deterioration of the condition in a large number of patients.

What associated abnormalities may be present?

Arnold–Chiari malformation, spina bifida, bony defects around the foramen magnum, hydrocephalus, spinal cord tumours.

What conditions may be present with a similar picture?

- Intramedullary tumours of the spinal cord.
- Arachnoiditis around the foramen magnum obstructing the CSF pathway.
- Haematomyelia.
- Craniovertebral anomalies.
- Late sequelae of spinal cord injuries (manifest as a painful ascending myelopathy).

What is the difference between hydromyelia and syringomyelia?

Hydromyelia is the expansion of the ependymal-lined central canal of the spinal cord, whereas syringomyelia is the formation of a cleft-like cavity in the inner portion of the cord. Both these lesions are associated with destruction of the white and grey matter and an accompanying reactive gliosis. In syringomyelia the process generally begins in the cervical cord, and with expansion of the cavity the brainstem and distal cord also become affected.

What are the clinical features of syringobulbia?

- Dissociated sensory loss of the face of the 'onion-skin' pattern (extending from behind forwards, converging on the nose and upper lip).
- Vertigo (common symptom).
- Wasting of the small muscles of the tongue (important physical sign).
- The process may be limited to the medullary region.
- The main cranial nerve nuclei involved are those of the fifth, seventh, ninth and tenth cranial nerves.

What does the cavity of the syrinx contain?

It contains a fluid similar to CSF but with a higher protein content.

What is the treatment available?

- Syringoperitoneal shunting (particularly in patients with basal arachnoiditis and without tonsillar descent).
- Direct drainage of the syrinx into the subarachnoid space (in post-traumatic cavitation).
- When there is an association with Arnold–Chiari malformation, the pressure is relieved by removing the lower central portion of the occipital bone and cervical laminectomy to restore normal CSF dynamics.

What other causes of Charcot's joints do you know?

- Diabetes mellitus, especially when toes and ankles are affected.
- Tabes dorsalis, especially when knee and hip joints are affected.

What do you know about Morvan's syndrome?

It was initially used to describe painless whitlows on the fingers but was subsequently applied to the progressive loss of pain sensation and its effects (such as ulceration, resorption of the phalanges and loss of soft tissue) in both hands and feet. These changes are now more commonly seen in leprosy.

The term 'syringomyelia' (from *syringx*, a pipe or tube) was first used by Ollivier in 1824, in his monograph on diseases of the spinal cord, to denote cavity formation. It denotes the presence of a large fluid-filled cavity in the grey matter of the spinal cord which is in communication with the central canal and contains CSF.
J Arnold (1835–1915), Professor of Pathology at Heidelberg.
H Chiari (1851–1916), an Austrian pathologist.

References

Batzdorf U (1988) Chiari I malformation with syringomyelia. Evaluation of surgical therapy by magnetic resonance imaging. *J Neurosurg* **68**: 726.

Logue V & Edwards MR (1981) Syringomyelia and its surgical treatment – an analysis of 75 patients. *J Neurol Neurosurg Psychiatry* **44**: 273–284.

Morvan AM (1883) De la parésie analgésique à panaris des extrémitiés supérieures ou paréso-analgésie des extrémitiés supérieures. *Gazette Hebdomadaire Médecine et de Chirurgie* **35**: 580.

CASE 72 Subacute Combined Degeneration of the Spinal Cord

Instruction

Carry out a neurological examination of the patient's legs.

Salient features

- Absent ankle jerks.
- Brisk knee jerks.
- Upgoing plantars.
- Diminished light touch, vibration and posterior column signs.
- Romberg's sign positive.

Proceed as follows:

- Examine the following:
    Mucous membranes for anaemia (pernicious anaemia).
    Abdomen for scars of previous gastrectomy (carcinoma of the stomach).
    Pupils (Argyll Robertson pupil because tabes is a differential diagnosis).
    Fundus for optic atrophy, seen in this condition.
- Tell the examiner that you would like to do the following investigations:
    Take a family history of pernicious anaemia.
    Do a mini-mental status examination for dementia.
    Take a history of alcohol consumption and previous gastrectomy.
    Take a history of chronic diarrhoea.

Diagnosis

This patient has absent ankle jerks, brisk knee jerks and upgoing plantars with posterior column signs (lesion) due to subacute combined degeneration of the spinal cord (aetiology) and due to paralysis (functional status).

Questions

Mention a few causes of vitamin B$_{12}$ deficiency.

- Vegan diet.
- Impaired absorption:
    From the stomach (pernicious anaemia, gastrectomy).
    From the small bowel (ileal disease, bacterial overgrowth, coeliac disease).

From the pancreas (chronic pancreatic disease).
As a result of fish tapeworm (rare).

Advanced-level Questions

What is the pathology of this condition?

There is degeneration of the axons in both the ascending tracts of the posterior columns and the descending pyramidal tracts (hence combined degeneration).

How would you investigate such a patient?

- FBC and reticulocyte count.
- Vitamin B_{12} and folate concentrations.
- Serum ferritin levels (since associated iron deficiency is common).
- Bone marrow examination.
- Parietal cell and intrinsic factor antibodies.
- Schilling test.

If this patient had a haemoglobin level of 6 g dl^{-1}, how would you treat it?

I would avoid giving packed cells before replacing vitamin B_{12} as this may irreversibly exacerbate the neurological manifestations. Furthermore, blood transfusion is reported to precipitate incipient heart failure and death.

What type of anaemia may be seen in such patients?

Macrocytic anaemia.

Mention a few other causes of macrocytic anaemia.

- With megaloblastic bone marrow: vitamin B_{12} deficiency, folate deficiency.
- With normoblastic marrow: haemolytic anaemias, post-haemorrhagic anaemia, severe hypoxia, myxoedema, hypopituitarism, bone marrow infiltration, acute leukaemia and aplastic anaemia.

What do you know about intrinsic factor antibodies?

Intrinsic factor antibodies are seen in about 50% of patients with pernicious anaemia. About 45% of the patients have no antibody to intrinsic factor. There are two types of antibody:

Type 1 – the blocking antibody which prevents vitamin B_{12} from binding to intrinsic factor and occurs in 55% of patients.

Type 2 – the binding or precipitating antibody, which reacts with intrinsic factor or with vitamin B_{12}–intrinsic factor complex and is seen in 35% of patients.

What is the relationship between pernicious anaemia and gastric carcinoma?

The incidence of gastric carcinoma in patients with pernicious anaemia is increased threefold compared with that in the general population.

What gastrointestinal investigations would you do in an asymptomatic patient with pernicious anaemia?

In the absence of gastrointestinal symptoms, gastroscopy or barium meal is not indicated, although many physicians tend to perform one of these investigations.

What do you understand by the term 'combined' degeneration of the cord?

This refers to the combined demyelination of both pyramids (or lateral columns) and posterior columns of the spinal cord.

What is the response of the neurological lesions to treatment with vitamin B_{12}?

The response to vitamin B_{12} therapy is variable: it may improve, remain unchanged or even deteriorate. Sensory abnormalities improve more than motor abnormalities and peripheral neuropathy responds to treatment better than myelopathy.

Subacute combined degeneration is also known as Putnam–Dana syndrome or Lichtheim's disease. James Jackson Putnam (1846–1918) and Charles Loomis Dana (1852–1935) were both US neurologists. Ludwig Lichtheim (1845–1928), a German physician.

Pernicious anaemia was usually fatal, until 1926 when Whipple, Minot and Murphy described the beneficial effects of feeding liver. The 1934 Nobel Prize in Medicine was awarded jointly to George Whipple (1878–1976) of University of Rochester, New York, and to George Minot (1885–1950) and William P Murphy (1892–1987) of Harvard Medical School and Peter Brent Brigham Hospital, Boston, for their discoveries concerning liver therapy in cases of anaemia.

William B Castle first found that oral adminstration of gastric juice (intrinsic factor) or beef (extrinsic factor, i.e. vitamin B_{12}) alone was not effective in the treatment of pernicious anaemia but that a mixture of both these factors rendered the patient erythropoietically active. Castle worked with Francis Peabody at the Harvard Medical School Unit at Boston City Hospital before he became Professor of Medicine at Harvard.

CASE 73   Tabes Dorsalis

Instruction

Examine this patient with lightning pains (lightning denotes that the pains are fleeting and does not necessarily mean they are excruciating).

Salient features

- Examine the eyes:
    Bilateral ptosis with frontalis overaction.
    Argyll Robertson pupil (irregular, small pupil which reacts sluggishly to light as compared with accommodation).
    Optic atrophy (primary).
- Examine the sensory system:
    Posterior column signs.
    Look for loss of pain sensation but with normal touch and temperature sensation over the nose, cheeks, inner aspects of the arms and legs, a band across the nipple and in the anal area.
    Squeeze calf muscles and the Achilles tendon (evokes no pain as deep sensation is lost).
- Examine
    The ankle jerks (absent) and plantar response (normal).
    The gait for ataxia (steppage gait) and Romberg's sign.
    The knees and hips for Charcot's joints.
    The feet for trophic ulcers.
- Tell the examiner that you would like to:
    Ask the patient about bladder sensation (lost), overflow incontinence and impotence (if male).
    Constipation (this is present as a rule).
    Check testicular sensation (usually lost early).

Note. Remember that, as a rule, the lower limbs are affected before the upper limbs. Very rarely, the upper limbs may be affected first – called 'cervical tabes'.

Diagnosis

This patient has posterior column signs and Argyll Robertson pupil (lesion) due to tabes dorsalis (aetiology), and has severe ataxia (functional status).

Advanced-level Questions

What do you know about neurosyphilis?

There are five clinical patterns of neurosyphilis:
- Meningovascular disease, which occurs 3–4 years after primary infection.
- Tabes dorsalis, which occurs 10–35 years after primary infection.
- Generalized paralysis of the insane (GPI), which occurs 10–15 years after primary infection.
- Taboparesis (a combination of the latter two).
- Localized gummata.

Tertiary syphilis of the nervous system never develops in those who have received appropriate therapy in the early stages.

What is the underlying pathology?

It is due to a combination of neuronal degeneration and/or arterial lesions.

How would you confirm the diagnosis?

The Wasserman reaction, Veneral Disease Reference Laboratory (VDRL) or *Treponema pallidum* haemagglutination assay (TPHA):
> Meningovascular syphilis – 70% positive, whereas CSF shows 90% positive.
> Tabes dorsalis – 75% positive.
> GPI – nearly 100% positive.

Mention a few conditions for which the Wasserman reaction may be falsely positive.

Rheumatoid arthritis, SLE, chronic active hepatitis, infectious mononucleosis.

How would you treat the active syphilitic infection?

A course of parenteral penicillin.

How would you manage other symptoms of tabes?

- Lightning pains: simple analgesics, carbamazepine.
- Sensory ataxia: re-educational exercises to improve limb co-ordination.
- Bladder symptoms: avoid anticholinergics, employ urodynamic studies and intermittent self-catheterization.

- Visceral crises: opiate analgesics; in recurrent cases, section of lower thoracic spinal dorsal roots.
- Perforating ulcer: well-fitting shoes and regular foot care.
- Charcot's arthropathy: symptomatic treatment, avoid insertion of prostheses as results are poor.

In which group of patients is syphilis now common?

In those with underlying human immunodeficiency virus (HIV) infection.

What is the Jarisch-Herxheimer reaction?

An acute hypersensitivity reaction seen when a patient with syphilis is treated with penicillin. Toxins from the killed spirochaetes cause this reaction, which can be fatal. Steroids are often given during the first few days of penicillin therapy.

How may this patient present to the surgeons?

With acute abdominal pain (lancinating pains).

What are the methods of eliciting deep pain?

- Abadie's sign is the loss of pain sense in the Achilles tendon.
- Biernacki's sign is the absence of pain on pressure on the ulnar nerve.
- Pitres' sign is loss of pain on pressure on the testes.
- Haenel sign is analgesia to pressure on the eyeballs.

Tabes was first recognized by Romberg and Duchenne. Fournier was the first to suspect that it was caused by syphilis.
AP Wassermann (1866–1925), a German physician.
A Jarisch (1850–1902), Professor of Dermatology in Austria.
K Herxheimer (1861–1944), a Jewish German dermatologist who died in a concentration camp.

References

Hook EW III & Marra CM (1992) Acquired syphilis in adults. *N Engl J Med* **326**: 1060.
Simon RP (1985) Neurosyphilis. *Arch Neurol* **42**: 606.

CASE 74 Ulnar Nerve Palsy

Instruction

Carry out a neurological examination of this patient's upper limbs.

Salient features

- Generalized wasting of the small muscles of the hand.
- There may be features of ulnar claw hand, i.e. hyperextension at the metacarpophalangeal joints and flexion at the interphalangeal joints of the fourth and fifth fingers.
- There is weakness of movement of the fingers, except that of the thenar eminence.
- There is sensory loss over the medial one and half fingers.

Proceed as follows:

- Examine the elbow for scars and signs of osteoarthrosis.

Diagnosis

This patient has wasting of the small muscles of the hand and claw hand with sensory loss over the medial one and half fingers (lesion) due to ulnar nerve palsy caused by trauma (aetiology). She is unable to button her clothes (functional status).

Advanced-level Questions

What are the muscles supplied by the ulnar nerve?

The ulnar nerve is derived from the eighth cervical and first thoracic spinal nerves. It gives no branches above the elbow and supplies:

In the forearm:
> Flexor carpi ulnaris.
> Medial half of the flexor digitorum profundus.

In the hand:
> Movers of the little finger – abductor digiti minimi, flexor digiti minimi and opponens digiti minimi.
> Adductor pollicis (oblique and transverse heads).
> Dorsal and palmar interossei.
> Third and fourth lumbricals.
> Palmaris brevis.
> Inner head of flexor pollicis brevis.

How would you differentiate between a lesion above the cubital fossa and a lesion at the wrist?

- In lesions above the cubital fossa the flexor carpi ulnaris is involved.
- In lesions at the wrist, the adductor pollicis is involved.

How would you test the flexor carpi ulnaris?

Ask the patient to keep her hand flat on a table with the palm facing upwards and then ask her to perform flexion and ulnar deviation at the wrist.

How would you test the adductor pollicis?

Ask the patient to grip a folded newspaper between the thumb and index finger of each hand so that the thumbs are uppermost – this causes the adductor to contract. When the muscle is paralysed, the thumb is incapable of adequate adduction and becomes flexed at the interphalangeal joint due to contraction of the flexor pollicis longus (innervated by the median nerve). This is known as Froment's sign.

What is ulnar paradox?

The higher the lesion in the upper limb, the lesser is the deformity. A lesion at or above the elbow causes paralysis of the ulnar half of the flexor digitorum profundus, interossei and lumbricals. Thus, the action of the paralysed profundus is not unopposed by the interossei and lumbricals; as a result the ring and little fingers are not flexed and hence there is no claw, whereas a lesion at the wrist causes an ulnar claw hand.

What causes the ulnar claw hand?

A lesion of the ulnar nerve at the wrist. The little and ring fingers are flexed at the interphalangeal joints and hyperextended at the metacarpo-phalangeal joints. The index and middle fingers are less affected as the first and second lumbricals are supplied by the median nerve.

What are the causes of claw hand?

True claw hand is seen in the following conditions:
Advanced rheumatoid arthritis.
Lesion of both the median and ulnar nerves, as in leprosy.
Lesions of the medial cord of the brachial plexus.
Anterior poliomyelitis.

Syringomyelia.
Polyneuritis.
Amyotrophic lateral sclerosis.
Klumpke's paralysis (lower brachial plexus, C7–8 involvement).
Severe Volkmann's ischaemic contracture.

How is the ulnar nerve affected at the wrist?

The deep branch of the ulnar nerve is motor and may be compressed in Guyon's canal, which runs between the pisiform and hook of the hamate. This results in wasting and weakness of the interossei, particularly the first and the adductor pollicis, but sensation is spared. Also the hypothenar muscles are usually spared, although the third and fourth lumbricals may be affected. The nerve may be compressed in Guyon's canal by a ganglion, neuroma or repeated trauma. Surgical exposure of the nerve may be necessary when there is no history of trauma.

What is the most common cause of an ulnar nerve lesion at the elbow?

It is due to compression of the nerve by the fibrous arch of the flexor carpi ulnaris (the cubital tunnel) which arises as two heads from the medial epicondyle and the olecranon.

What you understand by the term 'tardy ulnar nerve palsy'?

This occurs as a result of injuries or arthritic changes at the elbow causing a delayed or slowly progressive involvement of the ulnar nerve.

How would you rapidly exclude an injury to a major nerve in the arm?

- Radial nerve: test for wrist drop.
- Ulnar nerve: test for Froment's sign (see above).
- Median nerve: Ochsner's clasping test.

Jules Froment (1876–1946), Professor of Clinical Medicine, Lyons, France.
AJ Ochsner (b. 1896), a US surgeon, also investigated the role of tobacco in lung cancer.
Augusta Déjérine-Klumpke (1859–1927), a French neurologist, was the first woman to receive the title 'Internes des Hôpitaux' in 1877.
R von Volkmann (1830–1889), Professor of Surgery in Halle, Germany.

CASE 75

Lateral Popliteal Nerve Palsy, L4, L5 (Common Peroneal Nerve Palsy)

Instruction

Examine this patient's legs.
Test this patient's gait.

Salient features

- Wasting of the muscles on the lateral aspect of the leg, namely the peronei and tibialis anterior muscle.
- Weakness of dorsiflexion and eversion of the foot.
- Foot drop.
- High steppage gait.
- Loss of sensation on the lateral aspect of the leg and dorsum of the foot. If the deep peroneal branch is affected, the sensory loss may be limited to the dorsum of the web between the first and second toes.

Proceed as follows

- Test the ankle jerk:
  Absent ankle jerk: suspect an S1 lesion.
  Normal jerk: common peroneal nerve palsy.
  Brisk jerk: suspect an upper motor neuron lesion.
- Comment on calliper shoes by the bedside (if any).
- Tell the examiner that you would like to take a history of trauma at the head of the fibula.

Diagnosis

This patient has wasting of the lateral aspect of the leg and sensory loss (lesion) due to common nerve palsy caused by trauma to the head of the fibula (aetiology), and has to wear callipers (functional status).

Questions

Mention a few causes.

- Compression resulting from application of a tourniquet or plaster of Paris casts. The nerve is vulnerable at the head of the fibula, where it lies on the surface of the hard bone with a covering of only skin.
- Direct trauma to the nerve.

- Leprosy (commonest cause worldwide).
- Ganglion arising from the superior tibiofibular joint may compress the nerve.
- Compression of the nerve by the tendinous edge of the peroneus longus.

Advanced-level Questions

How would you manage such a patient?

- Nerve conduction studies: there may be a local conduction block or slowing in the region of the head of the fibula. There may denervation in the tibialis anterior and extensor digitorum profundus.
- If the intact nerve is severed: surgery.
- If the nerve is intact and concussed: 90-degree splint at night, calliper shoes with a 90-degree stop, and galvanic or faradic stimulation to maintain the bulk of the muscle until the nerve recovers.

What other types of nerve injury do you know?

- Neurapraxia, i.e. concussion of the nerve after which a complete recovery occurs.
- Axonotmesis, in which the axon is severed but the myelin sheath is intact; recovery may occur.
- Neurotmesis, in which the nerve is completely severed and the prognosis for recovery is poor.

What are the other causes of foot drop?

- Peripheral neuropathy (see page 160).
- L4, L5 root lesion.
- Motor neuron disease
- Sciatic nerve palsy.
- Lumbosacral plexus lesion.

CASE 76 Carpal Tunnel Syndrome

Instruction
Examine this patient's hands.

Salient features

- Wasting of the thenar eminence.
- Weakness of flexion, abduction and opposition of thumb.
- Diminished sensation over lateral three and half fingers.

Proceed as follows:

- Look carefully for scar of previous surgery (hidden by the crease of the wrist).
- Percuss over the course of the median nerve in the forearm: patient may experience tingling – this is Tinel's sign.
- Ask the patient to hyperextend the wrist maximally for 1 minute; this may bring on symptoms (dysaesthesia over the thumb and lateral two and half fingers).
- Tell the examiner that you would like to:
  Ask the patient about nocturnal pain (commonest cause of hand pain at night).
  Examine for underlying causes such as myxoedema, acromegaly and rheumatoid arthritis.
  Look for cervical spondylosis, frozen shoulder and tennis elbow (these may be associated).
  Take a family history (abnormally small size of carpal tunnel runs in families).
  Look for the Cimino–Brescia fistula for haemodialysis.

Diagnosis

This patient has median nerve involvement of the hand with Tinel's sign (lesion) due to carpal tunnel syndrome as a complication of chronic haemodialysis (aetiology). The patient has disabling tingling and pain at night (functional status).

Questions

Mention a few causes of carpal tunnel syndrome.

- Pregnancy.
- Oral contraceptives.
- Rheumatoid arthritis.
- Myxoedema.
- Acromegaly.
- If chronic renal failure patients on long-term dialysis it is due to β_2-microglobulin as amyloid deposition.
- Sarcoidosis.
- Hyperparathyroidism.

How would you treat this condition?

- Diuretics.
- Wrist splint.
- Local hydrocortisone injection.
- Surgical decompression.

Advanced-level Questions

How would you confirm the diagnosis?

Nerve conduction studies (increased latency at the wrist on stimulation of the median nerve. The muscle action potential from abductor pollicis brevis is a valuable diagnostic sign). Rarely, the proximal latency may be normal with a prolonged distal latency due to an anastomosis between the ulnar and median nerves in the forearm. A negative test thus does not rule the syndrome out absolutely but calls it into question.

Mention a few clinical diagnostic tests.

- Wrist extension test: the patient is asked to extend his wrists for 1 minute; this should produce numbness or tingling in the distribution of the median nerve.
- Phalen's test: the patient is asked to keep both hands with the wrist in complete palmar flexion for 1 minute; this produces numbness or tingling in the distribution of the median nerve.
- Tourniquet test: the symptoms are produced when the blood pressure cuff is inflated above the systolic pressure.
- Pressure test: if pressure is placed where the median nerve leaves the carpal tunnel, it causes pain.
- Luthy's sign: if the skinfold between the thumb and index finger does not close tightly around a bottle or cup because of thumb abduction paresis, this test is regarded as positive.
- Durkan's test: direct pressure over the carpal tunnel – the carpal compression test – is more sensitive and specific than the Tinel and Phalen sign.

Mention other entrapment neuropathies.

- Meralgia paraesthetica (lateral cutaneous nerve of the thigh trapped under the inguinal ligament).
- Elbow tunnel syndrome (ulnar nerve trapped in the cubital tunnel; see page 213).
- Common peroneal nerve trapped at the head of the fibula (see page 216).

- Morton's metatarsalgia (trapped medial and lateral plantar nerves causing pain between third and fourth toes).
- Tarsal tunnel syndrome (posterior tibial nerve is trapped).
- Suprascapular nerve trapped in the spinoglenoid notch.
- Radial nerve is trapped in the humeral groove.
- Anterior interosseous nerve trapped between the heads of the pronator muscle.

Jules Tinel (1879–1952), a French neurologist, described it as the 'sign of formication' in his book on nerve wounds. He took an active part in the French resistance.

TG Morton (1835–1903), a US surgeon, described this syndrome in 1876.

References

Brain WR, Wright AD & Wilkinson M (1947) Spontaneous compression of both median nerves. *Lancet* **i**: 277.

DeKrom MCTF, Knipschild PG, Kester ADM & Spaans F (1990) Efficacy of provocative tests for diagnosis of carpal tunnel syndrome. *Lancet* **335**: 393.

Danta G (1975) Familial carpal tunnel syndrome with onset in childhood. *J Neurol Neurosurg Psychiatry* **38**: 350.

Durkan JA (1991) A new diagnostic test for carpal tunnel syndrome. *J Bone Joint Surg* **73**: 535.

Harding AE & Le Fanu J (1977) Carpal tunnel syndrome related to antebrachial Cimino–Brescia fistula. *J Neurol Neurosurg Psychiatry* **40**: 511.

Iyer V & Fenichel GM (1976) Normal median nerve proximal latency in carpal tunnel syndrome: a clue to coexisting Martin–Gruber anastomosis. *J Neurol Neurosurg Psychiatry* **39**: 449.

Katz JN, Larson MG, Sabra A et al (1990) The carpal tunnel syndrome: diagnostic utility of the history and physical examination findings. *Ann Intern Med* **112**: 321.

Murray-Leslie CF & Wright V (1976) Carpal tunnel syndrome, human epicondylitis, and the cervical spine: a study of clinical and dimensional relations. *Br Med J* **1**: 1439.

CASE 77 Radial Nerve Palsy

Instruction

Perform a neurological examination of this patient's arms.

Salient features

- There is weakness of extension of the wrist and elbow (wrist flexion is normal).

- The patient is unable to straighten her fingers.
- However, if the wrist is passively extended, the patient is able to straighten her fingers at the interphalangeal joints (due to the action of interossei and lumbricals) but is unable to extend the metacarpophalangeal joint.
- There appears to be a weakness in abduction and adduction of the fingers, but this is not present when the hand is kept flat on a table and the fingers are extended.

Proceed as follows:

- Test the brachoradialis, looking for weakened elbow flexion. When the patient attempts to flex the elbow against resistance, the brachioradialis no longer springs up.
- Test the triceps.
- Check sensation over the first dorsal interosseous.

Note.
1. The radial nerve gives off two branches at the elbow:
   - Superficial radial (entirely sensory).
   - Posterior interosseous (entirely muscular).
2. If the injury is situated above the junction of the upper and middle thirds of the humerus, the action of triceps is lost.
3. If the lesion is situated in the middle third of the humerus (frequent site of fracture of the humerus), the brachioradialis is spared.

Diagnosis

This patient has features of radial nerve palsy with the brachioradialis remaining unaffected (lesion) resulting from a fracture located in the middle third of the humerus (aetiology); she is disabled by the deficits (functional status).

Advanced-level Questions

What is the cutaneous supply of the radial nerve?

Due to overlap in the areas supplied by the median and ulnar nerves, only a small area of skin over the first dorsal interosseous is exclusively supplied by the radial nerve.

What are the causes of radial nerve palsy?

- An intoxicated person sleeping with the head resting in the upper arm, causing compression of the nerve over the middle third of the humerus; this is known as Saturday night palsy.

- Trauma to the nerve while it courses through the axilla, e.g. crutch palsy, shoulder dislocation, fractures of humerus or radius.
- Lead neuropathy.

What do you know about the origin of the radial nerve?

The radial nerve is the termination of the posterior cord of the brachial plexus and is derived from the fifth, sixth, seventh and eighth cervical spinal nerves.

What muscles are supplied by the radial nerve?

The radial nerve supplies the triceps, anconeus, brachioradialis, extensor carpi radialis longus and, through the posterior interosseous nerve, extensor carpi radialis brevis, supinator, extensor digitorum, extensor digiti minimi, extensor ulnaris, the three extensors of the thumb and extensor indicis.

CASE 78 Chorea

Instruction

Patient 1: Sydenham's chorea
Look at this patient.

Salient features

- Irregular, jerking, ill-sustained, unpredictable, quasipurposive movements of the upper limbs.
- The patient is clumsy and keeps dropping objects. Patients with mild disease may show increased fidgeting or restlessness.

Proceed as follows:

- Check the grip of the hands – ask the patient to squeeze your fingers. A squeezing and relaxing motion occurs which has been described as a 'milkmaid's grip'.
- Look at the tongue for any involuntary movements – known as 'jack-in-the box' tongue or 'bag of worms'.
- Test deep tendon reflexes ('pendular' or 'hung-up' reflexes).
- Tell the examiner that you would like to make the following enquiries:
    Ask about sore throats if the patient is an adolescent, particularly if female; suspect Syndenham's chorea (St Vitus' dance) in rheumatic fever.

Take a family history (especially in the middle-aged adult) for Huntington's disease.

Assess mental status (to exclude premature dementia seen in Huntington's disease).

Take a history of oral contraceptive use in a young woman.

Diagnosis

This young patient has Sydenham's chorea (lesion) secondary to streptococcal sore throat (aetiology); this condition is usually self-limiting.

Advanced-level Questions

Mention a few more causes of chorea.

- SLE.
- Polycythaemia vera.
- Chorea gravidorum, seen in pregnancy.
- Idiopathic hypoparathyroidism.
- Following a stroke.
- Kernicterus.

What is the prognosis of patients with Sydenham's chorea?

Most patients recover within 1 month; a few may have relapses. A small proportion may develop valvular heart disease and hence should receive penicillin prophylaxis to prevent recurrence of rheumatic fever.

Is there any haematological disorder associated with chorea?

- Polycythaemia vera.
- Neuroacanthocytosis or 'chorea–acanthocystosis' where more than 15% of the red blood cells are acanthocytes.

Thomas Sydenham (1624–1689) was a Puritan from Dorset, and in 1666 published his first work on fevers which he dedicated to Robert Boyle.

Chorea in Greek means dance.

Reference

Hardie RJ, Pullon HWH, Harding AE et al (1991) Neuroacanthocytes: a clinical, haematological and pathological study of 19 cases. *Brain* **114**: 13.

Instruction

Patient 2: Huntington's disease
Look at this patient and ask him a few questions.

Salient features

- Young adult (aged 30–50 years).
- Chorea.
- Patient has dementia.

Proceed as follows:

- Tell the examiner that you would like to take a family history of dementia and chorea.

Diagnosis

This patient has chorea (lesion) due to Huntington's disease, and is severely limited by the disease and chorea.

Advanced-level Questions

What do you know about Huntington's disease?

It is an autosomal dominant disorder with a full penetrance characterized by progressive chorea and dementia in middle life. The defect is on the small arm of chromosome 4. There is associated random repetition of a sequence of trinucleotides (viz. CAG; normal chromosomes contain about 11–34 copies of this repeat). In Huntington's disease, the greater the number of CAG repeats, the earlier the onset of disease. The protein product for the gene has been termed huntingtin.

There is a marked reduction in acetylcholine, substance P and γ-aminobutyric acid (GABA) activity in corpus striatum, whereas dopamine activity is normal and somatostatin is increased.

Using neuropeptide immunochemistry, the chorea has been shown to be associated with damage to the lateral globus pallidus, whereas the parkinsonian signs are due to additional damage in projections of the medial globus pallidus.

What is the advantage of assessing CAG expansion in persons at risk for Huntington's disease?

It is a direct test allowing more accurate assessment of genetic risk, without the need to obtain DNA from family members. This also allows privacy and confidentiality to be maintained because of the reduced need for blood samples from relatives. However, since the misdiagnosis of other illnesses as Huntington's disease may occur, the testing of DNA from at least one affected relative is recommended to confirm that CAG expansion is present in other affected persons in the family. This finding will allow the correct interpretation of a normal number of CAG repeats in a person at risk.

Are any other diseases known to be associated with increased numbers of triplet repeats?

Yes, these include myotonic muscular dystrophy, spinocerebellar ataxia type 1, FRAXE mental retardation (a variant of fragile X syndrome) and hereditary dentatorubral pallidoluysian atrophy (DRPLA).

George Summer Huntington (1851–1916) first documented (in 1909) the clinical and hereditary features of this condition in a family from Suffolk settled in Long Island in New York.

References

Albin RL, Reiner A, Anderson KD et al (1990) Striatal and nigral neuron subpopulations in rigid Huntington's disease: implications for the functional anatomy of chorea and rigidity-kinesia. *Ann Neurol* **27**: 357.

Huntington's Disease Collaborative Research Group (1993) A novel gene containing a trinucleotide repeat that is expanded and unstable on Huntington's disease chromosomes. *Cell* **72**: 971.

CASE 79 **Hemiballismus**

Instruction

Look at this patient.

Salient features

● Unilateral, involuntary, flinging movements of the proximal upper limbs.

Diagnosis

This patient has hemiballismus (lesion) due to a stroke (aetiology), and has severe exhaustion (functional status).

Advanced-level Questions

Where is the lesion?

Ipsilateral subthalamic nucleus of Luys.

What is the underlying cause?

- Vascular event, usually an infarct.
- Rarely tumour, abscess, multiple sclerosis, arteriovenous malformation, cerebral trauma.

What investigations would you do?

- ECG for atrial fibrillation.
- CT scan, but this is usually unhelpful because the lesion is small.

What is the prognosis?

The prognosis for recovery is usually good and most patients recover within 1 month. Hemiballismus may occasionally prevent the patient from eating and can be exhausting or even life threatening.

Which drug is usually used in ameliorating this condition?

Tetrabenazine or haloperidol is usually effective. Prolonged and medically intractable hemiballism can be treated with contralateral thalamotomy or pallidectomy.

JB Luys (1828–1897), a French neurologist who also studied insanity, hysteria and hypnotism.

 CASE 80 Orofacial Dyskinesia

Instruction

Look at this patient.

Salient features

- Smacking, chewing or chomping movement of the lips seen particularly in elderly patients; it usually involves the masticatory, lower facial and tongue muscles.

Proceed as follows:

- Comment if the patient is edentulous.
- Tell the examiner that you would like to take a drug history, in particular for phenothiazines, L-dopa and related drugs.

Diagnosis

This patient has orofacial dyskinesia (lesion) due to phenothiazines (aetiology) and is in considerable distress (functional status).

Advanced-level Questions

What is Meige's syndrome?

A combination of blepharospasm, oromandibular dystonia and cranial dystonia. There is spastic dysarthria when the throat and respiratory muscles are affected. The neck muscles are invariably involved.

What do you understand by tardive dyskinesia?

It is a drug-induced dyskinesia which may appear long after drug therapy has been discontinued. It is troublesome and may resist all forms of treatment.

How would you manage such patients?

Anticholinergic drugs, baclofen, benzodiazepines and tetrabenazine, but pharmacotherapy is usually ineffective. Injection of botulinum toxin into the masseter, temporalis and internal pterygoid muscles results in improvement in chewing and speech in approximately 80% of patients with jaw closure due to oromandibular dystonia.

Mention a few other dystonias.

Blepharospasm, spasmodic torticollis, laryngeal dystonias, writer's cramp.

H Meige (1866–1940), a French physician, also wrote on ancient Egyptian diseases.

References

Koller WC (1983) Edentulous orodyskinesia. *Ann Neurol* **13**: 97.
Scott AB, Kennedy EG & Stubbs HA (1987) Use of botulinum toxin in the treatment of 100 patients with facial dyskinesias. *Ophthalmology* **2**: 237–254.

CASE 81 Internuclear Ophthalmoplegia

Instruction

Examine this patient's eyes.

Salient features

- Nystagmus is more prominent in the abducting eye (Harris' sign).
- Diverging squint.
- Abduction in either eye is normal, whereas adduction is impaired, i.e. there is dissociation of eye movements. On covering the abducting eye, the adduction in the other eye is normal.

Proceed as follows:

- Tell the examiner that you would like to look for other signs of demyelination: optic atrophy, pale discs, pyramidal signs.

Diagnosis

This patient has internuclear ophthalmoplegia (lesion) which is probably due to multiple sclerosis (aetiology).

Advanced-level Questions

Where is the lesion?

In the medial longitudinal bundle which connects the sixth nerve nucleus on one side to the third nerve nucleus on the opposite side of the brainstem. The eye will not adduct because the third nerve and, therefore, the medial rectus have been disconnected from the lateral gaze centre and sixth nucleus of the opposite side.

What are the causes?

- Multiple sclerosis.
- Vascular disease.
- Tumour (pontine glioma).
- Inflammatory lesions of the brainstem.

How would you investigate?

- MRI scan.
- Edrophonium (Tensilon) test to exclude myasthenia.

What are the mechanisms to elicit conjugate gaze?

There are four mechanisms for eliciting conjugate gaze in any direction:

1. The saccadic system involves voluntary gaze (even when the eyes are shut). Pathways mediating saccadic gaze arise in the frontal lobe and pass to the pontine gaze centre.
2. The pursuit system allows the subject to follow a moving object. Pathways mediating pursuit movements arise in the parieto-occipital lobe and pass to the pontine gaze centre.
3. The optokinetic system involves the restoration of gaze despite movements from the outside world, e.g. while a subject is sitting in a railway train and looking out of the window, the eyes move slowly as the train moves, to be followed by rapid corrective movement back to the initial position of gaze. This is tested with a hand-held drum bearing vertical black and white stripes. Optokinetic nystagmus is often disturbed even before damage to the pursuit system is apparent.
4. The vestibulo-ocular system involves correction of gaze for movements of the head. This is achieved by inputs from the labyrinths and neck proprioreceptors to the brainstem. The patient is asked to fixate to the examiner's face and the head is briskly rotated by the examiner from side to side or up and own (doll's head manoeuvre). In supranuclear gaze palsy, these vestibulo-ocular reflex eye movements are preserved, despite the absence of both saccadic and pursuit movements. Caloric tests are used to demonstrate the vestibulo-ocular reflex.

Note.
1. Diplopia is not a feature of defects in conjugate gaze.
2. The centres for saccadic and pursuit movements in the cerebral hemispheres control deviation of the eyes towards the opposite side of the body. These pathways descend towards the brainstem and cross before they reach the pons.
3. The centres for conjugate vertical gaze lie in the midbrain.
4. The centres for conjugate downward vertical gaze are not well localized and lesions both in the midbrain and at the level of the foramen magnum can cause defects of voluntary downgaze.

What do you know about 'Fisher's one and a half syndrome'?

It is a syndrome in which horizontal eye movement is absent and the other eye is capable only of abduction – one and half movements are paralysed.

The vertical eye movements and the pupils are normal. The cause is a lesion in the pontine region involving the medial longitudinal fasciculus and the parapontine reticular formation on the same side. This results in failure of conjugate gaze to the same side, impairment of adduction of the eye, and nystagmus on abduction of the other eye.

Internuclear ophthalmoplegia was first reported by Bielschowsky (1902) and then subsequently by Lhermitte in 1922. Spiller in 1924 described the necropsy findings, implicated the median longitudinal fasciculus and suggested the name 'ophthalmoplegia internuclearis anterior'.

CASE 82 Cerebellopontine Angle Tumour

Instruction

Examine this patient's cranial nerves.

Salient features

- Damage to the seventh and eighth cranial nerves is the hallmark of this lesion in this region.

Proceed as follows:

- Check the corneal reflex and test the trigeminal nerve (see page 98).
- Tell the examiner that you would like to look for the following:
    Cerebellar signs (see page 136).
    Signs of neurofibroma type 2 (see page 200).
    Papilloedema (seen uncommonly as a result of raised intracranial pressure).

Diagnosis

This patient has features of cerebellopontine angle tumour (lesion) usually due to an acoustic neuroma (aetiology), and has severe hearing loss (functional status).

Advanced-level Questions

Mention a few causes of cerebellopontine angle lesions.

- Acoustic neuroma.
- Meningioma, cholesteatoma, haemangioblastoma, aneurysm of the basilar artery.

- Pontine glioma.
- Medullablastoma and astrocytoma of the cerebellum.
- Carcinoma of the nasopharynx.
- Local meningeal involvement by syphilis and tuberculosis.

What do you understand by the term 'cerebellopontine angle'?

It is the shallow triangular fossa lying between the cerebellum, lateral pons and the inner third of the petrous temporal bone. It extends from the trigeminal nerve (above) to the glossopharyngeal nerve (below). The abducens nerve runs along the medial edge, whereas the facial and auditory cranial nerves transverse the angle to enter the internal auditory meatus.

What is the histology of acoustic neurofibroma?

It consists of elongated cells similar to spindle fibroblasts with much collagen and reticulum. They are believed to arise from Schwann cells and are also known as schwannomas.

How would you investigate such patients?

- Skull radiography, tomography of the internal auditory meatus, and CT head scan.
- Serology for syphilis.
- Audiography.
- Caloric test (which will reveal that the labyrinth is destroyed).
- Vertebral angiography.
- CSF may be abnormal or have raised protein concentration.

FT Schwann (1810–1882), a German anatomist, was Professor of Anatomy in the Louvain. He was one of the first to demonstrate that fermentation was associated with living organisms. Independently from Schleiden, he concluded that plants are formed of cells; this is known as the Schleiden–Schwann cellular theory. Schwann also discovered that the upper oesophagus contains striated muscle. He discovered pepsin and showed that bile was essential for digestion.

CASE 83 Jugular Foramen Syndrome

Instruction

Examine this patient's cranial nerves.

Salient features

- Sluggish movement of the palate when the patient says 'aah' on the affected side.
- Absent gag reflex on the same side.
- Flattening of the shoulder on the same side.
- Wasting of the sternomastoid.
- Weakness when the patient moves her chin to the opposite side.
- Difficulty in shrugging the shoulder on the same side.

Proceed as follows:

- Look for wasting and deviation of the tongue (12th cranial nerve palsy).
- Tell the examiner that you would like to check for two signs:
  Bovine cough.
  Husky voice.

Diagnosis

This patient has features of jugular foramen syndrome (lesion) which could be due to several causes including pharyngeal neoplasm (aetiology); she has difficulty in swallowing and requires a nasogastric tube (functional status).

Advanced-level Questions

Where is the jugular foramen located?

Between the lateral part of the occipital bone and the petrous portion of the temporal bones.

Which cranial nerves leave the skull through the jugular foramen?

The 9th, 10th and 11th cranial nerves.

Through which foramen does the 12th cranial nerve leave the skull?

The anterior condylar foramen.

Mention a few causes of jugular foramen syndrome.

- Carcinoma of the pharynx is the commonest cause.
- Fractured base of the skull.
- Paget's disease.
- Basal meningitis.
- Neurofibroma or any tumour.
- Thrombosis of jugular vein.

Do you know of any eponymous syndromes of the lower cranial nerves?

- Vernet's syndrome: paresis of the 9th, 10th and 11th cranial nerves due to extension of tumour into the jugular foramen.
- Collet–Sicard syndrome: fracture of the floor of the posterior cranial fossa, causing palsy of the last four cranial nerves.
- Villaret's syndrome: ipsilateral paralysis of the last four cranial nerves and cervical sympathetics.
- Syndrome of Schmidt: vagus and accessory nerve involvement.
- Syndrome of Hughlings Jackson: accessory and hypoglossal nerve involvement.

What is the cause of the unilateral 11th cranial nerve palsy?

- Trauma to the nerve in the neck.
- In hemiplegia.

How would you test for 11th cranial nerve palsy?

- Sternocleidomastoids are tested by having the patient turn her head forcibly against the examiner's hand in a direction away from the muscle being tested while the muscle is observed and palpated.
- Upper portion of the trapezii is tested by having the patient forcibly elevate (shrug) her shoulder while the examiner attempts to depress the shoulder.

M Vernet (b. 1887), a French neurologist, described this syndrome in 1916.
M Villaret (1877–1946), Professor of Neurology in France, described this syndrome in 1918.
FJ Collet (b. 1870), a French otolaryngologist, described his patient in 1915.
JA Sicard (1872–1929), a French physician and radiologist, was the first to perform myelography, use alcohol in trigeminal neuralgia and inject a sclerosing substance in varicose veins. He described his patient in 1917.

Reference

Davis JN, Thomas PK, Spalding JMK et al (1975). Disease of the ninth, tenth, and eleventh cranial nerves. In: Dyck PJ, Thomas PK & Lambert EH (eds) *Peripheral Neuropathy*, vol. 1, pp. 614–627. Philadelphia: WB Saunders.

CASE 84 Pseudobulbar Palsy

Instruction

Examine this patient's cranial nerves.

Salient features

- Spastic tongue.
- Donald Duck speech.
- Patient is emotionally labile.
- Sluggish movements of the palate when the patient is asked to say 'aah'.

Proceed as follows:

- Check the jaw jerk.
- Tell the examiner that you would like to do the following:
  Ask the patient whether he has difficulty in swallowing or nasal regurgitation.
  Check the gag reflex.
  Look for upper motor neuron signs in the limbs.

Diagnosis

This patient has pseudobulbar palsy (lesion) due to a stroke (aetiology); he has difficulty in swallowing and emotional lability (functional status).

Questions

What could be the underlying cause?

- Bilateral stroke.
- Multiple sclerosis.
- Motor neuron disease.

Advanced-level Questions

How would you differentiate bulbar palsy from pseudobulbar palsy?

	Pseudobulbar palsy	Bulbar palsy
Prevalence	Common	Rare
Type of lesion	Upper motor neuron	Lower motor neuron, muscular
Site of lesion	Bilateral, usually in the internal capsule	Medulla oblongata
Tongue	Small, stiff and spastic	Flaccid, fasciculations
Speech	Slow, thick and indistinct	Nasal twang
Nasal regurgitation	Not prominent	Prominent
Jaw jerk	Brisk	Normal or absent
Other findings	Upper motor neuron lesions of the limbs	Lower motor neuron lesions of the limbs
Effect	Emotionally labile	Normal effect
Causes	Stroke, multiple sclerosis, motor neuron disease, Creutzfeld–Jakob disease	Motor neuron disease, poliomyelitis, Guillain-Barré syndrome, myasthenia gravis myopathy

How would you manage the swallowing and speech difficulties?

The patient would initially require assessment by a speech therapist for the difficulty in swallowing and speech deficits. Barium swallow with videofluoroscopy may be required to 'visualize' the swallowing.

CASE 85 Bulbar Palsy

Instruction

Examine this patient's cranial nerves.
Ask the patient a few questions.
Test this patient's speech.

Salient features

- Nasal speech lacking in modulation, and great difficulty with all consonants.
- Wasting of the tongue with fasciculations.
- Weakness of the soft palate: ask the patient to say 'aah'.
- There may be accumulation of the saliva.

Proceed as follows:

- Check the jaw jerk (normal or absent).
- Tell the examiner that you would like to do the following:
  Ask the patient about nasal regurgitation, dysphagia.
  Check gag reflex.
  Examine the hands for fasciculations, dissociated sensory loss.

Diagnosis

This patient has bulbar palsy (lesion) due to motor neuron disease (aetiology) and has difficulty in swallowing (functional status).

Questions

What may be the underlying cause?

- Motor neuron disease (see page 195).
- Guillain–Barré syndrome.
- Syringomyelia (see page 203).
- Poliomyelitis.
- Nasopharyngeal tumour.
- Neurosyphilis.
- Neurosarcoid.

CASE 86 — Wallenberg's Syndrome (Lateral Medullary Syndrome)

Instruction

Examine this patient's cranial nerves.

Salient features

- Nystagmus.
- Ipsilateral involvement of fifth, sixth, seventh and eighth cranial nerves.
- Bulbar palsy: impaired gag, sluggish palatal movements.
- Horner's syndrome.

Proceed as follows:

- Tell the examiner that you would like to check for the following:
  Cerebellar signs on the same side.
  Pain and temperature sensory loss on the opposite side (dissociated sensory loss).

Diagnosis

This patient has lateral medullary syndrome (lesion) due to a stroke (aetiology) and has dysphagia (functional status).

Advanced-level Questions

Which vessel is occluded?

Any of the following five vessels:
    Posterior inferior cerebellar artery.
    Vertebral artery.
    Superior, middle or inferior lateral medullary arteries.

How may these patients present?

With sudden onset of vertigo, vomiting and ipsilateral ataxia, with contralateral loss of pain and temperature sensations.

Where is the lesion in lateral medullary syndrome?

It results from infarction of a wedge-shaped area of the lateral aspect of the medulla and inferior surface of the cerebellum. The deficits are due to involvement of one side of the nucleus ambiguus, trigeminal nucleus, vestibular nuclei, cerebellar peduncle, spinothalamic tract and autonomic fibres.

What is the medial medullary syndrome?

It is caused by occlusion of the lower basilar artery or vertebral artery. Ipsilateral lesions result in paralysis and wasting of the tongue. Contralateral lesions result in hemiplegia and loss of vibration and joint position sense.

Mention a few other eponymous syndromes with crossed hemiplegias.

- Weber's syndrome: contralateral hemiplegia with ipsilateral lower motor neuron lesion of the oculomotor nerve. The lesion is in the midbrain.
- Millard–Gubler syndrome: contralateral hemiplegia with lower motor neuron lesion of the abducens nerve. The lesion is in the pons.
- Foville's syndrome: as Millard–Gubler syndrome with gaze palsy.

What is Benedikt's syndrome?

It causes cerebellar signs on the side opposite the third nerve palsy (which is produced by damage to the nucleus itself or to the nerve fascicle). It is due to a midbrain vascular lesion causing damage to the red nucleus, interrupting the dentatorubrothalamic tract from the opposite cerebellar signs.

Auguste LJ Millard (1830–1915) and Adolphe Marie Gubler (1821–1879), Parisian physicians.
Achille LF Foville (1799–1878), a Parisian neurologist.
A Wallenburg (1862–1949), a German neurologist, described this syndrome in 1895.

CASE 87 Winging of the Scapula

Instruction

Look at this patient's back.

Salient features

- Winging of the scapula.
- Difficulty in raising the arms above the horizontal.

Proceed as follows:

- Check whether the winging is unilateral or bilateral.
- Ask the patient to push the outstretched arm firmly against your hand and check whether or not the winging is more prominent.
- Tell the examiner that you would like to examine the muscles in the arm to rule out muscular dystrophy.

Diagnosis

This patient has winging of the scapula (lesion) due to palsy of the long thoracic nerve of Bell (aetiology).

Advanced-level Questions

Which nerve lesion is responsible for these signs?

Long thoracic nerve of Bell arising from the anterior rami of C5, C6 and C7.

Which muscle is supplied by this nerve?

Serratus anterior.

What is the action of the serratus anterior?

It is responsible for the lateral and forward movement of the scapula, keeping it closely applied to the thorax.

Which other muscle palsy can cause winging of the scapula?

Paralysis of the trapezius.

How would you differentiate winging of the scapula caused by serratus anterior palsy from that of trapezius palsy?

In serratus anterior palsy, abduction of the arm laterally produces little winging of the scapula, whereas winging due to weakness of the trapezius is intensified by abduction of the arm against resistance.

What do you know about brachial neuritis?

Brachial neuritis (neuralgic amyotrophy, Parsonage–Turner syndrome) often follows an infection or surgery. Diagnosis may be difficult initially when the patients have only pain. Later the patients have muscular weakness, affecting particularly the deltoid and serratus anterior (winging of the scapula). Atrophy often becomes prominent. In this syndrome there is often more than one lesion. The white cell count in the cerebrospinal fluid is occasionally raised. Recovery occurs over the next year and may not be complete.

CASE 88 Becker Muscular Dystrophy

Instruction

Examine this patient's muscles.

Salient features

- Young adult male (> 15 years).
- Proximal weakness of the lower extremities (in later stages more generalized muscle involvement).

- Pseudohypertrophy of calves.
- Facial muscle weakness is characteristically absent or insignificant.
- Kyphoscoliosis in late stages.

Proceed as follows:

- Tell the examiner that you would like to:
    Check the IQ (mental retardation may be seen).
    Ask about shortness of breath (heart failure due to cardiomyopathy).
    Know whether there is a family history of the condition.

Diagnosis

This young patient has proximal muscle weakness and pseudohypertrophy (lesion) due to Becker's dystrophy (aetiology). The patient has mild disability and the condition is usually progressive (functional status).

Questions

What is the difference between Duchenne and Becker muscular dystrophy?

By definition, patients with Becker muscular dystrophy can ambulate beyond the age of 15 years. The onset in Becker is usually between the ages of 5 and 15 years, but onset can occur in the third or fourth decades or even later. The majority survive into the fourth or fifth decades.

Is there any difference between the genetics of Duchenne and Becker muscular dystrophy?

No, both Duchenne and Becker muscular dystrophy are caused by mutations in the same dystrophin gene, located at Xp21. Another protein, utrophin, closely related to dystrophin, is encoded by a second gene on chromosome 6. In normal muscle utrophin is located predominantly in the neuromuscular junction, whereas dystrophin is found in the sarcolemmal surface.

How would you confirm the clinical diagnosis of Becker dystrophy?

It requires Western blot analysis of muscle biopsy samples, demonstrating abnormal or reduced dystrophin.

Advanced-level Questions

Mention other X-linked myopathies?

- X-linked tubular myopathy linked to Xq28.
- McLeod syndrome where the responsible gene has been localized to Xp21 and the phenotype is characterized by mild, even subclinical, myopathy, acanthocytosis and haemolytic anaemia. The definitive diagnosis rests on determination of the Kell red cell antigen phenotype.
- Emery-Dreifuss muscular dystrophy, first described in a large family in Virginia by Emery and Dreifuss in 1966. Known association with deutan colour blindness led to localization of the gene on Xq28. The weakness presents in early childhood and is slowly progressive. The distribution of weakness is unique: an early humeral–peroneal pattern eventually evolves into a scapulo-humero-pelvo-peroneal distribution. Marked focal atrophy of the humeral and peroneal muscles is a consistent feature. Pseudohypertrophy is absent, except in extensor digitorum brevis.

PE Becker, Professor of Human Genetics at the University of Göttingen, Germany.
Edward Meryon described Duchenne muscular dystrophy in 1852, 10 years before the French neurologist Guillaume Benjamin Amand Duchenne, with remarkably prescient pathological observations: '. . . the sarcolemma or tunic of the elementary fibre was broken and destroyed'.
Duchenne is reported to have designed a version of the modern muscle biopsy needle which he kept in alcohol to prevent rusting. He could not have known that this also prevented sepsis.
Newton Morton, a geneticist, was the first to introduce discriminant and segregation analysis into modern human genetics as a part of a large population study of Duchenne muscular dystrophy. Tony Murphy used the disease to develop bayesian risk-analysis procedures.

Reference

Emery AEH & Emery MLH (1995) *The History of a Genetic Disease: Duchenne Muscular Dystrophy or Meryon's Disease*. London: Royal Society of Medicine.

CASE 89 Tetraplegia

Instruction

Carry out a neurological examination of this patient's lower limbs.

Salient features

- Increased or decreased tone in both lower limbs.

- Hyper-reflexia.
- Ankle clonus.
- Weakness in all four limbs.
- Wasted hands (cervical spondylosis, motor neuron disease or syringomyelia).

Proceed as follows:

- Remember to check the sensory level and examine the spine.
- Tell the examiner that you would like to do the following:
  Ask about bladder symptoms and check sacral sensation.
  Ask about radicular pain.
  Ask whether the weakness was sudden or gradual.
  Check for cerebellar signs (multiple sclerosis, Friedreich's ataxia).
  Check blood pressure (postural hypotension, autonomic dysreflexia)
- Try to localize the level of lesion using the following:
  Spasticity of all four limbs: lesion above the C4 spinal cord segment.
  Spasticity of the lower limbs with flaccid weakness of some muscles of the upper limb: lesion of cervical cord enlargement (C5–T2).
  Deep tendon reflexes – an absent biceps jerk with a brisk supinator jerk (inversion of the supinator jerk) or an absent biceps and supinator with a brisk triceps jerk localizes the lesion to C5–6.
  Radicular pain – useful early in the disease; with time becomes diffuse and ceases to have localizing value.
  Superficial sensation – not good for localizing as the level of sensory loss may vary greatly in different individuals and in different types of lesion.

Diagnosis

This patient has weakness in all four limbs (lesion) due to spinal trauma (aetiology), and is wheelchair bound (functional status).

Advanced-level Questions

What is autonomic dysreflexia?

It is bradycardia, sweating, rhinorrhoea, pounding headaches and severe paroxysmal hypertension which presents quickly and can rapidly precipitate seizures and death if not relieved. Precipitating factors include blockage of urinary catheter, visceral distension from full bowel, stimulation of the skin secondary to an irritative pressure sore and vesicoureteric reflux. Labour in a high-tetraplegic female may also be complicated by it.

Does ingestion of food affect blood pressure in tetraplegics?

The ingestion of food causes a small fall in blood pressure and this exacerbates the postural hypotension in these patients.

How would you manage spasticity in these patients?

- Drugs: diazepam, baclofen.
- Surgery: dorsal rhizotomy, neurectomy, myelotomy, orthopaedic procedures that divide and lengthen tendons of spastic muscles.

How do you localize the lesion to the fifth cervical root level?

- Muscular weakness: deltoid, supraspinatus, brachoradialis.
- Deep tendon reflexes affected: biceps and supinator jerks.
- Radicular pain/paraesthesia: neck, top of shoulder, outer aspect of the arm, forearm.
- Superficial sensory deficit: outer aspect of the upper arm.

How do you localize the lesion to the sixth cervical root level?

- Muscular weakness: biceps, brachioradialis, extensor carpi radialis longus.
- Deep tendon reflexes affected: biceps and supinator jerks.
- Radicular pain/paraesthesia: neck, shoulder, outer arm, forearm, thumb and index finger.
- Superficial sensory deficit: thumb and index finger.

How do you localize the lesion to the seventh cervical root level?

- Muscular weakness: triceps and most of the muscles on the dorsum of the forearm.
- Deep tendon reflexes affected: triceps jerk.
- Radicular pain/paraesthesia: neck, shoulder, arm, forearm to index and middle finger.
- Superficial sensory deficit: mostly middle and index fingers.

How do you localize the lesion to the eighth cervical root level?

- Muscular weakness: flexors of the forearm.
- Deep tendon reflexes affected: finger jerk.
- Radicular pain/paraesthesia: neck, shoulder, arm, ring and little fingers.
- Superficial sensory deficit: ring and little fingers.

How do you localize the lesion to the first thoracic root level?

- Muscular weakness: small muscles of the hand.
- Deep tendon reflexes affected: finger jerk.
- Radicular pain/paraesthesia: neck, axilla, medial aspect of the arm and forearm, little and ring finger.
- Superficial sensory deficit: medial arm and little finger.

What precautions would you take when transporting patients with acute high spinal injuries by air?

- Lung function should be stable before transfer.
- Air humidifier and supplemental oxygen should be available.
- Patient should be accompanied by someone trained in manoeuvres to clear airway secretions. Tracheal suction should be done regularly; this may be complicated by reflex bradycardia and cardiac arrest, and so atropine and orciprenaline should be readily available.

What is the mode of onset in patients with the classical syndrome of foramen magnum?

First, there is weakness of the shoulder and arm, followed by weakness of the ipsilateral leg, then contralateral leg and, finally, contralateral arm. Neoplasms in this region can cause suboccipital pain spreading to the neck and shoulders.

What is Raymond-Cestan syndrome?

Raymond–Cestan syndrome is due to the obstruction of twigs of the basilar artery causing lesions of the pontine region; it is characterized by tetraplegia, nystagmus and anaesthesia.

Sir Ludwig Guttman, FRS, fled from Nazi persecution and worked at the National Spinal Injuries Centre in Stoke Mandeville Hospital, Aylesbury. He was entrusted to look after the paraplegics and tetraplegics of the war. He was the first to show that pressure sores can be avoided by 2-hourly turning of patients.

Hans L Frankel, OBE, contemporary Physician, National Hospital of Spinal Injuries, Stoke Mandeville Hospital, Aylesbury.

References

Armitage JM, Pyne A, Williams SJ & Frankel H (1990) Respiratory problems of air travel in patients with spinal cord injuries. *Br Med J* **300**: 1498.

Baliga RR, Catz AB, Short DJ, Frankel HL & Mathias CJ (1993) Postprandial cardiovascular haemodynamics in tetraplegics and paraplegics. *J Am Coll Cardiol* **21**: 259A.

Geisler FH, Dorsey FC & Coleman WP (1991) Recovery of motor function after spinal-cord injury – a randomised, placebo-controlled trial with GM-1 ganglioside. *N Engl J Med* **324**: 1829–1838.

CASE 90 Brown-Séquard Syndrome

Instruction

Examine this patient's neurological system.

Salient features

Deficits below the level of the lesion include:
- Ipsilateral monoplegia or hemiplegia.
- Ipsilateral loss of joint position and vibration sense.
- Contralateral loss of spinothalamic (pain and temperature) sensation. The latter is sometimes localized to one or two segments below the anatomical level of the lesion.

Deficits in the segment of the lesion:
- Ipsilateral lower motor neuron paralysis.
- Ipsilateral zone of cutaneous anaesthesia and a zone hyperaesthesia just below the anaesthetic zone.
- Segmental signs such as muscular atrophy, radicular pain or decreased tendon reflexes are usually unilateral.

Proceed as follows:

- Tell the examiner that you would like to take a history for bladder and bowel symptoms.

Diagnosis

This patient has Brown-Séquard syndrome (or hemisection of the spinal cord) at the level of T8 (lesion) and is probably due to a compressive or destructive lesion of the spinal cord (aetiology). The patient is limited by the weakness in one limb (functional status).

Advanced-level Questions

What are the causes of hemisection of the spinal cord?

- Syringomyelia (see page 203).
- Cord tumour.

- Haematomyelia.
- Bullet or stab wounds.

CE Brown-Séquard (1817–1884) was Professor of Physiology in Virginia, USA, at the National Hospital, Queen Square, London, at Harvard, and finally in Paris. He was the first physician-in-chief of the National Hospital in Queen Square which was founded in 1860. In 1899 he is said to drawn much attention and criticism for injecting himself with a testicular extract. Several nations lay claim to Brown-Séquard: he was born in Mauritius, then a British colony, the son of a French woman and an American sea captain.

Reference

Aminoff MJ (1993) *Brown-Séquard: A Visionary of Science*. New York: Raven Press.

CASE 91 Cauda Equina Syndrome

Instruction

This patient has bowel and bladder dysfunction; examine the lower limbs.

Salient features

- Flaccid, asymmetrical paraparesis.
- Knee and ankle jerks are diminished or absent.
- Saddle distribution of sensory loss up to the L1 level.
- Plantars downgoing.

Proceed as follows:

- Ask the patient whether there is pain (usually projected to the perineum and thighs).
- Determine whether there is a history of trauma and 'neural claudication' (where the patient develops root pain and leg weakness, usually a foot drop while walking; this rapidly recovers by resting).

Diagnosis

This patient has flaccid paraparesis with saddle anaesthesia due to cauda equina syndrome (lesion) caused by a compressive lesion (aetiology).

Advanced-level Questions

What is the relationship of the spinal cord to the vertebra?

The spinal cord extends from the foramen magnum to the interspace between the 12th thoracic (dorsal) and first lumbar spines, although the thecal membranes may extend down the body of the second sacral vertebra. To determine the spinal segments in relation to the vertebral body: For cervical vertebrae add 1, for thoracic 1–6 add 2, for thoracic 7–9 add 3, and the lumbar segments lie opposite the 10th and 11th thoracic spines and the next interspinal space. The first lumbar arch overlies the sacral and coccygeal segments. (Remember that the sacral segments are compressed into the last inch of the cord known as the conus medullaris; the latter is located behind the ninth thoracic to the first lumbar vertebra.)

At which vertebral level is the lesion in cauda equina syndrome?

A lesion in the spinal canal at any level below the tenth thoracic (dorsal) vertebra can cause cauda equina syndrome.

How would you differentiate between cauda equina and conus medullaris syndrome?

The cauda equina consists of lower spinal roots (T12 to S5) and hence a lesion causes lower motor neuron signs, whereas the conus medullaris is the lowest part of the spinal cord and lesions result in upper motor neuron signs. Both conus and cauda lesions result in a mixed picture.

What are the causes of cauda equina syndrome?

- Centrally placed lumbosacral disc or spondylolisthesis at the lumbo-sacral junction.
- Tumours of the cauda equina (ependymoma, neurofibroma).

What are the types of cauda equina syndrome in adults?

- The lateral cauda equina syndrome: pain in the anterior thigh, wasting of the quadriceps muscle, weakness of the foot invertors (due to L4 root lesion) and an absent knee jerk. Causes include neurofibroma, a high disc lesion.
- The midline cauda equina syndrome: bilateral lumbar and sacral root lesions. Causes include disc lesion, primary sacral bone tumours (chordomas), metastatic bone disease (from prostate) and leukaemia.

CASE 92 — Torsion Dystonia (Dystonia Musculorum Deformans)

Instruction

Look at this patient.

Salient features

- Dystonic movements of head and neck.
- Torticollis.
- Blepharospasm.
- Facial grimacing.
- Forced opening or closing of the mouth.
- Limbs may adopt abnormal but characteristic postures.

Proceed as follows:

- Tell the examiner that you would like to take a history of:
    Perinatal anoxia, birth trauma or kernicterus.
    Family history.
    Drug history (neuroleptics).
    The age of onset of clinical features (abnormal movements are
        usually present before the age of 5 years in birth anoxia).

Diagnosis

This patient has torsion dystonia (lesion) which may be due to birth anoxia (aetiology), and is confined to a wheelchair because of the disability (functional status).

Questions

What do you understand by the term dystonia?

It implies a movement caused by a prolonged muscular contraction when a part of the body is thrown into spasm.

Advanced-level Questions

What is the inheritance of idiopathic torsion dystonia?

Idiopathic torsion dystonia can occur sporadically, or on a hereditary basis with autosomal dominant (where the gene is on chromosome 9q), X-linked recessive and autosomal recessive inheritance. There is normal birth and developmental history in idiopathic torsion dystonia.

What are the other causes of dystonia?

- Birth anoxia (abnormal movements develop before the age of 5 years; often associated with a history of seizures and mental disability).
- Wilson's disease, Huntington's disease or parkinsonism.
- Drugs.

How would you treat such patients?

- Drugs: patients respond poorly to drugs. Occasionally helpful medications include diazepam, levodopa, amantidine, carbamezapine, tetrabenazine, phenothiazines and haloperidol.
- Stereotactic thalamotomy may be useful in predominantly unilateral dystonia.

CASE 93 Epilepsy

Instruction

This patient is suspected to have seizures; ask her a few questions. The eye-witness (usually the spouse) of the suspected event is next to the patient and you may ask him or her any relevant questions.

Salient features

Proceed as follows:

- Ask the patient about aura, whether she bit her tongue, whether she was incontinent during the attack, any hallucinations (*déjà vu* phenomenon). Ask the patient about triggering factors (including television, disco strobes, hypoglycaemia and alcohol ingestion) and whether they are recurrent. Take a family history (about 30% of patients with epilepsy have a history of seizures in relatives), and past history of head injury.
- Confirm this by asking the eye-witness about the description of seizures (note whether they were tonic–clonic), frothing at the mouth, whether the patient was unconscious or incontinent, how long the whole 'episode' lasted and how long she was unconscious after the attack, and whether there was any weakness after the attack (Todd's paralysis).

Diagnosis

This patient has recent-onset grand mal epilepsy (lesion) which could be due to an intracranial tumour (aetiology). The patient will have to give up her job as a truck-driver as a consequence of this (functional status).

Questions

How would you investigate the patient?

- Full blood count, urea and electrolytes, blood glucose, liver function tests.
- Chest radiography.
- EEG.
- CT scan.

Mention some metabolic abnormalities found in these patients.

Hypoglycaemia, hyponatraemia (e.g. syndrome of inappropriate anti-diuretic hormone secretion (SIADH)), hypocalcaemia, hepatic failure, uraemia.

How would you classify seizures?

- Generalized seizures: grand mal (tonic–clonic) seizures, absence seizures (petit mal and atypical absences), myoclonus, akinetic seizures.
- Partial or focal seizures: simple partial seizures (no impairment of consciousness), complex partial seizures, partial seizures evolving to tonic–clonic.

Advanced-level Questions

What is jacksonian epilepsy?

It is a simple partial seizure which usually originates in one portion of the prefrontal motor cortex so that fits begin in one part of the body (e.g. thumb) and then proceed to involve that side of the body and then the whole body. It suggests a space-occupying lesion.

What is Todd's paralysis?

Paresis of a limb or hemiplegia occurring after an epileptic attack, which may last up to 3 days.

How would you manage epilepsy?

- General advice: avoid ladders, heights, unsupervised swimming and cycling for 2 years from the last episode.
- Antiepileptic drugs: phenytoin (in generalized tonic–clonic seizures), sodium valproate (petit mal or partial seizures) and carbamazepine (partial seizures).
- Advice about driving: those who have had more than one seizure are unable to hold a driving licence in the UK unless they have been free from any form of epileptic attack whilst awake for a period of 2 years before the issue of a licence or, in the case of attacks whilst asleep, these attacks must have occurred only whilst asleep and the person must have been free from an attack for at least 3 years before the issue of a licence. Drivers of heavy goods vehicles and public service vehicles are automatically barred from holding such a licence following any attack after the age of 3 years.

RB Todd (1809–1860), FRS, an Irish physician, graduated from Pembroke College, Oxford, and was Professor of Physiology at King's College, London. He was founder of King's College Hospital.
J Hughlings Jackson (1835–1911), an English neurologist, worked at the National Hospital, Queen Square, London.

CASE 94 Guillain–Barré Syndrome

Instruction

Examine this patient's lower limbs whose weakness began distally.

Salient features

- Weakness of distal limb muscles.
- Distal numbness.
- Areflexia.

Proceed as follows:

- Tell the examiner that you would like to:
    Assess respiratory function (forced vital capacity).
    Check blood pressure (for labile blood pressure).
    Ascertain whether the onset was preceded by a trivial viral illness.

Diagnosis

This patient has Guillain–Barré syndrome (lesion) and is currently experiencing weakness of the distal limb muscles (functional status).

Questions

What is the pathology?

It is a demyelinating neuropathy.

Advanced-level Questions

How is the diagnosis confirmed?

- Nerve conduction studies demonstrate slowing of conduction or conduction block.
- CSF shows albumino-cytological dissociation, i.e. a normal cell count but the protein concentration is frequently raised.

What is Miller – Fisher syndrome?

A rare proximal variant of Guillain–Barré syndrome which initially affects the ocular muscles and in which ataxia is prominent.

What is the differential diagnosis?

Poliomyelitis, botulism, primary muscle disease or other neuropathy (porphyric, diphtheric heavy metal or organophosphorous poisoning).

How would you treat such patients?

- High-dose intravenous γ-globulin during the acute phase to reduce the severity and duration of symptoms.
- Ventilatory support if respiratory muscles are affected.
- Physiotherapy and occupational therapy for muscle weakness.

C Guillain (1876–1961), Professor of Medicine in Paris.
JA Barré (1880–1967), Professor of Neurology in Strasbourg, trained in Paris.

References

Ropper AH (1992) The Guillain–Barré syndrome. *N Engl J Med* **326**: 1130.
van der Meché FGA, Schmitz PIM and the Dutch Guillain–Barré Group (1992) A randomized trial comparing intravenous immune globulin and plasma exchange in Guillain–Barré syndrome. *N Engl J Med* **326**: 1123–1129.

CASE 95 Multiple System Atrophy

Instruction

Perform a neurological examination on this patient.

Salient features

- Mask-like facies and other features of bradykinesia.
- Increased tone (rigidity).
- Cerebellar signs.

Proceed as follows:

- Ask the patient about dysphagia.
- Tell the examiner that you would like to:
    Look for postural hypotension, the hallmark of this condition (due to autonomic failure).
    Look for signs of autonomic dysfunction (pupillary asymmetry, Horner's syndrome).
    Ask about incontinence, impotence and anhidrosis.

Diagnosis

This patient has cerebellar and Parkinson's signs (lesion) due to multiple system atrophy, a degenerative disorder (aetiology), and has marked disability including incontinence (functional status).

Advanced-level Questions

What is the pathology in this condition?

In 1960, Shy and Drager described changes in the brainstem and ganglia; subsequently, loss of neurons has been shown in the autonomic nervous system and in the cells of the intermediolateral column of the spinal cord. Positron emission tomography shows decreased uptake of dopamine in the putamen and caudate lobe.

What factors can lower blood pressure in these patients?

Standing up (orthostatic hypotension, a hallmark of this condition), food- and exercise-induced hypotension. Food and exercise can produce hypotension even in the supine position.

What is the morbidity of this condition?

It is tends to disable most patients severely by the end of 5–7 years.

How would you treat these patients?

Treatment is symptomatic and supportive for hypotension and neurological deficits. Symptoms of postural hypotension may be ameliorated by antigravity stockings and fluorohydrocortisone.

GM Shy (1919–1967), a US neurologist who obtained his MRCP in London in 1947.
GA Drager (1917–1967), a US neurologist.
Bradbury and Eggleston in 1925 first described the combination of postural hypotension, incontinence, impotence and abnormality of sweating (anhidrosis). Neurological manifestations develop later.
Christopher J Mathias, FRCP, DSc, contemporary Professor of Medicine, St Mary's Hospital Medical School and National Hospital, Queen Square, London, whose chief interest is the autonomic control of the cardiovascular system.

References

Brooks DJ, Salmon EP, Mathias CJ et al (1990) The relationship between locomotor disability, autonomic dysfunction, and integrity of the striatal dopaminergic system in patients with multiple system atrophy, pure autonomic failure, and in Parkinson's disease, studied with PET. *Brain* **113**: 1539.

Baliga RR & Mathias CJ (1990) Exercise-induced hypotension in autonomic failure. *J Neurol* **237**(suppl 1): S24.

Baliga RR, Watson L & Mathias CJ (1993) Supine exercise induces profound hypotension in patients with autonomic dysfunction. *J Am Coll Cardiol* **21**: 97A.

CASE 96 Neurological Bladder

Instruction

This patient is suspected to have difficulty in micturition accompanying paraparesis. Would you like to ask him a few questions?

Salient features

Proceed as follows:

Ask the patient the following questions:
- Do you get a sensation when the bladder is full?
- Do you feel the urine passing?
- Are you able to stop urine passing in midstream at your own will?

- Does the bladder leak continually?
- Do you suddenly pass large volumes?
- Is there any difficulty in defaecation?
- Is there any numbness in the perineal region?

- Tell the examiner that in male patients you would like to take a history of impotence and examine the neurological system and spine.

Diagnosis

This patient has a spastic bladder (lesion) accompanying his paraparesis which occurred as a result of trauma (aetiology) and requires an indwelling urinary catheter (functional status).

Advanced-level Questions

What are the types of neurogenic bladder?

- Spinal or spastic bladder: the bladder is small and spastic and holds less than 250 ml. It is seen in lesions of the spinal cord secondary to trauma, multiple sclerosis, and spinal cord tumour (upper motor neuron lesion). Bladder fullness is not appreciated and the bladder tends to empty reflexly and suddenly – the automatic bladder. Evacuation may be incomplete unless it is massaged by pressure in the suprapubic region.
- The autonomous bladder: this results from damage to the cauda equina, i.e. lower motor neuron lesion (see page 246). The patient is incontinent with continual dribbling and there is no sensation of bladder fullness. Despite the dribbling there is considerable residual urine. There is loss of perineal sensation and sexual dysfunction. (In conus medullaris–cauda equina lesions, it is possible to have a flaccid lower motor neuron detrusor, with a spastic sphincter. The reverse may also occur.)
- The sensory bladder: similar to autonomous bladder and seen in tabes dorsalis, subacute combined degeneration of the cord and multiple sclerosis. There is loss of awareness of bladder fullness with a loss of spinal reflex. This results in retention of large quantities of urine, incontinence with dribbling, high volume of residual urine which can be voided by considerable straining.
- The uninhibited bladder: occurs to lesions affecting the second gyrus of the frontal lobe, e.g. frontal lobe tumours, parasagittal meningiomas, aneurysms of the anterior communicating arteries and dementia. Patient has urgency despite low bladder volumes and has sudden uncontrolled evacuation. There is no residual urine. When there is deterioration of the intellect, the patient may pass urine at any time without concern.

What do you know about the neurological control of the bladder?

- Micturition follows activation of the parasympathetic pathways to the detrusor muscle and inhibition of the somatic input to the external urethral sphincter. The parasympathetic reflex is based in the S3 roots and S3 segments of the cord.
- The sympathetic system promotes urinary storage by increasing urethral resistance and depressing detrusor contractions. The sympathetic supply descends into the pelvis from the hypogastric reflex.
- A cortical representation of the bladder is present in the paracentral lobule, stimulation of which may evoke bladder contractions. It may play a part in initiating voluntary contractions and in stopping micturition by initiating contraction of the external sphincter.

What investigations are done to evaluate bladder function?

Cystometry, sphincter electromyography, uroflowmetry with measurement and recording of urinary flow, urethral pressure profiles, and electrophysiological tests of bladder wall innervation.

What are the different types of urinary incontinence?

Urinary continence is dependent on a compliant reservoir (the bladder) and sphincteric efficiency which depends on its two components: the involuntary smooth muscle of the bladder neck and the voluntary skeletal muscle of the external sphincter. Urinary incontinence occurs when urine leaks involuntarily and is of five types:
- Total incontinence where the patient loses urine at all times and in all positions. It occurs when the sphincter is damaged (surgery, cancerous infiltration and nerve damage) or when there is a fistula between the urinary tract and the skin, or ectopic ureters.
- Stress incontinence: occurs when there is an increase in intra-abdominal pressure (on coughing, sneezing, lifting, exercising). It is seen in patients with a lax pelvic floor (e.g. multiparous women, patients who have undergone pelvic surgery). Patients do not lose urine in the supine position.
- Urge incontinence: loss of urine preceded by a strong, unexpected urge to void urine. It occurs with inflammation or neurogenic disorders.
- Overflow incontinence occurs in chronic urinary retention from a chronically distended bladder.
- Enuresis: a form of involuntary nocturnal incontinence. It is usually seen in children.

RESPIRATORY SYSTEM

EXAMINATION OF THE CHEST

1. Introduce yourself to the patient.
2. Place the patient in a sitting position and ask whether he or she is comfortable.
3. Examine the sputum cup and comment on the sputum.
4. Examine the patient from the foot end of the bed and comment as follows:
   - Whether the patient is breathless at rest.
   - On wasting, if any, in the infraclavicular region.
   - On diminished movement on the right or left side.
   - Count the respiratory rate.
5. Examine the hands:
   - Clubbing.
   - Cyanosis.
   - Tar staining (the yellow 'nicotine' staining is actually due to tar).
   - Examine the pulse for bounding pulse and asterixis (signs of carbon monoxide narcosis).
6. Examine the face:
   - Comment on the tongue, looking for central cyanosis.
   - Comment on the eyes, looking for pallor and evidence of Horner's syndrome.
7. Examine the neck:
   - Comment on neck veins.
   - Check for cervical lymphadenopathy.
   - Comment on the trachea:
     Whether or not it is deviated.
     The distance between the cricoid cartilage and suprasternal notch.
8. Palpate:
   - Apex beat.
   - Movements on both sides with the fingers symmetrically placed in the intercostal spaces on both sides.
   - Vocal fremitus (tell the examiner that you would prefer to do vocal resonance because it gives the same information and is more reliable).

9. Percussion:
   - Percuss over supraclavicular areas, clavicles, upper, middle and lower chest on both sides.
10. Auscultation:
   - Over supraclavicular areas, upper, middle and lower chest on both sides – comment on breath sounds (whether vesicular or bronchial) and on adventitious sounds (wheeze, crackles or pleural rub). If crackles are heard, ask the patient to cough and then repeat auscultation. It is important to time the crackles to ascertain whether they are early, mid or late inspiration.
   - While auscultating the front of the chest, seize the opportunity to listen to the second pulmonary sound.
   - Check for vocal resonance by asking the patient to repeat 'one, one, one'.
   - Check for forced expiratory time (FET) if your diagnosis is chronic obstructive airways disease (COAD) by asking the patient to exhale forcefully after full inspiration while you are listening over the trachea: if the patient takes more than 6 seconds, airway disease is indicated.
11. Ask the patient to sit forward:
   - Palpate – assess expansion posteriorly.
   - Percuss – on both sides including axillae.
   - Auscultate – posteriorly including the axillae.
12. Remember to look for signs of middle lobe disease in the right axilla.

CASE 97 Pleural Effusion

Instruction

Examine this patient's chest.
Examine this patient's chest from the back.
Examine this patient's chest from the front.

Salient features

- Decreased movement on the affected side.
- Tracheal deviation to the opposite side.
- Stony dull note on the affected side.
- Decreased vocal resonance and diminished breath sounds on the affected side.

Proceed as follows:

- Comment on aspiration marks.
- Percuss for the upper level of effusion in the axilla.
- Listen for bronchial breath sounds.
- Listen for aegophony at the upper level of the effusion.
- It is important to elicit any evidence of an underlying cause, such as clubbing, tar staining, lymph nodes, radiation burns and mastectomy, raised JVP, rheumatoid hands or butterfly rash.

Diagnosis

This patient has a pleural effusion (lesion) probably due to bronchogenic carcinoma and is short of breath at rest (functional status).

Questions

How would you investigate this patient?

- CXR: standard posteroanterior and lateral chest radiographs detect pleural fluid in excess of 175 ml.
- Pleural tap:
  Pleural fluid for determination of the levels of protein, albumin, LDH, glucose, cholesterol and cytology. A simultaneous blood sample should be obtained for estimation of glucose, protein, albumin and LDH.
  When empyema is suspected or seen, pleural fluid pH should be obtained.
  When tuberculosis is suspected, pleural fluid adenosine deaminase or lysozyme levels should be determined and Ziehl–Neelsen staining and pleural fluid mycobacterial cultures should be done.
  Pleural fluid amylase levels should be estimated when malignancy, pancreatitis or oesophageal rupture is suspected.
  In autoimmune disorders, pleural fluid rheumatoid factor or antinuclear antibodies should be tested.
- Pleural biopsy: the biopsy specimen is sent for histopathological examination and mycobacterial culture.

What are the causes of dullness at a lung base?

- Pleural effusion.
- Pleural thickening.
- Consolidation and collapse of the lung.
- Raised hemidiaphragm.

How would you differentiate between the above?

- Pleural effusion: stony dull note; trachea may be deviated to the opposite side in large effusions.
- Pleural thickening: trachea not deviated; breath sounds will be heard.
- Consolidation: vocal resonance increased; bronchial breath sounds and associated crackles.
- Collapse: trachea deviated to the affected side; absent breath sounds.

How would you differentiate between an exudate and a transudate?

- The protein content of an exudate is more than 3 g l^{-1}. However, if this criterion alone is applied, about 10% of the exudates and 15% of the transudates will be wrongly classified. A more accurate diagnosis is made when Light's criteria for an exudate are applied: (1) the ratio of the pleural fluid to serum protein is greater than 0.5; (2) the ratio of pleural fluid to serum lactic dehydrogenase (LDH) is greater than 0.6; (3) pleural fluid LDH is greater than two-thirds the upper normal limit for blood LDH levels. Roth et al (1990) found that, although Light's criteria had a sensitivity of 100%, they had a low specificity of 72%. This was due to the fact that many patients with effusion due to chronic cardiac failure have protein values in the exudate range, particularly when on chronic diuretic therapy. They found that the serum-effusion albumin gradient (i.e. serum albumin minus pleural fluid albumin) was 95% sensitive but a more specific (100%) marker of exduative effusion. A gradient of less than 1.2 g dl^{-1} indicates an exudative effusion whereas a gradient greater than 1.2 g dl^{-1} indicates a transudative effusion.
- The pleural fluid cholesterol level is below 60 mg dl^{-1} in transudates. All malignant effusions have a pleural cholesterol level greater than this value, and therefore this test is useful to separate these two categories of effusion.

Mention a few causes for an exudate and a transudate.

- Causes for an exudate:
   Bronchogenic carcinoma (presence of effusion is an ominous sign).
   Secondaries in the pleura (lung, breast, ovary and pancreas).
   Pneumonia.
   Pulmonary infarction.
   Tuberculosis.
   Rheumatoid arthritis.
   SLE.
   Lymphoma (in young individuals).
   Mesothelioma.

- Causes of a transudate:
    Nephrotic syndrome.
    Cardiac failure.
    Liver cell failure.
    Hypothyroidism.

Advanced-level Questions

Mention a few conditions in which the pleural fluid pH and glucose levels are low with a raised LDH concentration.

Empyema, malignancy, tuberculosis, rheumatoid arthritis, systemic lupus erythematosus and oesophageal rupture.

What is the value of measuring pleural fluid pH and glucose concentrations in cases of malignant effusions?

It is of value in determining the prognosis. Patients with a low pleural fluid pH (< 7.3) or low glucose concentration (< 60 mg dl^{-1}) have a shorter life expectancy than those with higher values: 2.1 months versus 9.8 months. The low pH group tends have more extensive pleural involvement as determined by thoracoscopy and a higher failure rate for chemical pleurodesis.

What further investigation would you do to determine the underlying cause of the pleural effusion?

- Pleural biopsy.
- CT chest scan.
- Magnetic resonance imaging of the chest: although this technique has limited value owing to motion artefacts caused by cardiac and respiratory movements, radiologists were able to differentiate transudates, simple exudates and complex exudates.

What is the role of pleural fluid cytology in the diagnosis of pleural effusion?

- Pleural fluid usually contains about 1500 cells per μl (predominantly mononuclear cells). Counts above 50 000 are seen in parapneumonic effusions, whereas transudates usually have counts of less than 1000 cells per μl.
- Pleural fluid eosinophilia, i.e greater than 10%, suggests a benign disease, including pneumothorax, asbestos-related effusions and post-haemothorax, although malignancy cannot be excluded.
- Pleural fluid lymphocytosis is seen in about one-third of transudates, in

malignancy, tuberculosis, lymphoma, collagen vascular diseases and sarcoidosis.

- Computerized interactive morphometry (analyses the size and nuclei of cells in a stained centrifuged specimen) differentiates between malignant cells and reactive lymphocytosis. This method is particularly useful when differentiating between benign reactive mesothelial cells from malignancy.

What characteristics of the pleural fluid in a parapneumonic effusion indicate a need for closed-tube drainage?

A pleural fluid glucose concentration of less than 40 mg dl^{-1} or a pH < 7.0 indicates the need for closed-tube drainage.

What does a pleural fluid total neutral fat level greater than 400 mg dl^{-1} suggest?

It suggests chylothorax and is seen most often in patients with lymphomas, solid tumours, nephrotic syndrome and cirrhosis, and occasionally in rheumatoid arthritis.

What is the significance of pleural fluid amylase levels?

A pleural fluid amylase level greater than the serum amylase concentration is seen in patients with pancreatitis, carcinoma, bacterial pneumonia and oesophageal rupture. In malignant effusions, when cytology cannot differentiate adenocarcinoma from mesothelioma, a raised amylase level suggests the presence of the former. Amylase-rich pleural effusions occur frequently, and pleural fluid isoamylase determination can be useful; the finding of a pleural effusion rich in salivary isoamylase should prompt an evaluation for carcinoma (particularly a lung primary), but may also be seen in other pleural inflammatory conditions.

What are the causes of an exudate with negative cytology findings and pleural fluid lymphocytosis?

Possible causes include tuberculosis, collagen vascular diseases and tumours, including lymphoma.

In such patients what other tests could you perform on the pleural fluid to determine the underlying cause?

- Pleural fluid adenosine deaminase concentration (an enzyme involved in purine metabolism and found in T lymphocytes) is markedly

raised in tuberculous and rheumatoid effusions compared with malignant effusions.
- Increased pleural fluid lysozyme concentration (muramidase) is used to differentiate tuberculosis, rheumatoid arthritis and empyema from malignant effusions.
- Combined use of the latter two tests yields a sensitivity and specificity of 100% for tuberculous effusions if empyema is excluded.
- γ Interferon and soluble interleukin 2 receptor levels are also raised in tuberculous effusions compared with malignant effusions.
- Estimation of pleural fluid rheumatoid factor and antinuclear antibodies is useful in confirming the diagnosis of rheumatoid and lupus erythematosus respectively.

In which conditions is the pleural fluid bloody?

Haemorrhagic fluid is seen in malignancy, pulmonary embolus, tuberculosis and trauma to the chest.

What are the earliest radiological signs of pleural fluid?

The earliest radiological signs are blunting of the costophrenic angle on the anterior–posterior view or loss of clear definition of the diaphragm posteriorly on the lateral view.

When in doubt of a small effusion, how would you confirm your suspicions?

Either by a lateral decubitus view (which shows a layering of the fluid along the dependent chest wall unless the fluid is loculated) or by ultrasonography.

What are the other uses of ultrasonography in the diagnosis of pleural effusion?

Ultrasonography is also useful for loculated effusions, for guided thoracocentesis, closed pleural biopsy or insertion of a chest drain, and to differentiate pleural fluid from pleural thickening.

What is a pseudotumour?

It is the accumulation of fluid between the major or minor fissure or along the lateral chest wall, and can be mistaken for a tumour on the radiograph. Such loculated effusions can be confirmed with ultrasonography.

What do you know about pleural disease in rheumatoid arthritis?

About 70% of patients with rheumatoid arthritis have pleural inflammation at autopsy and about 5% have radiological evidence of pleural inflammation at some time. Pleural involvement is associated with male sex, rheumatoid factor in serum, the presence of nodules and other systemic manifestations. The effusion is thought to develop as an inflammatory response to the presence of multiple subpleural nodules. For reasons that are entirely unclear, the left side is the more common site of unilateral rheumatoid pleural effusions. The pleural fluid glucose level is characteristically low and is said to be due to an 'entrance block' in which glucose is unable to enter the pleural space, unlike in empyema and malignant effusions where the low pleural fluid glucose concentration is attributed to the increased use of glucose by cells. Cytological appearances of slender and elongated macrophages, round giant multinucleated macrophages, presence of very few mesothelial cells and necrotic background material are thought to be pathognomonic of rheumatoid pleuritis.

What are the complications of thoracocentesis?

Pneumothorax, haemothorax, intravascular collapse and unilateral pulmonary oedema (the latter after withdrawal of large quantities of fluid).

What do you know about Meigs' syndrome?

Meigs' syndrome comprises pleural effusion (usually right sided and a transudate) and ovarian malignancy (usually benign ovarian fibroma).

Mention some causes of drug-induced pleural effusion.

Practolol, procarbazine, methysergide, bromocriptine, methotrexate and nitrofurantoin.

The patient used to be a shipbuilder: what diagnosis would you consider?

It is most likely that this patient has malignant mesothelioma. If the diagnosis is confirmed, I would advise him to apply for industrial injuries benefit.

What are the mechanisms for abnormal accumulation of pleural fluid?

There are three main mechanisms:
- An abnormality of the pleura itself, such as neoplasm or inflammatory process, usually associated with increased permeability.
- Disruption of the integrity of a fluid-containing structure within the

pleural cavity, such as the thoracic duct, oesophagus, major blood vessels or tracheobronchial tree, with leakage of the contents into the pleural space.

- Abnormal hydrostatic or osmotic forces operating on an otherwise normal pleural surface and producing a transudate.

References

Berkman N & Kramer MR (1993) Diagnostic tests in pleural effusion – an update. *Postgrad Med J* **69**: 12–18.

Hamm H, Brohan U, Bohmer R & Missmahl HP (1987) Cholesterol in pleural effusions. A diagnostic aid. *Chest* **92**: 296–302.

Hirsch A, Ruffie P, Nebut M et al (1979). Pleural effusion: laboratory tests in 300 cases. *Thorax* **304**: 106.

Joseph J, Viney S, Beck P, Strange C, Sahn SA & Basran GS (1992) A prospective study of amylase-rich pleural effusions with special reference to amylase isoenzyme analysis. *Chest* **102**: 1455–1459.

Light RW, MacGregor MI, Luchsinger PC & Ball WC (1972) Pleural effusions: the diagnostic separation of transudates and exudates. *Ann Intern Med* **77**: 507–513.

Prakash UBS & Reiman HM (1985) Comparison of needle biopsy with cytologic analysis for evaluation of pleural effusion. Analysis of 414 cases. *Mayo Clin Proc* **60**: 158.

Roth BJ, O'Meara TF & Cragun WH (1990) The serum-effusion albumin gradient in the evaluation of pleural effusion. *Chest* **98**: 546–549.

Sahn SA & Good JT (1988) Pleural fluid pH in malignant effusions. Diagnostic, prognostic and therapeutic implications. *Ann Intern Med* **108**: 345–349.

Seaton A (1990) Asbestos diseases and compensation. *Br Med J* **301**: 453.

Valdes L, Pose A, Suarez J et al (1991) Cholesterol: a useful parameter for distinguishing between pleural exudates and transudates. *Chest* **99**: 1097–1102.

CASE 98 Pleural Rub

Instruction

This patient presented with sudden onset of lateral chest pain aggravated by deep inspiration and coughing. Listen to this patient's chest. Examine her chest.

Salient features

- Pleural rub (superficial, scratchy, grating sound heard on deep inspiration).

Proceed as follows:

- Differentiate between pleural rub and crackles by asking the patient to cough and check whether or not there is any change in the nature. (**Note.** No change with the pleural rub.)
- Tell the examiner that you would like to proceed as follows:
  Listen for tachycardia and right ventricular gallop.
  Take a history of the nature of the sputum (purulent expectoration in a patient with chest infection, haemoptysis in pulmonary embolism).
  Take a drug history (oral contraceptives).

Diagnosis

This patient has a pleural rub (lesion) which is due to either underlying infection or pulmonary embolism (aetiology). You would like to analyse blood gases to determine whether she is hypoxic (functional status).

Questions

How would you investigate this patient?

- FBC.
- Sputum cultures.
- Blood gases.
- ECG.
- CXR.
- Ventilation–perfusion scan.

Advanced-level Questions

What would you expect to see in the ventilation–perfusion scan in a patient with pulmonary embolism?

In acute pulmonary embolism the area of decreased perfusion usually has normal ventilation, whereas in pneumonia there are abnormalities in both the ventilation and perfusion scan.

How would you treat a patient with pulmonary embolism?

- Initially with heparin and then with oral anticoagulants for at least 3 months.
- Pain relief for pleurisy.

CASE 99 Asthma

Instruction

Examine this patient's chest.

Salient features

- Bilateral scattered wheeze.

Proceed as follows:

- Tell the examiner that you would like to know whether the following apply:
  It is a reversible airway obstruction (by taking history).
  There is a history of atopy (eczema, hay fever).

Diagnosis

This patient has a history of hay fever and bilateral scattered wheeze (lesion) due to bronchial asthma (aetiology), and is breathless at rest (functional status).

Questions

Mention a few trigger factors known to aggravate asthma.

- Infection.
- Emotion.
- Exercise.
- Drugs, e.g. beta-blockers.
- External allergens.

What are the symptoms of asthma?

- Wheeze.
- Recurrent cough.
- Exacerbation of the above symptoms at night or after exercise.
- Improvement of the above symptoms with bronchodilator therapy.

What do you understand by the term 'asthma'?

Asthma is an inflammatory disorder characterized by hyper-responsiveness of the airway to various stimuli, resulting in widespread narrowing of the airway. The changes are reversible, either spontaneously or as a result of therapy.

Advanced-level Questions

What do you understand by the term 'intrinsic asthma'?

Intrinsic asthma is of non-allergic aetiology and usually begins after the age of 30 years. It tends to be more continuous and more severe; status asthmaticus is common in this group.

What do you understand by the term 'extrinsic asthma'?

Extrinsic asthma has a clearly defined history of allergy to a variety of inhaled factors and is characterized by a childhood onset and seasonal variation.

What are the indications for steroids in chronic asthma?

- Sleep is disturbed by wheeze.
- Morning tightness persists until midday.
- Symptoms and peak expiratory flows progressively deteriorate each day.
- Maximum treatment with bronchodilators.
- Emergency nebulizers are needed.

What is the effect of reducing or discontinuing inhaled budesonide in patients with mild asthma?

Early treatment with inhaled budesonide results in long-lasting control of mild asthma (i.e. FEV_1 more than 85% of predicted value). Maintenance therapy can usually be given at a reduced dose, but discontinuation of treatment is often accompanied by exacerbation of the disease.

How would you manage a patient with acute asthma?

- Nebulized β-agonists, e.g. terbutaline or salbutamol.
- Oxygen, using a high concentration.
- High-dose steroids: intravenous hydrocortisone or oral prednisolone or both.
- Blood gases.
- CXR to rule out pneumothorax.

When life-threatening features are present:
- Add ipratropium to nebulized β-agonist.
- Intravenous aminophylline or salbutamol or terbutaline.

What do you know about the BritishThoracic Society step care regimen for the management of chronic asthma in adults?

- Step 1: Inhaled short-acting β-agonists used as required for symptom relief. If required more than once, go to step 2.
- Step 2: Step 1 plus regular inhaled anti-inflammtory agents (such as beclomethasone, budesonide, cromoglycate or nedocromil sodium).
- Step 3: Step 1 plus high-dose inhaled steroids (using a large-volume spacer).
- Step 4: Step 1 plus high-dose inhaled steroids and regular broncho-dilators (long-acting inhaled or oral β-agonists, sustained-release theophylline, inhaled ipratropium).
- Step 5: Step 4 plus addition of oral steroids.

Patients should be started on treatment at the step most appropriate to the initial severity. A rescue course of prednisolone may be needed at any time and at any step. Stepwise reduction in treatment should be undertaken after the asthma has been stable over a 3–6 month period.

What are the features of acute severe asthma?

- Inability to complete a sentence in one breath.
- Respiration rate greater than 25 per minute.
- Pulse rate greater than 110 beats per minute.
- Peak expiratory flow rate less than 50% of predicted or best.

What are the life-threatening indicators in acute asthma?

- Peak expiratory flow rate less than 33% of predicted or best.
- Exhaustion, confusion, coma.
- Silent chest, cyanosis or feeble respiratory effort.
- Bradycardia or hypotension.

Note. Arterial blood gases should be measured if *any* of these features are present.

What are the indicators of a very severe, life-threatening attack?

- Normal (5–6 kPa, 36–45 mmHg) or increased carbon dioxide tension.
- Severe hypoxia of less than 8 kPa (60 mmHg).
- Low pH.

What is the value of assessing pulsus paradoxus in a patient with acute severe asthma?

It is a poor guide to the severity of acute asthma as it compares poorly with the measurement of peak flow.

In which other conditions is wheeze a prominent sign?

Chronic obstructive airway disease, left ventricular failure (cardiac asthma), polyarteritis nodosa, eosinophilic lung disease, recurrent thromboembolism, tumour causing localized wheeze.

What are the indications for mechanical ventilation with intermittent positive pressure ventilation?

- Worsening hypoxia (Pao_2 < 8 kPa) despite 60% inspired oxygen.
- Hypercapnia ($Paco_2$ > 6 kPa).
- Drowsiness.
- Unconsciousness.
- Intermittent positive pressure ventilation.

Professor Peter J Barnes, contemporary chest physician, National Institute for Heart and Lung Diseases, London; his major interest is asthma.

References

British Thoracic Society (1993) Guidelines for the management of asthma: a summary. *Br Med J* **306**: 776–782.

British Thoracic Society (1993) Guidelines for the management of asthma. *Thorax* **48**(suppl): S1–24.

Haahtela T, Järvinen M, Kava T et al (1994) Effects of reducing or discontinuing inhaled budesonide in patients with mild asthma. *N Engl J Med* **331**: 700–705.

Pearson MG, Spence DPS, Ryland I & Harrison BDW (1993) Value of pulsus paradoxus in assessing acute severe asthma. *Br Med J* **307**: 659.

Rees J & Price J (1995) Chronic asthma – general management. *Br Med J* **310**: 1400–1401.

CASE 100 Chronic Bronchitis

Instruction

Examine this patient's chest.

Salient features

Proceed as follows:

- Begin with examination of the *sputum pot*.
- Observe the patient from the end of the bed – for obvious breathlessness, pursed lip breathing and symmetrical chest movements – and count respiratory rate.
- Look for nail changes such as tar staining.
- Feel the palms for warmth and the pulse for rapid bounding pulse (signs of carbon dioxide retention).
- Look at the lips and tongue for central cyanosis.

In the neck:

- Comment on the active contractions of the accessory muscles of respiration such as sternocleidomastoids, scaleni and trapezii.
- Palpate for tracheal deviation and measure the distance between the cricoid cartilage and suprasternal notch (less than three fingers' breadth in emphysema).
- Comment on the raised JVP.

Palpate for:

- Apex beat.
- Chest expansion.
- Vocal fremitus.

Percussion:

- Look for hyper-resonance and obliteration of cardiac and liver dullness.

Auscultate for:

- Breath sounds.
- Vocal resonance.
- FET: normal individuals can empty their chest from full inspiration in 4 seconds or less. The end-point of FET is detected by auscultating over the trachea in the suprasternal notch. Prolongation of the FET to more than 6 seconds indicates airflow obstruction.

Diagnosis

This patient has features of chronic obstructive airway disease (COAD) (lesion) due to cigarette smoking (aetiology) and is very cyanosed at rest (functional status).

Questions

What do you understand by the term 'chronic bronchitis'?

Chronic bronchitis is cough with mucoid expectoration for at least 3 months in a year for 2 successive years.

What is the definition of emphysema?

Emphysema is the abnormal permanent enlargement of the airway distal to the terminal respiratory bronchioles with destruction of their walls. Clinical, radiological and lung function tests give an imprecise picture in an individual case but a combination of all these features gives a reasonable picture.

Advanced-level Questions

What is the role of high-resolution CT in the diagnosis of emphysema?

It is the most sensitive (but expensive) technique for the diagnosis of emphysema. It is useful in evaluating symptomatic patients with almost normal pulmonary function except for a low carbon monoxide diffusing capacity – a combination of findings that occurs in emphysema, interstitial lung disease and pulmonary vascular disease.

How would you differentiate emphysema from chronic bronchitis?

	Emphysema	Chronic bronchitis
	Pink puffer	Blue bloater
Cyanosis	Absent	Prominent
Dyspnoea	++	+
Hyperinflation	++	+
Cor pulmonale	–	Common
Respiratory drive	High	Low

If the patient was between the ages of 30 and 45 years, what would you consider to be the underlying cause of the emphysema?

Smoking, a_1-antitrypsin (AAT) deficiency.

How would you treat an acute exacerbation?

- Nebulized bronchodilators (terbutaline, ipratropium bromide).
- Intravenous antibiotics.
- Oxygen (24%).
- Intravenous hydrocortisone and oral steroids.
- Antibiotics: initially with amoxycillin and, if no clinical response, then with a second-generation cephalosporin, quinoline or co-amoxiclav.

What are the organisms commonly associated with exacerbations of COAD?

Haemophilus influenzae and *Streptococcus pneumoniae* are the commonest organisms identified in the sputum during exacerbations of COAD, accounting for 43% and 25% respectively of positive cultures in one study. *Moraxella* (previously *Branhamella*) *catarrhalis* is also frequently isolated from sputum during exacerbations. Less commonly, *Chlamydia pneumoniae* or *Pseudomonas aeruginosa* have been associated with some exacerbations.

What clinical features would suggest that this patient is suitable for long-term domiciliary oxygen therapy?

- COAD: forced expiratory volume in 1 second (FEV_1) less than 1.5 litres; forced vital capacity less than 2 litres; stable chronic respiratory failure ($Pao_2 < 7.3$ kPa) in patients who have (1) had peripheral oedema or (2) not necessarily had hypercapnia or oedema.
- Terminally ill patients of whatever cause with severe hypoxia ($Pao_2 < 7.3$ kPa).

How can the sensation of breathlessness be reduced?

By the use of either promethazine or dihydrocodeine.

How would you treat acute respiratory failure?

If Pao_2 is less than 8 kPa, administer 24% oxygen. There is no need for oxygen when Pao_2 is greater than 8 kPa. Monitor blood gases after 30 minutes. If $Paco_2$ is rising (by 1 kPa), monitor blood gases hourly. If $Paco_2$ continues to rise, administer doxapram. If, in spite of this, the patient continues to deteriorate, artificial ventilation may be called for.

What do you know about non-invasive ventilation?

Non-invasive ventilation is an alternative approach to endotracheal intubation to treat hypercapnic ventilatory failure which occurs in COAD. It thus reduces the complications of endotracheal intubation such as infection and injury to the trachea. Non-invasive ventilation is pressure-support ventilation delivered with a face mask and a piece of white foam placed in the face mask to reduce the amount of internal dead space. In a recent randomized trial, non-invasive ventilation was shown to reduce the need for endotracheal intubation, length of hospital stay and in-hospital mortality rate in selected patients with acute exacerbations of COAD.

What do you know about α_1-antitrypsin deficiency?

- It was first described in Sweden. The patient is deficient in α_1-antitrypsin, with activity approximately 15% that of the normal value; concentrations of 40% or more are required for health. The patient is homozygous for protease inhibitor (Pi) ZZ gene. Other genetic combinations and their percentage normal activity are PiMS (80%), PiMZ (60%), PiSS (60%), PiSZ (40%). Six per cent of the population is heterozygous for S(PiMS) and 4% for Z(PiMZ), making an overall frequency of 1 in 10 for the carriage of the defective gene. Liver transplantation results in conversion to the genotype of the donor.
- In the lung α_1-antitrypsin inhibits the excessive actions of neutrophil and macrophage elastase, which cigarette smoke promotes. When the lung is heavily exposed to cigarette smoke, the protective effect of α_1-antitrypsin may be overwhelmed by the amount of elastase released or by a direct oxidative action of cigarette smoke on the α_1-antitrypsin molecule. The emphysema is panacinar and is seen in the lower lobes of the lungs. Smoking increases the severity and decreases the age of onset of emphysema. Liver disease is a much less common complication. Human α_1-antitrypsin prepared from pooled plasma from normal donors is recommended for patients over 18 years with serum levels below 11 μmol l^{-1} and abnormal lung function.
- The siblings of an index case should be screened for this disorder. Their identification should be followed by counselling to avoid smoking and occupations with atmospheric pollution. Children of homozygotes will inherit at least one Z gene and hence will be heterozygotes. They should avoid pairing with another heterozygote if they wish to avoid the risk of producing an affected homozygote.

What are the general indications for lung transplantation?

The general indication is end-stage lung disease without alternative forms of therapy. Patients should be below 60 years of age and should have a life expectancy of less than 12 or 18 months; they should not have an underlying cancer or other serious systemic illness. The most common lung diseases are pulmonary fibrosis, emphysema (particularly α_1-antitrypsin deficiency), bronchiectasis, cystic fibrosis and primary pulmonary hypertension.

What is the role of lung transplantation in COAD?

It has been successful for at least 3–4 years in patients with COAD. Single-lung transplantation is currently recommended in most cases. The criteria for selecting patients for transplantation have not been established.

What is the role of bullectomy in COAD?

Bullectomy may improve gas exchange and airflow, and reduce dyspnoea in selected patients with bullae larger than one-third of the hemithorax and accompanying lung compression. Although laser ablation of bullae has been reported, the risks and benefits have not been determined.

What is the role of nutrition in COAD?

Undernutrition is associated with reduced respiratory muscle function and an increased mortality rate. A high dietary intake of n-3 fatty acids may protect cigarette smokers against COAD.

Peter Howard, contemporary chest physician, Sheffield; his chief interest is long-term domiciliary oxygen therapy.

References

Brochard L, Mancebo J, Wysocki M et al (1995) Noninvasive ventilation for acute exacerbations of chronic obstructive pulmonary disease. *N Engl J Med* **333**: 817–822.

Hosker H, Cooke NJ & Hawkey P (1994) Antibiotics in chronic obstructive pulmonary disease. *Br Med J* **308**: 871–872.

Klein JS, Gamsu G, Webb WR, Golden JA & Müller NL (1992) High resolution CT diagnosis of emphysema in symptomatic patients with normal chest radiographs and isolated low diffusing capacity. *Radiology* **182**: 817–821.

Medical Research Council Working Party (1981) Long term domiciliary oxygen therapy in chronic hypoxic cor pulmonale complicating chronic bronchitis and emphysema. *Lancet* **i**: 681–686.

Nocturnal Oxygen Therapy Trial Group (1980) Continuous or nocturnal oxygen therapy in hypoxaemic chronic obstructive lung disease: a clinical trial. *Ann Intern Med* **93**: 391–398.

Patterson GA, Maurer JR, Williams TJ et al (1991) Comparison of outcome of double and single lung transplantation of obstructive lung disease. *J Thorac Cardiovasc Surg* **101**: 623–632.

CASE 101 Bronchiectasis

Instruction

Examine this patient's chest.
Listen to this patient's chest.

Salient features

- Copious purulent expectoration (remember to check the sputum cup in a chest case).
- Finger clubbing.
- Bilateral coarse, late, inspiratory crackles.

Proceed as follows:

- Comment on kyphoscoliosis if any.
- Tell the examiner that you would like to know whether the bronchiectasis is long standing; if so, you would like to examine the abdomen for splenomegaly (amyloidosis).

In addition there may be signs of collapse, fibrosis or pneumonia.

Diagnosis

This patient has bilateral, coarse, late inspiratory crackles with purulent sputum (lesion) due to bronchiectasis (aetiology), and is cyanosed.

Questions

What do you understand by the term 'bronchiectasis'?

It is a chronic necrotizing infection of the bronchi and bronchioles leading to abnormal, permanent dilatation of the airways.

Mention the causes of bronchiectasis.

- Postpneumonic, measles, pertussis, tuberculosis (TB).
- Mechanical bronchial obstruction, as in TB, carcinoma, nodal compression.
- Allergic bronchopulmonary aspergillosis.

- γ-Globulin deficiency – congenital, acquired.
- Immotile cilia syndrome (Kartagener's syndrome).
- Cystic fibrosis.
- Neuropathic disorders (namely Riley–Day syndrome, Chagas' disease).
- Idiopathic.

What investigations would you do in such a patient?

FBC, sputum culture, CXR, bronchography, CT scan of the chest.

Advanced-level Questions

How can CT assess bronchiectasis?

High-resolution CT performed at the end of expiration suggests that small airways disease may be an early feature of bronchiectasis, which leads to more progressive injury and bronchiolar distortion. Larger studies with long-term follow-up are required to confirm this. Conventional CT has a sensitivity of 60–80% for detecting bronchiectasis, whereas high-resolution CT has a sensitivity of more than 90%, using bronchography as the 'gold standard'.

What is the difference between standard and high-resolution CT?

In standard CT the resolution is 10 mm thick whereas with high-resolution CT the slices are 1–2 mm thick and high spatial resolution algorithms are used to reconstruct images.

What do you know about spiral CT?

This is a rapidly evolving technique to image the chest with the advantages of truly contiguous sections; consequently totally seamless reconstructions are possible. This may allow virtual-reality bronchoscopy imaging.

What are the complications of bronchiectasis?

- Pneumonia, pleurisy, pleural effusion, pneumothorax.
- Sinusitis.
- Haemoptysis.
- Brain abscess.
- Amyloidosis.

What are the major respiratory pathogens in bronchiectasis?

Staphylococcus aureus, Haemophilus influenzae, Pseudomonas aeruginosa.

How would you treat such patients?

- Postural drainage.
- Antibiotics.
- Bronchodilators.
- Surgery in selected cases.

What abnormalities may be associated with bronchiectasis?

- Congenital absence of bronchial cartilage (Williams–Campbell syndrome).
- Tracheobronchomegaly (Mounier–Kuhn syndrome).
- Obstructive azoospermia and chronic sinopulmonary infection (Young's syndrome), said to be due to mercury intoxication. It was first described from the north of England by Young in 1970.
- Congenital kyphoscoliosis.
- Situs inversus and paranasal sinusitis (Kartagener's syndrome).
- Unilateral absence of pulmonary artery.

What is the indication for surgery in bronchiectasis?

Bronchiectasis localized to a single lobe or a segment without clinical, bronchographic or CT evidence of bronchiectasis or bronchitis affecting other parts of the lung.

What are the common sites for localized disease?

Left lower lobe and lingula.

What do you understand by the term bronchiectasis sicca?

Bronchiectasis or 'dry' bronchiectasis is that which presents with recurrent dry cough associated with intermittent episodes (months or years apart) of haemoptysis. The haemoptysis can be life threatening as bleeding is from bronchial vessels with systemic pressures. There is usually a past history of granulomatous infection, particularly tuberculosis. The upper lobes are often primarily affected, allowing good drainage.

What do you know about bronchiectasis in allergic bronchopulmonary aspergillosis?

The bronchial dilatation occurs in more proximal bronchi as a result of type III immune complex reactions.

What do you know about Reid's classification of bronchiectasis?

In 1950 Reid correlated pathological changes with bronchography and described three different appearances. All the three types can be present in the same patient; they are:

- Cylindrical bronchiectasis: refers to bronchi that are uniformly dilated and do not taper, but rather end abruptly. This is due to plugging of smaller bronchi by thick mucus and casts. The bronchi are dilated to greater than 2 mm but can be so large as to admit a finger.
- Varicose bronchiectasis: refers to dilated bronchi with irregular bulging contours similar to a varicose vein. They do not taper and terminations are bulbous. Bronchial subdivisions are reduced.
- Cystic or saccular bronchiectasis is the most severe form and is characterized by sharply reduced bronchial subdivisions and dilated bronchi ending in cystic pus-filled cavities.

Laennec was the first to describe bronchiectasis in 1819.
M Kartagener (b. 1897), a Swiss physician.
CM Riley and RL Day, both US paediatricians. Riley–Day syndrome consists of dysautonomia and lack of co-ordination in swallowing.
CJR Chagas (1879–1934) a Brazilian physician.

References

Hansell DM, Wells AU, Rubens MB & Cole PJ (1994) Bronchiectasis: functional significance of areas of decreased attenuation at expiratory CT. *Radiology* **193**: 369–374.
Paranjape DV & Bergin CJ (1994) Spiral CT of the lungs: optimal technique and resolution compared with conventional CT. *Am J Roentgenol* **162**: 561–567.

CASE 102 Cor Pulmonale

Instruction

Examine this patient's chest.

Salient features

- Patient is short of breath at rest and is centrally cyanosed.
- Tar staining of the fingers.
- JVP is raised: both 'a' and 'v' waves are seen, 'v' waves being prominent if there is associated tricuspid regurgitation.

- On examination of the chest there is bilateral wheeze and other signs of chronic bronchitis (see page 271).

Proceed as follows:

- Tell the examiner that you would like to examine the cardiovascular system for signs of pulmonary hypertension:
  Left parasternal heave (often absent when the chest is barrel shaped).
  Right ventricular gallop rhythm.
  Loud P_2 and a loud ejection click.
  Pansystolic murmur of tricuspid regurgitation.
  Early diastolic Graham Steell murmur in the pulmonary area.
- Look for signs of:
  Hepatomegaly.
  Pedal oedema.

Diagnosis

This patient has chronic cor pulmonale (lesion) due to long-standing COAD (aetiology) and is in congestive cardiac failure (functional status).

Questions

What do you understand by the term 'cor pulmonale'?

Cor pulmonale is right ventricular enlargement due to the increase in afterload that occurs in diseases of the lung, chest wall or pulmonary circulation.

Mention a few causes of cor pulmonale.

Respiratory disorders:
- Obstructive:
  COAD.
  Chronic persistent asthma.
- Restrictive:
  Intrinsic – interstitial fibrosis, lung resection.
  Extrinsic – obesity, muscle weakness, kyphoscoliosis, high altitude.

Pulmonary vascular disorders:
- Pulmonary emboli.
- Vasculitis of the small pulmonary arteries.
- Adult respiratory distress syndrome.
- Primary pulmonary hypertension.

Advanced-level Questions

How would you manage a patient with cor pulmonale?

- Treat the underlying cause.
- Treat respiratory failure. If Pao_2 is less than 8 kPa, administer 24% oxygen. There is no need for oxygen if Pao_2 is more than 8 kPa. Monitor blood gases after 30 minutes. If Pco_2 is rising (by 1 kPa), monitor blood gases hourly. If Pco_2 continues to rise, administer doxapram. If, in spite of this, the deterioration continues, the patient may merit artificial ventilation.
- Treat cardiac failure with frusemide.
- Consider venesection if the haematocrit is more than 55%.

What is the prognosis in cor pulmonale?

Approximately 50% of patients succumb within 5 years.

Reference

Editorial (1989) Polycythaemia due to hypoxaemia: advantage or disadvantage. *Lancet* **ii**: 20–21.

CASE 103 Consolidation

Instruction

Examine this patient's chest.

Salient features

- Purulent sputum (if bacterial in aetiology).
- Tachypnoea.
- Reduced movement of the affected side.
- Trachea central.
- Impaired percussion note.
- Bronchial breath sounds.
- Crackles.

Diagnosis

This patient has left lower lobe consolidation with purulent sputum (lesion) indicating a bacterial pneumonia (aetiology).

Questions

What is the aetiology?

- Bacterial pneumonia.
- Bronchogenic carcinoma.
- Pulmonary infarct.

How would you investigate suspected bacterial pneumonia?

- Full blood count, serum urea, electrolytes and liver function tests.
- Sputum and blood cultures.
- Arterial blood gases.
- CXR.
- Tests for *Legionella* (culture, direct fluorescent-antibody test, or urinary antigen assay), mycoplasma immunoglobulin M.
- Consider serological testing for human immunodeficiency virus (for patients 15–54 years old, particularly when there is lymphopenia or a low CD4 cell count).

Advanced-level Questions

What are the causes of a poorly resolving or recurrent pneumonia?

- Carcinoma of the lung.
- Aspiration of a foreign body.
- Inappropriate antibiotic.
- Sequestration (rare; suspect if left lower lobe is involved).

What do you know about atypical pneumonias?

Typical pneumonia is due to pneumococcus (*Streptococcus pneumoniae*), whereas atypical pneumonia is that *not* due to pneumococcus; the latter may be caused by *Mycoplasma, Legionella, Chlamydia, Coxiella*, etc. The clinical picture in atypical pneumonia is dominated by constitutional symptoms, such as fever and headache rather than respiratory symptoms.

What do you know about mycoplasma pneumonia?

Mycoplasma pneumoniae is an important cause of atypical pneumonia. It is important community-acquired pneumonia and epidemics are seen every 4 years or so. Its incubation is 2–3 weeks and it is usually seen in children and young adults. Reinfection can occur in older patients with detectable *M. pneumoniae* antibody. Like all other pneumonias, mycoplasma pneumonia is common in winter months.

What are the extrapulmonary manifestations of mycoplasma pneumonia?

- Arthralgia and arthritis.
- Autoimmune haemolytic anaemia.
- Neurological manifestations involving both central and peripheral systems.
- Pericarditis, myocarditis.
- Hepatitis, glomerulonephritis.
- Non-specific rash, erythema multiforme and Stevens–Johnson syndrome.
- Disseminated intravascular coagulation (DIC).

Which antibiotics would you use in a patient with community-acquired pneumonia where the pathogen is not known?

The British Thoracic Society recommends that empirical therapy 'should always cover' *Strep. pneumoniae*. The preferred regimen is amoxycillin or pencillin; when *Legionella* or *M. pneumoniae* is specifically suspected, erythromycin should be given, and antibiotics directed against *Staphylococcus aureus* should be considered during epidemics of influenza.

What are the poor prognostic factors in patients with community-acquired pneumonia?

- Age > 65 years.
- Coexisting conditions such as cardiac failure, renal failure, chronic obstructive pulmonary disease, malignancy.
- Clinical features: respiratory rate > 30 per min, hypotension (systolic blood pressure < 90 mmHg or diastolic pressure < 60 mmHg), temperature > 38.3°C, impaired mental status (stupor, lethargy, disorientation or coma), extrapulmonary infection (e.g. septic arthritis, meningitis).
- Investigations: haematocrit < 30%, white cell count < 4000 or > 30 000 per mm^3, azotaemia, arterial blood gas < 60 mmHg while breathing room air, chest radiograph showing multiple lobe involvement, rapid spread or pleural effusion.
- Microbial pathogens: *Staph. aureus*, *Legionella*, *Strep. pneumoniae*.

What do you know about pulmonary eosinophilic disorders?

Crofton et al (1952) described five classes of pulmonary eosinophilic disorder:
- Löffler's syndrome: characterized by transient pulmonary infiltrates and peripheral eosinophilia. It is associated with parasitic infections, drug

allergies and exposure to inorganic chemicals such as nickel carbonyl. The course is benign and respiratory failure almost unknown.

• Eosinophilia in asthmatics: the most common cause is allergic bronchopulmonary aspergillosis. This condition is benign but chronic.

• Tropical eosinophilia which is secondary to filarial infection (*Wuchereria bancrofti* or *W. malayi Brug*).

• Churg–Strauss syndrome: Diagnosis requires four of the following features: asthma; eosinophilia greater than 10%, mononeuropathy or polyneuropathy, paranasal sinus abnormality; non-fixed pulmonary infiltrates visible on chest radiographs and blood vessels with extravascular eosinophils found on biopsy.

• Chronic eosinophilic pneumonia: chronic debilitating illness characterized by malaise, fever, weight loss and dyspnoea. The chest radiograph shows a peripheral alveolar filling infiltrate predominantly in the upper lobes (the 'photographic negative' of pulmonary oedema).

What do you know about bronchopulmonary sequestration?

It is an uncommon congenital lesion in which a portion of non-functioning lung tissue is detached from the normal lung and supplied by an anomalous systemic artery, usually arising from the aorta or one of its branches. The tissue has no communication with the bronchopulmonary tree. Two types of sequestration have been described: extralobar and intralobar. An extralobar sequestration has its own pleural lining, which separates it from the remaining lung tissue, and the intralobar type shares its pleura with the adjacent normal lung. Patients usually present in childhood with cough and recurrent pneumonia, and occasionally present with haemoptysis.

References

Bartlett JG & Mundy LM (1995) Community-acquired pneumonia. *N Engl J Med* **333**: 1618–1624.

British Thoracic Society (1992) Optimal duration of anticoagulation for deep-vein thrombosis and pulmonary embolism. *Lancet* **340**: 873–876.

British Thoracic Society (1993) Guidelines for the management of community-acquired pneumonia in adults admitted to hospital. *Br J Hosp Med* **49**: 346–350.

British Thoracic Society and the Public Health Laboratory Service (1992) The aetiology, management and outcome of severe community-acquired pneumonia on the intensive care unit. *Respir Med* **86**: 7–13.

Crofton JW, Livingstone JL, Oswald NC & Roberts ATM (1952) Pulmonary eosinophilia. *Thorax* **7**: 1–35.

CASE 104 Bronchogenic Carcinoma

Instruction

Examine this patient's chest.

Salient features

- *Patient 1* has clubbing and tar staining the fingers.
  Dull percussion note at the apex with absent breath sounds.
  Look for Horner's syndrome and wasting of the small muscles of the hand.
- *Patient 2* has signs of pleural effusion on one side.
- *Patient 3* shows signs of unilateral collapse or consolidation of the upper lobe on one side.

Note. If you suspect bronchogenic carcinoma, always look for clubbing, tar staining, cervical lymph nodes and radiation marks, and comment on cachexia.

Diagnosis

This patient with marked clubbing and large pleural effusion (lesion) probably has bronchogenic carcinoma (aetiology) and is very short of breath due to the large effusion (functional status).

Questions

How may patients with bronchogenic carcinoma present?

- Cough (in 80% of cases), haemoptysis (70%) and dyspnoea (60%); loss of weight, anorexia.
- Skeletal manifestations: clubbing (in 30% of cases).
- Local pressure effects: recurrent laryngeal palsy, superior vena caval obstruction, Horner's syndrome.
- Endocrine manifestations (12% of the tumours) – in particular small cell tumours – present with syndrome of inappropriate antidiuretic hormone (SIADH), hypercalcaemia, adrenocorticotrophic hormone (ACTH) secretion, gynaecomastia.
- Neurological manifestations: Eaton–Lambert syndrome, cerebellar degeneration, polyneuropathy, dementia, proximal myopathy.
- Cardiovascular: thrombophlebitis migrans, atrial fibrillation, pericarditis, non-bacterial thrombotic endocarditis.
- Cutaneous manifestations: dermatomyositis, acanthosis nigricans, herpes zoster.

- Anaemia, disseminated intravascular coagulation, thrombotic thrombo-cytopenic purpura.

How would you investigate this patient?

- Sputum cytology.
- CXR.
- Pleural fluid cytology.
- Bronchoscopy.
- CT scan of the chest.
- Bone scan for metastases (helpful in staging).

Advanced-level Questions

What is the role of surgery in lung carcinoma?

Surgery is beneficial in peripheral non-small cell carcinoma. Its role is limited in small cell carcinoma as over 90% would have metastasized by the time of diagnosis.

Which tumours respond well to chemotherapy?

Small cell carcinoma: cyclophosphamide, doxorubicin, cisplatin, etoposide and vincristine are some of the drugs used. The combination of etoposide and cisplatin appears to have the best therapeutic index of any regimen. A meta-analysis on the role of chemotherapy in non-small cell lung cancers suggested that the benefits are small.

What are the indications for radiotherapy?

- Pain – either local or metastatic.
- Breathlessness due to bronchial obstruction.
- Dysphagia.
- Haemoptysis.
- Superior venal caval obstruction.
- Pancoast's tumour.
- Before and after operation in selected patients.

What are the contraindications for surgery?

- Metastatic carcinoma.
- FEV_1 less than 1.5 litres.
- Transfer factor less than 50%.
- Severe pulmonary hypertension.

- Uncontrolled major cardiac arrhythmias.
- Carbon dioxide retention.
- Myocardial infarction in the past 3 months.

Is the progression of cancer associated with genetic change?

Yes: it is accompanied by a mutation in the p53 gene and loss of a portion of the short arm of chromosome 3 in small cell cancer; the functional significance of this is not clear.

Robert Souhami, Professor of Clinical Oncology, University College and Middlesex School of Medicine, London.

References

Non-small Cell Lung Cancer Collaborative Group (1995) Chemotherapy in non-small cell lung cancer: a meta-analysis using updated data on individual patients from 52 randomised trials. *Br Med J* **311**: 899–909.
Souhami R (1992) Lung cancer. *Br Med J* **304**: 1298.
Spiro G (1990) Management of lung cancer. *Br Med J* **301**: 1287.

CASE 105 Cystic Fibrosis

Instruction

Examine the chest of this male patient who has had a good appetite, poor weight gain and foul fatty stool.

Salient features

- Sputum is purulent.
- Patient is short of breath.
- Central cyanosis.
- Finger clubbing.
- Bilateral coarse crackles.

Proceed as follows:

- Tell the examiner that you would like to check the following levels:
    Urine sugar.
    Faecal fat.
    Sweat sodium.

Diagnosis

This patient has bilateral coarse crackles, asthenia and foul fatty stool (lesion) due to cystic fibrosis (aetiology) and requires continuous oxygen indicating respiratory failure (functional status).

Questions

What are the chances of this male patient having a child?

Males are sterile owing to the failure of development of the vas deferens and epididymis.

What are the clinical manifestations of this condition?

- Neonates: recurrent chest infections, failure to thrive, meconium ileus and rectal prolapse.
- In childhood and young adults:
    Respiratory: infection, bronchiectasis, pneumothorax, haemoptysis, nasal polyps, allergic bronchopulmonary aspergillosis, deterioration during and after pregnancy.
    Cardiovascular: cor pulmonale.
    Gastrointestinal: rectal prolapse, distal ileal obstruction (meconium ileus equivalent), cirrhosis, gallstones, intussusception.
    Miscellaneous: male infertility, diabetes mellitus, hypertrophic pulmonary osteoarthropathy.

How would you treat steatorrhoea?

- Low fat diet.
- Pancreatic supplements.
- H_2-receptor antagonist.

How would you treat chest complications?

- Postural drainage.
- Antibiotics.
- Bronchodilators.
- Heart–lung transplantantion.

What is the role of physiotherapy?

Physiotherapy has shown to be useful, but there remains considerable debate regarding the effectiveness of different techniques including traditional postural drainage and percussion, forced expiratory technique, positive expiratory pressure masks, autodrainage and flutter valves.

Advanced-level Questions

What is the inheritance in cystic fibrosis?

Autosomal recessive. On the long arm of chromosome 7 resides the gene coding for a 1480-amino-acid protein, now called the cystic fibrosis transmembrane conductor regulator (CFTR). This gene is carried by 1 in 20 Caucasians and its incidence is about 1 in 2000 live births. There is a mutation on the long arm of chromosome 7 in 70% of patients. There is a deletion of the codon for phenylalanine at position 508 (Δ508). This defect leads to a failure of the chloride channel to open in response to cyclic AMP. More than 175 other types of lesion in the cystic fibrosis gene are responsible for the disease in the remaining 30% of patients.

How is this condition diagnosed in infancy?

Immunoreactive trypsin assay in dried blood.

What do you know about sweat testing?

A sweat sodium concentration over 60 mmol l^{-1} is indicative of cystic fibrosis. It identifies over 75% by the age of 2 years and about 95% by the age of 12 years. It is more difficult to interpret in older children and adults.

What is the basic defect in the airways of these patients?

The opening of chloride channels at the luminal surface of the airway epithelial cells in normal individuals allows the passive transport of chloride along an electrochemical gradient from the cytoplasm to the lumen. In patients with cystic fibrosis there is a defect in these channels which prevents the normal secretion of chloride into the airway lumen. Simultaneously, there is a threefold increase in the reabsorption of sodium from the airway lumen into the cytoplasm of the epithelial cell. As the movement of water into airway secretions follows the movement of salt, it is believed that a decreased secretion of chloride into the airway lumen and the increased reabsorption of sodium from the airway lumen combine to reduce water content and increase the viscosity and tenacity of the airway secretions.

If the patient has persistent purulent cough which organisms are usually responsible?

Staphylococcus aureus, Haemophilus influenzae, Burkholderia cepacia and *Pseudomonas aeruginosa*. The latter is associated with poor prognosis as this organism is almost impossible to eradicate.

Which antibiotics are usually used to treat pseudomonal infections?

Intravenous or aerosol carbenicillin and gentamicin in combination.

What is the risk of cancer in patients with cystic fibrosis?

The overall risk of cancer is similar to that of the general population, but there is an increased risk of digestive tract cancers. Persistent or unexplained gastrointestinal symptoms in these patients ought to be investigated carefully.

What is the life span in such patients?

The median age of survival is currently in the early 30s. It is estimated that at least half of those with cystic fibrosis will be adults by the year 2000.

What is the cause of death in cystic fibrosis?

Death occurs from pulmonary complications, such as pneumonia, pneumothorax or haemoptysis, or as a result of terminal chronic respiratory failure.

What parameters can predict death in cystic fibrosis?

Prediction of death within 2 years can be made for 50% of the patients whose forced expiratory volume in 1 second (FEV_1) is less than 30%. Thus the necessity for referral for transplantation can be anticipated about 1 year in advance of death.

How would you manage a patient who has been accepted for transplantation?

The aim is to sustain life by aggressive therapy with nocturnal oxygen, continuous intravenous antibiotics, enteral feeding, respiratory stimulants and nasal intermittent positive pressure ventilation.

If this patient requires lung transplantation, which type of transplantation is the treatment of choice?

Bilateral lung transplantation is necessary for patients with chronic bronchial infection such as cystic fibrosis (or bronchiectasis) to avoid contamination of the donor lung by spill-over of infected material from the recipient's remaining lung.

What are the complications of lung transplantation?

Early post-transplantation lung oedema, infection and rejection (including obliterative bronchiolitis).

What are the indications for a combined heart – lung transplantation?

The combined heart–lung transplantation has relatively few indications, the primary one being congenital heart disease with Eisenmenger's syndrome.

What are the new methods of treatment available?

- High-dose ibuprofen in patients with mild disease (FEV_1 of at least 60% of the predicted value), taken consistently for 4 years, significantly slows the progression of lung disease without serious adverse effects.
- Aerosolized recombinant human DNAse, which is capable of degrading DNA in the bronchial secretion, has been shown to improve forced expiratory flow rates when given by aerosol.
- Gene therapy: the gene is transferred in a 'carrier' (either in a cationic lipid envelope known as a liposome, or in an adenovirus). On transferring the gene for cystic fibrosis to the nasal epithelium using a cationic liposome, the deficit was partly restored without provoking a local inflammatory response.
- Improvement of the hydration of secretion:
  - a) By blocking the reabsorption of sodium from the airway lumen with amiloride.
  - b) By stimulating the secretion of chloride with triphosphate nucleotides (ATP or uridine triphosphate) through nucleotide receptors by a pathway independent of cylic AMP metabolism.
- Immunization to various components of *Pseudomonas*.

What advice would you give a patient with cystic fibrosis who wishes to become pregnant?

- The couple will be offered genetic counselling and the man will be offered testing to determine his genetic status. If he is a carrier, chorionic villous sampling will be considered as the risk of the couple conceiving an infant with cystic fibrosis is 1 in 2 and they may wish to consider selective termination in the first trimester. The hazards of general anaesthesia (as lung function is impaired) for termination of pregnancy will be brought to their attention. Termination of pregnancy either with spinal anaesthesia or medications is an alternative.

- Women with severe disease will be informed that they may be unable to complete pregnancy and that their premature demise may leave a motherless child.
- In women with an FEV_1 less than 60% of the predicted value there is an increased risk of premature delivery, an increased rate of caesarean section, some loss of lung function and risk of respiratory complications, and early death of the mother.
- Pregnancy after heart–lung transplantation offers better health and increased longevity in the mother, but the risk of organ rejection and exposure of the fetus to potentially teratogenic immunosuppressants means that pregnancy should not be attempted by women with transplants.

What is the 'forme fruste' of cystic fibrosis?

Increasingly, with the availability of neonatal screening with immuno-reactive trypsin and thorough diagnosis by genetic studies, milder forms of disease have been recognized without the increase in sweat sodium. It is predicted that a considerable number will present with a pattern of disease in adult life that has not been recognized in the past as being due to cystic fibrosis.

Sir Magdi H Yacoub, contemporary Egyptian-born cardiothoracic surgeon at Harefield Hospital, London, popularized cardiac transplantation in the UK.
The first successful pregnancy in a woman with cystic fibrosis was reported in 1960.

References

Caplen NJ, Alton EW, Middleton PG et al (1995) Liposome-mediated CFTR gene transfer to the nasal epithelium in patients with cystic fibrosis. *Nature Medicine* **1**: 39–46.

Collins FS (1992) Cystic fibrosis: molecular biology and therapeutic implications. *Science* **256**: 774–779.

Davis PB (1991) Cystic fibrosis from bench to bedside. *N Engl J Med* **325**: 575–577.

Edenborough FP, Stableforth DE & Mackenzie WE (1995) Pregnancy in women with cystic fibrosis. *Br Med J* **311**: 822–823.

Fuchs HL, Borowitz DS, Christiansen DH et al for the Pulmozyme Study Group (1994) Effect of aerosolized recombinant human DNAse on exacerbations of respiratory symptoms and on pulmonary function in patients with cystic fibrosis. *N Engl J Med* **331**: 637–642.

Hodson ME, Madden BP, Steven MH, Tsang VT & Yacoub MH (1991) Non-invasive mechanical ventilation for cystic fibrosis patients – a potential bridge to transplantation. *Eur Respir J* **4**: 524–527.

Kerem E, Corey M, Kerem B et al (1990) The relation between genotype and phenotype in cystic fibrosis – analysis of the most common mutation (D508). *N Engl J Med* **323**: 1517.

Kerem E, Reisman J, Corey M, Canney GJ & Levison H (1992) Prediction of mortality in patients with cystic fibrosis. *N Engl J Med* **326**: 1187–1191.

Knowles MR, Clarke LL & Boucher RC (1991) Activation by extracellular nucleotides of chloride secretion in the airway epithelia of patients with cystic fibrosis. *N Engl J Med* **322**: 1189–1194.

Konstan MW, Byard PJ, Hoppel CL & Davis PB (1995) Effect of high-dose ibuprofen in patients with cystic fibrosis. *N Engl J Med* **332**: 848–854.

Neglia JP and the Cystic Fibrosis and Cancer Study Group (1995) The risk of cancer among patients with cystic fibrosis. *N Engl J Med* **332**: 494–499.

Ramirez JC, Patterson GA, Winton TL et al (1992) Bilateral lung transplantation for cystic fibrosis. *J Thorac Cardiovasc Surg* **103**: 287–294.

CASE 106 Fibrosing Alveolitis

Instruction

Examine this patient's chest.
Examine the respiratory system from the back.

Salient features

- Clubbing.
- Central cyanosis.
- Bilateral, basal, fine, end-inspiratory crackles which disappear or become quieter on leaning forwards. Furthermore, the crackles do not disappear on coughing (unlike those of pulmonary oedema). The crackles have been called 'Velcro' or 'Cellophane' crackles.
- Tachypnoea (in advanced cases).

Proceed as follows:

- Examine the following:
  Hands (for rheumatoid arthritis, systemic sclerosis).
  Face (for typical rash of SLE, heliotropic rash of dermatomyositis, typical facies of systemic sclerosis, lupus pernio of sarcoid).
  Mouth (for aphthous ulcers of Crohn's disease, dry mouth of Sjögren's syndrome).
  (Talk during this examination step so that the examiner knows what you are looking for.)
- Look for signs of pulmonary hypertension: 'a' wave in the JVP, left parasternal heave and P_2.
- Tell the examiner that you would like to take a drug history (amiodarone, nitrofurantoin and busulphan).

Diagnosis

This patient has bilateral, basal, fine, end-inspiratory crackles (lesion) due to fibrosing alveolitis (aetiology) and is tachypnoeic at rest (functional status).

Questions

In which other conditions is clubbing associated with crackles?

- Bronchogenic carcinoma (crackles are localized).
- Bronchiectasis (coarse crackles).
- Asbestosis (history of exposure to asbestos).

Advanced-level Questions

Mention other conditions which have similar pulmonary changes.

- Rheumatoid arthritis, SLE, dermatomyositis, chronic active hepatitis, ulcerative colitis, systemic sclerosis.
- Pneumoconiosis.
- Granulomatous disease: sarcoid, TB.
- Chronic pulmonary oedema.
- Radiotherapy.
- Lymphangitis carcinomatosa.
- Extrinsic allergic alveolitis: farmer's lung, bird fancier's lung.

What is the pathology in fibrosing alveolitis?

Fibrosing alveolitis is characterized by the presence of connective tisse matrix proteins within the acinar regions of the lung in association with a variable cellular infiltrate within the alveoli and in the interstitium.

What are the types of interstitial pneumonitis?

Liebow and Carrington in 1969 described five subgroups depending on histology:
- Classical (usual) interstitial pneumonia (UIP), characterized by thickening of the alveolar interstitium by fibrous tissue and mononuclear cells; characteristically varying in severity from one focus to another.
- Desquamative interstitial pneumonia (DIP) where there is a marked accumulation of macrophages in the alveolar airspaces associated with a relatively mild but uniform thickening of the interstitial space caused by mononuclear inflammatory cells.

- A diffuse lesion similar to UIP but with superimposed bronchiolitis obliterans.
- Lymphoid interstitial pneumonia (LIP) in which there is marked infiltration of interstitium by lymphocytes that may be indistinguishable from lymphoma.
- Giant-cell interstitial pneumonia consisting of a mononuclear cell infiltrate in the interstitium associated with large numbers of multinucleated giant cells.

How would you investigate this patient?

- CXR typically shows bilateral basal reticulonodular shadows which progress upwards as the disease progresses. In advanced cases there is marked destruction of the parenchyma, causing 'honeycombing' (due to groups of closely set ring shadows), and nodular shadows are not conspicuous. The mediastinum may appear broad as a result of a decrease in lung volume.
- Blood gases: arterial desaturation worsens while upright and improves on recumbency. There is arterial hypoxaemia and *hypocapnia*.
- Pulmonary function tests: in the early stages lung volumes may be normal, but there is arterial desaturation following exercise. Typically there is a restrictive defect with reduction of both the gas transfer factor and gas transfer coefficient.
- High ESR; raised immunoglobulins; raised antinuclear factor; rheumatoid factor is positive.
- Bronchial lavage: a large number of lymphocytes indicates a good response to steroids and a good prognosis. A large number of neutrophils and eosinophils indicates a poor prognosis (5-year survival rate of 60% for to steroid responders versus 25% for nonresponders). The patients are more likely to respond to cyclophosphamide if the number of neutrophils is increased.
- Lung biopsy: in early stages there is mononuclear cell infiltration in the alveolar walls, progressing to interstitial fibrosis – known as usual interstitial pneumonitis (UIP); in later stages fibrotic contraction of the lung, honeycombing, bronchial dilatation and cysts are seen. DIP – alveolar macrophages with little mononuclear infiltration or fibrosis – has a better prognosis than UIP as it responds to steroids.
- MRI is useful in determining disease activity without ionizing radiation but it is an expensive method.
- High-resolution CT is useful to assess the pattern and extent of disease. Patients with a predominantly ground-glass appearance are treated whereas those with a predominantly reticular appearance undergo technetium diethylenetriamine penta-acetate scanning to assess the probability of deterioration.

- Technetium-99m diethylenetriamine penta-acetate scanning in non-smokers is of value in identifying which patients are more likely to deteriorate. Therapy can be postponed when there is slow clearance, whereas those with fast clearance should receive treatment.

Mention some prognostic factors.

Short duration of disease, young age of patient at onset, and presence of little fibrosis on lung biopsies are good prognostic factors.

How would you manage this patient?

- All patients should receive a course of steroids (unless there are contraindications): prednisolone 40 mg per day for 6 weeks. Monitor symptoms, CXR, lung function tests. If response is good, continue; if no response then taper over 1 week.
- Steroid non-responders may benefit from a course of cyclophosphamide. Occasionally, patients who are unresponsive to prednisolone and cyclophosphamide will respond to prednisolone and azathioprine.
- Identify the underlying cause and manage accordingly.

What is the prognosis?

The 5-year overall survival rate is 50%, 65% in steroid responders and 25% in steroid non-responders.

What are the causes of death in such patients?

- Respiratory failure or cor pulmonale precipitated by chest infection.
- Tenfold increase in bronchogenic carcinoma compared with normal controls.

What is the role for lung transplantation?

Single lung transplantation is now an established and effective form of treatment for certain individuals. Current survival rate at 1 year is approximately 60%.

What do you know about the Hamman—Rich syndrome?

The Hamman–Rich syndrome is a rapidly progressive and fatal variant of interstitial lung disease described by Hamman and Rich.

Mention indications for transbronchial and open lung biopsy?

- Transbronchial: sarcoidosis, tuberculosis, berylliosis, lymphangitis carcinomatosa, extrinsic allergic alveolitis.
- Open lung biopsy: fibrosing alveolitis, rheumatological disease, pulmonary vasculitis, lymphangioleiomyomatosis, Langerhan's cell histiocytosis.

LV Hamman (1877–1946), physician, and AR Rich (1893–1968), pathologist, worked at the Johns Hopkins Hospitals, Baltimore.

Dame Margaret Turner-Warwick, contemporary chest physician, was the first woman President of the Royal College of the Physicians of London; her chief interest is fibrotic lung disease.

References

Fulmer JD (1982) An introduction to the interstitial lung disease. *Clin Chest Med* **3**: 457.

Hamman L & Rich AR (1944) Acute diffuse interstitial fibrosis of the lungs. *Bull Johns Hopkins Hosps* **74**: 177.

Liebow AA & Carrington CB (1969) The interstitial pneumonias. In: Simon M, Potchen EJ, LeMay M (eds) *Frontiers of Pulmonary Radiology*, pp. 102–141. New York: Grune and Stratton.

McFadden RG, Carr TJ & Wood TE (1987) Proton magnetic resonance imaging to stage activity of interstitial lung disease. *Chest* **92**: 31.

Tenholder MF, Russel MD, Knight E et al (1987) Orthodexia: a new finding in interstitial fibrosis. *Am Rev Respir Dis* **136**: 170.

Toronto Lung Transplant Group (1986) Unilateral lung transplantation for pulmonary fibrosis. *N Engl J Med* **314**: 1140–1145.

Turner-Warwick M & Haslam PL (1987) The value of serial bronchoalveolar lavages in assessing clinical progress of patients with cryptogenic fibrosing alveolitis. *Am Rev Respir Dis* **135**: 26.

Turner-Warwick M, Lebowitz M, Burrows B & Johnson A (1980) Cryptogenic fibrosing alveolitis and lung cancer. *Thorax* **35**: 496.

Wells AU, Hansell DM, Harrison NK, Lawrence R, Black CM & du Bois RM (1993) Clearance of inhaled 99m-Tc DTPA predicts the clinical course of fibrosing alveolitis. *Eur Respir J* **6**: 797–802.

CASE 107 Pulmonary Fibrosis

Instruction

Examine this patient's chest.

Salient features

- The fibrosis is usually apical.

- Flattening of the chest on the affected side.
- Tracheal deviation to the affected side.
- Reduced expansion on the affected side.
- Dull percussion note.
- Presence of localized crackles; bronchial breathing may be present.

Proceed as follows:

- Look for the following signs:
     Scars of phrenic nerve crush, plombage, thoracotomy.
     Radiation scars.

Diagnosis

This patient has flattening of the R/L side of the chest with diminished movements on that side, tracheal deviation and localized crackles (lesion) due to pulmonary fibrosis secondary to tuberculosis (aetiology), and is comfortable at rest (functional status).

Questions

Mention a few causes of upper lobe fibrosis.

- Tuberculosis.
- Ankylosing spondylitis.
- Radiation-induced fibrosis.

Advanced-level Questions

Which is the best imaging procedure for the upper lobe lesions?

MRI is better for upper lobe lesions than CT of the chest.

What is the role of MRI of the thorax?

MRI of the thorax is less useful than CT scanning because of poorer imaging of the pulmonary parenchyma and inferior spatial resolution. However, MRI can provide images in multiple planes (e.g. sagittal, coronal as well as transverse) which CT cannot. MRI is excellent for evaluating processes near the lung apex, spine and thoracoabdominal junction.

On 8 November 1895 Röntgen discovered what he called X-rays. In the subsequent 7 weeks he meticulously performed experiments, and an X-ray picture of his wife's hand convinced him about the potential role of the new ray. In 1901 he was awarded the Nobel Prize for physics.

Hounsfield's work on CT in the EMI laboratories at Hounslow made it possible to obtain detailed cross-sectional views of the soft tissues, particularly brain. Sir Godfrey N Hounsfield (1919–) and Alan M Cormack (1924–), the latter of Tufts University, Boston, were jointly awarded the 1979 Nobel Prize for Medicine for the development of computer-assisted tomography.

CASE 108 Pneumothorax

Instruction

Examine this patient's chest.

Salient features

- Decreased movement of the affected side.
- Trachea may be central (small pneumothorax) or deviated to the affected side (underlying collapse of lung) or the opposite side (large pneumothorax).
- Increased vocal resonance with diminished breath sounds.

Proceed as follows:

- Look for clues regarding aetiology:
  Pleural aspiration site.
  Infraclavicular region for a bruise of the central line.
  Comment if the patient is thin or has marfanoid features.
  Inhaler or peak flow meter by the bedside (asthma, COAD).
- Tell the examiner that you would like to take a history of wheeze (bronchial asthma, COAD).

Diagnosis

This patient has diminished breath sounds and hyper-resonant note on R/L side of the chest (lesion) due to pneumothorax secondary to Marfan's syndrome (aetiology), and is not breathless at rest (functional status).

Questions

What do you understand by the term 'pneumothorax'?

Air in the pleural cavity.

How would you investigate this patient?

- CXR, both inspiratory and expiratory.
- Blood gases if the patient is breathless.

Advanced-level Questions

How would you grade the degree of collapse?

British Thoracic Society of grading:
- Small: where there is a small rim of air around the lung.
- Moderate: when the lung is collapsed towards the heart border.
- Complete: airless lung, separate from the diaphragm (aspiration is necessary).
- Tension: any pneumothorax with cardiorespiratory distress (rare and requires immediate drainage).

How would you manage this patient?

- Small pneumothoraces (less than 20% in size) spontaneously resolve within weeks.
- Larger ones (irrespective of size) with normal lungs are managed by simple aspiration rather than an intercostal tube as the initial drainage procedure. Aspiration is less painful than intercostal drainage, leads to a shorter admission and reduces the need for pleurectomy with no increase in recurrence rate at 1 year.
- When there is rapid re-expansion following simple aspiration, an intercostal tube with underwater seal drainage is used. The tube should be left in for at least 24 hours. When the lung re-expands, clamp the tube for 24 hours. If repeat radiography shows that the lung remains expanded, the tube can be removed. If not, suction should be applied to the tube. If it fails to resolve within 1 week, surgical pleurodesis should be considered.

What are the causes of pneumothorax?

- Spontanenous (usually in thin males).
- Trauma.
- Bronchial asthma.
- COAD – emphysematous bulla.
- Carcinoma of the lung.
- Cystic fibrosis.
- TB.
- Mechanical ventilation.
- Marfan's syndrome, Ehlers–Danlos syndrome.

- Catamenial pneumothorax, i.e. pneumothorax that occurs in association with menstruation.

How would you do a pleurodesis?

By injecting talc into the pleural cavity via the intercostal tube.

In which patients would you avoid doing a pleurodesis?

In patients with underlying cystic fibrosis. These patients may require lung transplantation in the future and pleurodesis may make this procedure technically not feasible.

When would you suspect a tension pneumothorax?

Tension pneumothorax should be suspected in the presence of any of the following:
- Severe progressive dyspnoea.
- Severe tachycardia.
- Hypotension.
- Marked mediastinal shift.

When should open thoracotomy be considered?

It should be considered if there is one of the following present:
- A third episode of spontanenous pneumothorax.
- Any occurrence of bilateral pneumothorax.
- Failure of the lung to expand after tube thoracostomy for the first episode.

OK Williamson (1866–1941), an English physician, described the Williamson sign, i.e. blood pressure in the leg is lower than that in the upper limb on the affected side in pneumothorax.
The use of simple aspiration to manage pneumothorax was first reported by OG Raja in 1981 when he was a medical registrar.

References

Harvey J, Prescott RJ & The British Thoracic Society (1994) Simple aspiration versus intercostal tube drainage for management of spontaneous pneumothorax in patients with normal lungs. *Br Med J* **309**: 1338–1339.

Miller KS & Sahn SA (1987) Chest tubes: indications, techniques, management and complications. *Chest* **91**: 258.

Miller AC, Harvey JE & The British Thoracic Society. (1993) Guidelines for the management of spontaneous pneumothorax. *Br Med J* **307**: 114–115.

Raja OG & Lalor AJ (1981) Simple aspiration of spontaneous pneumothorax. *Br J Dis Chest* **75**: 207–208.

Spencer Jones J (1985) A place for aspiration in the treatment of spontaneous pneumothorax. *Thorax* **40**: 66–67.

Wong PS (1993) Never clamp a chest drain. *Br Med J* **307**: 443.

CASE 109 Old Tuberculosis

Instruction

Examine this patient's chest.

Salient features

These patients tend to have signs of common chest diseases which are not cut and dried. There are several reasons for this, such as pleural thickening, thoracotomy and pneumonectomy, associated COAD, associated chest infection, plombage or phrenic nerve crush.

Following are some examples:

Patient 1
The candidate was asked to examine the chest from the front, as a result of which the old thoracotomy scar was not seen. The patient was wheezy. The trachea was deviated to the right. Percussion note was stony dull from the right second intercostal space downwards. Wheeze was present on the left side. This patient had a right pneumonectomy with COAD in the left lung. The candidate's diagnosis of right-sided pleural effusion with underlying collapse and left-sided COAD was accepted.

Patient 2
The trachea was central. A phrenic nerve crush scar was seen. Percussion note was dull in the left infra-axillary region and there were associated crackles. The diagnosis of pleural thickening with associated chest infection was accepted; that of pleural effusion was not.

Questions

How would you manage a patient with old tuberculosis?

Old tuberculosis requires no antituberculosis treatment. However, the patient may require symptomatic treatment for wheeze and shortness of breath.

In which groups of patients is the risk of tuberculosis high?

- Asian and Irish immigrants.
- The elderly.
- Immunocompromised individuals, particularly AIDS patients.
- Alcoholics.
- Occupations at risk: doctors, nurses, chest physiotherapists.

Advanced-level Questions

Would you isolate a patient with newly diagnosed, sputum-positive, pulmonary TB?

Yes. Segregation in a single room for 2 weeks is recommended for patients with smear-positive tuberculosis. Barrier nursing, however, is unnecessary. Adults with smear-negative or non-pulmonary disease may be in a general ward. A child with TB should be segregated until the source case is identified as this person may be visiting the child.

How are contacts investigated?

Contacts are investigated by inquiry into bacille Calmette–Guérin (BCG) vaccination site, Heaf testing and CXR examination.

To whom would you offer BCG vaccination?

BCG vaccination is offered to previously unvaccinated, persistently Heaf test-negative or grade 1 contacts aged under 35 years unless there is a special occupational, travel or ethnic risk. Patients with known or suspected HIV infection should not be offered the vaccination.

What are the indications for chemoprophylaxis?

- Chemoprophylaxis may be given to those with strongly positive Heaf test reactions but no clinical or radiological evidence of TB.
- Chemoprophylaxis should be given to children under 5 years who are close contacts of a smear-positive adult irrespective of their tuberculin test result.
- If chemoprophylaxis is not undertaken, follow-up with periodic CXR examinations for 2 years is recommended in all these groups.

Which rapid test allows early diagnosis of tuberculosis?

Polymerase chain reaction (PCR).

Robert Koch (1843–1910), Institute for Infectious Diseases, Berlin, was awarded the 1905 Nobel Prize for Medicine for his investigations and discoveries in relation to tuberculosis.

Kary Mullis of the USA was awarded the Nobel Prize for developing the technique of polymerase chain reaction.

Reference

British Thoracic Society (1994) Control and prevention of tuberculosis in the United Kingdom: Code of practice 1994. *Thorax* **49**: 1193–1200.

CASE 110 Pickwickian Syndrome

Instruction

Look at this patient.

Salient features

- Obese patient who is plethoric and cyanosed.
- Short of breath at rest.
- May be nodding off to sleep.

Proceed as follows:

- Look for signs of pulmonary hypertension and right heart failure.
- Tell the examiner that you would like to take a history of the following:
  Snoring.
  Daytime somnolence.
  Headache.
  Poor concentration.

Diagnosis

This patient has marked obesity and hypersomnolence with signs of pulmonary hypertension (lesion) which indicate she has pickwickian syndrome. The patient is in cardiac failure (functional status).

Advanced-level Questions

What is the cause of cyanosis in such a patient?

A mixture of obstructive apnoea and sleep-induced hypoventilation. The blood gas picture is hypoxia and carbon dioxide retention.

Where is the obstruction?

It is caused by the apposition of the tongue and the palate of the posterior pharyngeal wall.

How would you treat such a patient?

- Weight reduction.
- Avoidance of smoking and alcohol.
- Progesterone (enhances respiratory drive).
- Continuous nasal positive airway pressure delivered by a nasal mask.

Mr Pickwick is a character in the novel *Pickwick Papers*, written by Charles Dickens, and this term was applied by Sir William Osler.

References

Semple SJG & Gibson GJ (1993) Sleep apnoea and related conditions: summary of a report of a working party of the Royal College of Physicians. *J R Coll Phys (Lond)* **27**: 363–364.

Toff NJ (1993) Hazards of air travel for the obese: Miss Pickwick and the Boeing 747. *J R Coll Phys (Lond)* **27**: 375.

CASE III **Collapsed Lung**

Instruction

Examine this patient's chest.

Salient features

- Trachea deviated to the affected side.
- Movements decreased on the affected side.
- Percussion note dull on the affected side.
- Breath sounds diminished on the affected side.

Proceed as follows:

- Tell the examiner that you would like to look for tar staining (tobacco smoking), clubbing and cachexia (bronchogenic carcinoma; see page 285).

Diagnosis

This patient has a collapsed lung (lesion); you would like to exclude malignancy (aetiology). He is breathless at rest (functional status).

Questions

What are the causes of lung collapse?

These include:
- Bronchogenic carcinoma.
- Mucus plugs (asthma, allergic bronchopulmonary aspergillosis).
- Extrinsic compression from hilar adenopathy (e.g. primary TB).
- Tuberculosis (Brock's syndrome).
- Other intrabronchial tumours including bronchial adenoma.

What are the chest X-ray findings of collapse of the right middle lobe?

The loss of definition of the right heart border reflects collapse (or consolidation) affecting the right middle lobe.

What is Brock's syndrome?

It is collapse due to compression of the right middle lobe bronchus by an enlarged lymph node.

Sir Russel C Brock (1903–1980) graduated from Guy's Hospital and was surgeon at Guy's and Brompton Hospitals. His interests included both thoracic and cardiac surgery. He was the President of the Royal College of Surgeons, 1963–1966.

Reference

Berkin KE, Vernon DRH & Kerr JW (1982) Lung collapse caused by allergic bronchopulmonary aspergillosis in non-asthmatic patients. *Br Med J* **285**: 552.

ABDOMEN

EXAMINATION OF THE ABDOMEN

1. Ensure the patient is lying flat (remove any extra pillows, if present, with the permission of the patient); the hands should lie by his or her side with the abdomen exposed from the inframammary region to just above the genitalia. Do not expose the genitalia.

2. Begin with the hands, looking for the following signs:
   - Clubbing, leuconychia (white chalky nails).
   - Palmar erythema.
   - Duputryen's contracture (feel for thickening of the fascia).
   - Hepatic flap.

3. Examine the arms:
   - Look for arteriovenous fistula, haemodialysis catheters, spider naevi.

4. Comment on the skin:
   - Pigmentation.
   - Scratch marks.

5. Examine the following:
   - Supraclavicular and cervical lymph nodes.
   - Tongue for pallor.
   - Eyes for anaemia, jaundice, xanthelasma.
   - Upper chest and face for spider naevi.
   - Axilla for hair loss, acanthosis nigricans.
   - Breast for gynaecomastia.

6. Inspect the abdomen, looking for the following signs:
   - Movements.
   - Any obvious mass.
   - Visible veins (check direction of flow, which is usually away from the umbilicus).
   - Visible peristalsis.

- Hernial orifices (ask the patient to cough at this stage).
- Expansile pulsations of aortic aneurysm.

7. Ask the patient whether the abdomen is sore at any part.

8. Palpation: kneel on the floor or sit on a chair before you begin palpation. At all times look at the patient's eyes to check whether he or she winces in pain. Begin with superficial pain and begin in the least tender area. Palpate in all the quadrants (remember that there are four quadrants).

9. Palpate:
   - For mass – determine its characteristics.
   - Liver (percuss for upper border using heavy percussion, for lower border using light percussion).
   - Kidneys (bimanual palpation, demonstrate ballottement).
   - Groin for lymph nodes.
   - Check hernial orifices.
   - Test for expansile pulsation of an aortic aneurysm.

10. Percuss, looking for shifting dullness (at this stage, when the patient is lying on his or her right side, seize the opportunity to examine for a small spleen and for pitting oedema over the sacral region). Remember that abdominal percussion should follow adequate inspection and percussion.

11. Auscultate:
    - Over an enlarged liver for bruit.
    - Over a suspected aortic aneurysm.
    - For bowel sounds.

12. Tell the examiner that you would like to perform a rectal examination and examine the external genitalia.

13. Examine the legs for oedema.

CASE 112 Hepatomegaly

Instruction

Examine this patient's abdomen.

Salient features

- Enlarged liver: comment on its size, tenderness, surface (smooth or irregular); percuss the upper border (normally in the fifth intercostal space in the right mid-clavicular line) and auscultate for bruit.

Note. By percussion, the mean liver size is 7 cm for women and 10.5 cm for men. A liver span 2–3 cm larger or smaller than these values is considered abnormal. The liver size depends on several factors including age, sex, body size, shape and the examination technique utilized (e.g. palpation versus percussion versus radiographic).

Proceed as follows:

- Look for the following signs:
  Spleen for ascites.
  Signs of cirrhosis.
  Lymph nodes.
  Raised JVP.
- At this stage you may be asked to look for nervous system signs of alcoholism (peripheral neuropathy, proximal myopathy, cerebellar syndrome, bilateral sixth cranial nerve palsy as in Wernicke's encephalopathy, recent memory loss and confabulation in Korsakoff's psychosis).

Diagnosis

This patient has a nodular, hard hepatomegaly (lesion) which indicates secondaries in the liver. I would like to look for a primary, particularly in the gastrointestinal tract (aetiology).

Questions

What does a tender liver indicate?

A stretch of its capsule due to a *recent* enlargement, as in cardiac failure or acute hepatitis.

What are the common causes of a palpable liver in the UK?

- Cardiac failure (firm, smooth, tender, mild to massive enlargement).
- Cirrhosis (non-tender, firm; in later stages the liver decreases in size).
- Secondaries in the liver (enlarged with rock-hard or nodular consistency).

Advanced-level Questions

Mention some less common causes of hepatomegaly.

- Leukaemia and other reticuloendothelial disorders.
- Infections – glandular fever, infectious hepatitis.
- Primary biliary cirrhosis.
- Haemochromatosis.
- Sarcoid, amyloid.
- Tumours – hepatoma, hydatid cysts.

Note. The liver may be felt without being enlarged in the following circumstances: increased diaphragmatic descent, presence of emphysema with an associated depressed diaphragm, thin body habitus with a narrow thoracic cage, presence of a palpable Riedel's lobe and right-sided pleural effusion.

In which condition does a pulsatile liver occur?

Tricuspid regurgitation.

What does a hepatic arterial bruit over the liver indicate?

The hepatic arterial bruit has been described in alcoholic hepatitis, primary or metastatic carcinoma. Although reported to occur in cirrhosis, it is rare without associated alcoholic hepatitis.

What does the presence of an abdominal venous hum indicate?

It is virtually diagnostic of portal venous hypertension (usually due to cirrhosis). When present together with the hepatic arterial bruit in the same patient, it suggests cirrhosis with either alcoholic hepatitis or cancer.

What do you know about Cruveilhier-Baumgarten syndrome?

It is the presence of the abdominal venous hum in portal hypertension secondary to cirrhosis.

What does a hepatic friction rub indicate?

In a young woman it could be due to gonococcal perihepatitis (Fitz–Hugh–Curtis syndrome) and in others it could indicate hepatic neoplasm with inflammatory changes or infection in or adjacent to the liver. The presence of a hepatic rub with a bruit usually indicates cancer of the liver, whereas the presence of the hepatic rub, bruit and abdominal venous hum indicates that a patient with cirrhosis has developed a hepatoma.

Dame Sheila Sherlock, Emeritus Professor of Medicine, Royal Free Hospital, London, is a doyen of liver diseases.
Hans Popper (1903–1988), Professor of Pathology at Chicago and the founding dean of Mount Sinai School of Medicine in New York; he is regarded as the founding father of hepatology.
Howard Clarence Thomas, contemporary Professor of Medicine, St Mary's Hospital, London; his main interest is viral hepatitis.

References

Bloom HJG (1950) Venous hums in hepatic cirrhosis. *Br Heart J* **12**: 343–350.
Castell DO & Frank BB (1977) Abdominal examination: role of percussion and auscultation. *Postgrad Med* **62**: 131–134.
Castell DO, O'Brien DK, Myench H & Chalmers TC (1969) Estimation of liver size by percussion in normal individuals. *Ann Intern Med* **70**: 1183–1189.
Cheng TO, Sutton GC & Sutton DC (1954) Cruveilhier–Baumgarten syndrome. *Am J Med* **17**: 143–150.
Clain D, Wartnaby K & Sherlock S (1966) Abdominal arterial murmurs in liver disease. *Lancet* **ii**: 516–519.
Fred HL & Brown GR (1962) The hepatic friction rub. *N Engl J Med* **266**: 554–555.
Goldstein LT (1968) Enlarged tortuous arteries and hepatic bruit. *JAMA* **206**: 2518–2520.
Sherman HI & Hardison JE (1979) The importance of a coexistent hepatic rub and bruit. A clue to the diagnosis of cancer in the liver. *JAMA* **241**: 1495.
Simpson JA (1971) Liver friction rub. A useful sign in the diagnosis of hepatic metastases. *Am J Dig Dis* **16**: 39–40.

CASE 113   Cirrhosis of the Liver

Instruction

Examine this patient's abdomen.

Salient features

• In the hands:
  Clubbing, leuconychia.

      Dupuytren's contracture, palmar erythema.
      Spider naevi, tattoos, hepatic flap, pallor.
      Scratch marks, generalized pigmentation.
- Eyes and face:
  Icterus, cyanosis, parotid enlargement.
- Chest:
  Spider naevi, loss of axillary hair, gynaecomastia.
- Abdomen:
  Splenomegaly (seldom more than 5 cm below the costal margin).
  Ascites.
  Hepatomegaly (particularly in alcoholic liver disease).
- Leg oedema.

Diagnosis

This patient has spider naevi, gynaecomastia, splenomegaly, parotid enlargement (lesions) due to cirrhosis of the liver caused by alcohol abuse (aetiology). The patient has hepatic flap indicating liver cell failure (functional status).

Questions

What is cirrhosis?

Cirrhosis is defined pathologically as a diffuse liver abnormality characterized by fibrosis and abnormal regenerating nodules.

Mention a few causes of cirrhosis of the liver.

- Alcohol dependence.
- Hepatitis B virus infection (look for tattoos).
- Lupoid hepatitis.
- Primary biliary cirrhosis.
- Haemochromatosis.
- Drugs – methyldopa, amiodarone, methotrexate.
- Metabolic: Wilson's disease, α_1-antitrypsin deficiency.
- Cryptogenic.

How would you investigate this patient?

- FBC including haemoglobin and platelet count.
- Liver function tests including γ-glutamyl transpeptidase (GGT).
- Prothrombin time.
- Hepatitis B markers.
- Serum autoantibodies.

- Serum iron and ferritin.
- Serum α-fetoprotein.
- Ascitic fluid analysis.
- Ultrasonography of the liver.

Why does this patient have a low serum albumin concentration?

Albumin is synthesized in the liver and in cirrhosis there is liver cell failure, causing impaired synthesis.

What are the major sequelae of cirrhosis?

- Portal hypertension.
- Variceal haemorrhages.
- Hepatic encephalopathy.
- Ascites and spontaneous bacterial peritonitis.
- Hepatorenal syndrome.
- Coagulopathy.
- Hepatocellular carcinoma.

Advanced-level Questions

What are the poor prognostic factors?

- Encephalopathy.
- Low serum sodium concentration, less than 120 mmol l^{-1} (not due to diuretic therapy).
- Low serum albumin level, less than 25 g l^{-1}.
- Prolonged prothrombin time.

What factors can precipitate hepatic encephalopathy in a patient with previously well-compensated hepatic cirrhosis?

- Infection.
- Diuretics, electrolyte imbalance.
- Diarrhoea and vomiting.
- Sedatives.
- Upper gastrointestinal haemorrhage.
- Abdominal paracentesis.
- Surgery.

CASE 114   Jaundice

Instruction

Would you like to ask this patient (*Patient 1*) a few questions?

Salient features

Proceed as follows:

- Ask the patient about the following:
    His or her age (hepatitis is more common in the young and carcinoma in the elderly).
    Sore throat and rash (infectious mononucleosis).
    Occupation (Weil's disease in sewerage and farm workers).
    Contact with jaundice (hepatitis A).
    Drug history (oral contraceptives, phenothiazines).
    Blood transfusions, injections, arthritis, urticaria (hepatitis B).
    Alcohol consumption.
    Pruritus (cholestasis due to hepatitis A, primary biliary cirrhosis).
    Colour of the urine.
    Colour of the stools (pale stools in obstructive jaundice).
    Abdominal pain (cholecystitis, gallstones, cholangitis, carcinoma of the pancreas).
    Past history (recurrent jaundice, as in Dubin–Johnson syndrome).

Instruction

Would you like to examine this icteric patient (*Patient 2*)?

Salient features

Proceed as follows:

- Examine the following:
    Hands (clubbing, palmar erythema, Duputryen's contracture).
    Sclera (to confirm the icterus).
    Conjuctiva (for pallor).
    Neck (lymph nodes).
    Upper chest (spider naevi, loss of axillary hair and gynaecomastia).
    Abdomen (hepatomegaly, splenomegaly, Murphy's sign, palpable gallbladder, ascites).
    Legs (for pitting oedema).
- Tell the examiner that you would like to investigate as follows:

Examine the urine.

Do a per rectal examination.

Remember: the most important question to answer in the evaluation of any jaundiced patient is 'Will this patient require surgery to relieve biliary obstruction?'

Diagnosis

This patient is markedly icteric and has spider naevi and gynaecomastia (lesions) due to alcoholic liver disease (aetiology).

Questions

What do you understand by the term jaundice?

It is the yellowish discoloration of skin, sclera and mucous membrane due to the accumulation of bile pigments. It is usually clinically manifest when the serum bilirubin concentration is at least 7–8 mg dl^{-1}.

How would you differentiate jaundice from carotenaemia?

The discoloration of carotenaemia is differentiated from jaundice by the absence of yellow colour in the sclera and mucuous membranes, normal urine colour and the presence of yellow–brown pigmentation of carotenoid pigment in the palms, soles and nasolabial folds.

What is Murphy's sign and what does it indicate?

It is the tenderness elicited on palpation at the midpoint of the right subcostal margin on inspiration. It is a sign of cholecystitis.

Have you heard of Courvoisier's law?

It states that in a patient with obstructive jaundice a palpable gallbladder is unlikely to be due to chronic cholecystitis.

What is Charcot's fever?

Intermittent fever associated with jaundice and abdominal discomfort in a patient with cholangitis and biliary obstruction.

How would you investigate this patient?

- Urine for bile pigments.
- FBC.

- Serum haptoglobulin, reticulocyte count and Coomb's test (if you suspect haemolysis).
- Liver function tests (serum albumin, bilirubin, enzymes).
- Prothrombin time.
- Viral studies (hepatitis antigen and antibodies, Epstein–Barr virus antibodies).
- Ultrasonography of the abdomen (if you suspect cholestatic jaundice).
- Special investigations: mitochondrial antibodies, endoscopic retrograde cholangiopancreatography (ERCP), CT of the abdomen, liver biopsy.

Advanced-level Questions

What do you know about Dubin-Johnson syndrome?

It is a rare benign condition characterized by jaundice and pigmentation secondary to a failure of excretion of conjugated bilirubin. The liver is stained by melanin in the centrilobular zone. The bromsulphthalein test shows a late secondary rise at 90 minutes.

Mention a few causes of post-operative jaundice.

Causes of postoperative jaundice (usually occurring in the first 3 postoperative weeks) include:
- Resorption of haematomas, haemoperitoneum, haemolysis of transfused erythrocytes (particularly when stored blood products are used), haemolysis due to glucose-6-phosphate dehydrogenase deficiency.
- Impaired hepatocellular function due to halogenated anaesthetics, sepsis, hepatic ischaemia secondary to perioperative hypotension.
- Extrahepatic biliary obstruction due to biliary stones, unsuspected injury to biliary tree.

How does estimation of serum bilirubin concentration help in discerning the aetiology of jaundice?

Normal serum bilirubin concentration is no greater than 1.5 mg dl^{-1} and consists of predominantly unconjugated form. When jaundice is primarily due to haemolysis or a disorder of bilirubin conjugation, the unconjugated form is at least 85% of the total. With normal liver function, haemolysis alone does not produce a serum bilirubin level greater than 4 mg dl^{-1}. A rise in serum bilirubin levels of up to 2 mg dl^{-1} day^{-1} is compatible with extrahepatic cholestasis, but a greater rate indicates haemolysis, hepatitis or hepatic cell necrosis. The serum bilirubin level of patients with pure biliary obstruction seldom exceeds 30 mg dl^{-1}; a greater value indicates that there is associated hepatocellular jaundice as well.

A Gilbert (1858–1927), Professor of Medicine at l'Hôtel Dieu in Paris.

PSA Weil (1848–1916), Professor of Medicine in Tartu, Estonia and Berlin.

JB Murphy (1857–1916), Professor of Surgery at Northwestern University in Chicago.

J Courvoisier (1843–1918), Professor of Surgery, Basel, Switzerland.

IN Dubin, Professor of Pathology, Pennsylvania, and FB Johnson, pathologist, Veterans Adminstration Hospital, Washington.

CASE 115 Ascites

Instruction

Examine this patient's abdomen.

Salient features

- Full flanks, and umbilicus.
- Presence of shifting dullness (always percuss with your finger parallel to the level of fluid).
- If the ascites is gross, use the 'dipping' method of palpation to feel the liver and spleen.

Proceed as follows:

- Check for sacral oedema and swollen ankles.

Diagnosis

This patient has marked ascites and leg oedema with splenomegaly (lesions) due to portal hypertension, the cause of which needs to be investigated (aetiology).

Questions

What are the causes of a distended abdomen?

Fat, fluid, faeces, flatus and fetus.

What do you understand by the term ascites?

It is the pathological accumulation of fluid in the peritoneal cavity.

What are the common causes of ascitic fluid?

- Portal hypertension with cirrhosis.
- Abdominal malignancy.
- Congestive cardiac failure.

What investigations would you do to determine the underlying cause?

Diagnostic paracentesis for proteins and malignant cells, ultrasonography of the abdomen, peritoneal biopsy or laproscopy if the cause remains unclear.

What is the difference between an exudate and a transudate?

An exudate has a protein content of over 25 g l^{-1}.

Advanced-level Questions

What are the mechanisms of ascites formation in cirrhosis?

- It is due to a combination of liver failure and portal hypertension. Liver failure decreases renal blood flow, resulting in retention of salt and water.
- Secondary hyperaldosteronism due to increased renin release and decreased metabolism of aldosterone by the liver.
- Decreased metabolism of aldosterone by the liver.
- Decreased metabolism of antidiuretic hormone.
- Hypoalbuminaemia which decreases colloid oncotic pressure.
- Lymphatic obstruction, resulting in a 'weeping' liver.

What is the relation between ascites and chronic liver disease?

- Ascites indicates decompensation of previously asymptomatic chronic liver disease.
- Ascites occurs in about half of the patients within 10 years of a diagnosis of compensated cirrhosis.
- The development of fluid retention in patients with chronic liver disease is a poor prognostic sign – only half of these patients survive beyond 2 years.

What do you know about the serum – ascites albumin gradient?

It is calculated by subtracting the ascitic fluid albumin concentration from the serum albumin concentration from samples obtained at the same time. This gradient correlates directly with portal pressure; those whose gradient exceeds 1.1 g dl^{-1} have portal hypertension and those with gradients of less than 1.1 g dl^{-1} do not. The accuracy of such determinations is 97%.

How would you manage a patient with cirrhosis and ascites?

The most important treatments are sodium restriction and diuretics:
- Sodium restriction to 88 mmol per day; only 15% of these patients lose weight or have a reduction in ascitic fluid with this therapy alone.
- Fluid restriction is usually not necessary unless the serum sodium concentration drops below 120 mmol l^{-1}.
- When the patient has tense ascites, 5 litres or more of ascitic fluid should be removed to relieve shortness of breath, to diminish early satiety and to prevent pressure-related leakage of fluid from the site of a previous paracentesis.
- Diuretic therapy should be initiated immediately, before which the serum sodium concentration of a random urine sample should be measured. Serial monitoring of urinary sodium concentration helps to determine the optimal dose of diuretic; doses are increased until a negative sodium balance is achieved. The most effective diuretic regimen is a combination of spironolactone and frusemide. More than 90% of patients respond to this therapy.
- Diuretic-resistant ascites:
    Therapeutic paracentesis with infusion of salt-free albumin (reported to decrease hospital stay).
    Peritoneovenous shunting, e.g. Le Veen shunt, limited by the high rate of infection and disseminated intravascular coagulation.
    Transjugular intrahepatic portasystemic stent shunt (TIPS) is a non-surgical side-to-side shunt consisting of a stented channel between a main branch of the portal vein and the hepatic vein. The stent shunt is associated with an operative mortality rate of 1% compared with 5–39% for surgical shunts.
    Extracorporeal ultrafiltration of ascitic fluid with reinfusion.
    Liver transplantation.

What are the complications of ascites?

- Respiratory embarrassment may complicate large amounts of ascites.
- Spontaneous bacterial peritonitis is seen in cirrhotics (suspect when there is an ascitic fluid leukocyte count of 500 cells per μl, or more than 250 polymorphonuclear cells per μl; empirical therapy with a non-nephrotoxic broad-spectrum antibiotic should be initiated immediately).

Mention some uncommon causes for ascitic fluid.

- Nephrotic syndrome.
- Constrictive pericarditis.

- Tuberculous peritonitis.
- Chylous ascites.
- Budd–Chiari syndrome.
- Meigs' syndrome.

What do you know about the pathogenesis of ascites in cirrhotics?

Two theories have been proposed:
- Underfilling theory: this suggests that the primary abnormality is inappropriate sequestration of fluid within the splanchnic vascular bed due to portal hypertension. This results in a decrease in intravascular volume and the kidney responds by retaining salt and water.
- Overflow theory: this suggests that the primary abnormality is inappropriate retention of salt and water by the kidney in the absence of volume depletion.

G Budd (1808–1882), Professor of Medicine at King's College, London.
H Chiari (1851–1916), Professor of Pathology at the German University in Prague.
JV Meigs (1892–1963), Professor of Gynaecology at Harvard, Massachusetts General Hospital.
Le Veen, gastroenterologist at the Veterans Adminstration Hospital in New York.

References

Epstein FM (1982) Underfilling versus overfilling in hepatic ascites. *N Engl J Med* **307**: 1577.
Ochs A, Rössle M, Haag K et al (1995) The transjugular intrahepatic portosystemic stent–shunt procedure for refractory ascites. *N Engl J Med* **332**: 1192–1197.
Runyon BA (1994) Current concepts: care of patients with ascites. *N Engl J Med* **330**: 337–342.

CASE 116   Haemochromatosis

Instruction

Examine this patient's abdomen.
Look at this patient.

Salient features

- The patient is a pigmented male over 30 years of age.
- Palmar erythema, spider naevi.

- Jaundice.
- Ascites, hepatomegaly (firm, regular).
- Loss of secondary sexual hair.

Proceed as follows:

- Tell the examiner that you would like to investigate as follows:
    Look for testicular atrophy (due to iron deposition affecting hypothalamopituitary function).
    Take a history of joint pain (present in 50% of cases): pseudogout usually affects the second and third metacarpophalangeal joints.
    Any of small joints may be involved.
    Examine the heart for dilated cardiomyopathy, cardiac failure.
    Check urine for sugar, looking for evidence of diabetes mellitus (present in 80% of cases).

Remember that such patients develop cirrhosis and hepatocellular carcinoma.

Diagnosis

This male patient has generalized hyperpigmentation, hepatomegaly and signs of liver cell disease (lesions) due to haemochromatosis which may be hereditary (aetiology).

Advanced-level Questions

Does this disease run in families?

Yes, and it is an autosomal recessive condition. It is closely associated with human leukocyte antigen HLA-A3 and to a lesser extent with HLA-B14 antigen. The responsible alleles are on the short arm of chromosome 6. Asymptomatic close relatives of patients with hereditary haemochromatosis, in particular siblings, should be advised to undergo screening, i.e. measurements of serum ferritin and iron, and saturation of iron binding capacity.

What is the benefit of early identification?

Early venesection has shown benefits, particularly in those who have not developed diabetes mellitus or cirrhosis. Early venesection prevents progression of hepatic disease and may consequently prevent complication of hepatocellular carcinoma.

How would you confirm your diagnosis?

- Transferrin saturation is increased.
- Serum ferritin levels are raised.
- Liver biopsy to measure iron stores is a definitive test.

How would you manage such a patient?

- Avoidance of alcohol and Indian balti curries which are prepared in cast iron cookware.
- Venesection prolongs life and often reverses tissue damage. Initially, weekly venesection for 2 years (as 50 g iron or more is removed) and then once every 3 months. Many manifestations improve (insulin requirements often diminish) except for testicular atrophy and chrondrocalcinosis.

What is the commonest cause of death in patients with hereditary haemochromatosis?

The most common cause of death is hepatocellular carcinoma for which the risk is 200-fold greater than that in the general population. Depletion of iron, and even reversal of cirrhosis, do not totally prevent the occurrence of this fatal neoplasm. Patients diagnosed in the subclinical, precirrhotic stage and treated by regular phlebotomy have a normal life expectancy.

Mention a few causes of generalized pigmentation.

Common causes are sun tan and race.
Uncommon causes are as follows:
- Liver disease: haemochromatosis in males; primary biliary cirrhosis in females.
- Addison's disease.
- Uraemia.
- Chronic debilitating conditions such as malignancy.

The term haemochromatosis was first used by von Recklinghausen (see page 202) in 1889 to describe autopsy findings in men with cirrhosis associated with massive deposition of iron in the hepatocytes.
The inherited nature of haemochromatosis was first recognized by Sheldon in 1935.

References

Edwards CQ & Kushner JP (1993) Screening for haemochromatosis. *N Engl J Med* **328**: 1617–1620.

Fairweather SJ, Fox TE & Mallillion A (1995) Balti curries and iron. *Br Med J* **310**: 1368.

Finlayson NDC (1990) Hereditary (primary) haemochromatosis. *Br Med J* **309**: 351

Niederau C, Fischer R, Sonnenberg A et al (1985) Survival and causes of death in cirrhotic and in non-cirrhotic patients with primary haemochromatosis. *N Engl J Med* **313**: 1256–1262.

Sheldon JH (1935) *Haemochromatosis*. London: Oxford University Press.

von Recklinghausen FD (1889) Ueber Hämochromatose. *Tageblatt Versamml Dtsch Naturforsch Aertze Heidelberg* **62**: 324–325.

CASE 117 Primary Biliary Cirrhosis

Instruction

Examine this patient's abdomen.

Salient features

- Usually occurs in middle-aged women.
- Clubbing.
- Generalized pigmentation.
- Xanthelasmata.
- Icterus.
- Scratch marks.
- Hepatosplenomegaly.

Proceed as follows:

- Look for xanthomata over joints, skin folds and sites of trauma to the skin.
- Remember that there may be clinical features of other autoimmune diseases such as rheumatoid arthritis, dry mouth of Sjögren's syndrome, systemic sclerosis, CREST syndrome (see page 359), Hashimato's thyroiditis, dermatomyositis.
- Tell the examiner that you would like to investigate as follows:
  Take a history of steatorrhoea.
  Check for proximal muscle weakness due to osteomalacia.
  Examine for peripheral neuropathy.
  Test for high serum levels of alkaline phosphatase and anti-mitochondrial antibodies (present in 95% of the patients, with the M2 antibody being more specific; it is almost always negative in extrahepatic obstruction).

Diagnosis

This middle-aged woman has generalized pigmentation, jaundice, xanthelasmata and pruritus with hepatosplenomegaly (lesions) due to primary biliary cirrhosis (aetiology). She is in liver cell failure as evidenced by the hepatic flap (functional status).

Advanced-level Questions

How does primary biliary cirrhosis present?

Classically, it presents with itching in a middle-aged woman. However, in 50% of cases there may be no liver symptoms.

Is there a cure for primary biliary cirrhosis?

Liver transplantation is the only known cure.

When is liver transplantation indicated?

It is indicated in patients with liver failure and pronounced jaundice.

What drugs have been used to control pruritus?

Cholestyramine, colestipol, rifampicin and opiates.

What drugs have been used to treat this condition?

Steroids, azathioprine, chlorambucil, cyclosporin, bile salts.

What is the rationale behind bile salt therapy?

Hepatocytes affected by autoimmune processes are further injured by endogenous bile acids (such as chenodeoxycholic acid and cholic acid) which accumulate due to associated cholestasis. Partial replacement of water-soluble bile acids such as ursodeoxycholic acid may reduce pruritus and damage to the liver cell.

What do you understand by secondary biliary cirrhosis?

It is that which occurs secondary to large duct obstruction and is usually due to extrahepatic obstruction such as bile duct stricture, gallstones and sclerosing cholangitis.

Peter Brunt, contemporary gastroenterologist and liver physician, Aberdeen Royal Infirmary, is also the personal physician to the Queen and is an astute clinician. He is the President of the Association of Physicians of Great Britain, a society founded by Osler.

Roger Williams, Professor at King's College, London, and Sir Roy Calne, Professor of Surgery, Cambridge, pioneered liver transplantation in the UK.

Thomas E Starzl, surgeon, Pittsburgh, USA, is an internationally known pioneer in liver transplantation.

References

Bateson MC (1990) New directions in primary biliary cirrhosis. *Br Med J* **301**: 1290.

Kaplan MM (1993) Primary biliary cirrhosis. *N Engl J Med* **328**: 1236. (Classic histopathological pictures of this condition.)

CASE 118 Wilson's Disease

Instruction

Look at this patient's eyes.

Salient features

- Greenish yellow to golden-brown pigmentation at the limbus of the cornea, called the Kayser–Fleischer ring. The ring is most marked at the superior and inferior poles of the cornea and is due to the deposition of copper in the Descemet's membrane in the cornea. (It is often apparent only on slit-lamp examination. It may be absent in patients with hepatic manifestations only but is present in those with neuropsychiatric disease.)

Proceed as follows:

- Look for the following:
  Jaundice (look at the sclera).
  Sunflower cataracts.
  Hepatomegaly.
  Signs of liver cell failure.
  Neurological manifestations – tremor, chorea, mask-like facies with a vacuous smile.

Diagnosis

This patient has a classical Kayser–Fleischer ring with jaundice and hepatomegaly (lesions) due to Wilson's disease (aetiology) and does not have a hepatic flap (functional status).

Advanced-level Questions

Is Kayser – Fleischer ring pathognomonic of Wilson's disease?

No, it is also seen in primary biliary cirrhosis, chronic active hepatitis with cirrhosis, cryptogenic cirrhosis and long-standing intrahepatic cirrhosis of childhood.

At what age do the neurological manifestations usually manifest?

They usually appear between 12 and 30 years of age. The most frequent first neurological symptom is a difficulty in speaking or writing while in school.

What do you know about the inheritance of the disease?

Autosomal recessive inheritance with the gene located on chromosome 13, often associated with a family history of consanguinity.

What do you know about the pathophysiology of this disease?

The precise defect is not known. The major aberration is excessive absorption of copper from the small intestine with decreased excretion of copper by the liver, resulting in an increase in tissue deposition, particularly in the brain, cornea, liver and kidney.

What are the biochemical changes in Wilson's disease?

- Low serum ceruloplasmin level (ceruloplasmin is the copper-carrying protein).
- Serum copper concentration may be high, low or normal.
- Orally administered radiolabelled copper is incorporated into ceruloplasmin.
- Increased urinary excretion of copper.

How is the diagnosis of a suspected case confirmed?

By the demonstration of one of the following:
- Kayser–Fleischer rings and a serum ceruloplasmin level lower than 20 mg l^{-1}.
- Serum ceruloplasmin concentration of less than 200 mg l^{-1} and copper concentration in a liver biopsy sample greater than 250 µg g^{-1} on a dry-weight basis.

How would you treat such a patient?

Pencillamine, which removes and detoxifies deposits of copper. Treatment is lifelong and continuous.

Samuel Alexander Kinnier Wilson (1877–1937) qualified in Edinburgh and worked at the National Hospital, Queen Square, London, as a neurologist.
Bernard Kayser (1869–1954) and Bruno Fleischer, both German ophthalmologists, described the same condition in 1902 and 1903 respectively.

References

Anonymous (1984) Case records – 44. *N Engl J Med* **311**: 1171.
Biglan AW & Taylor SL (1993) Kayser–Fleischer ring in a patient with Wilson's disease. *N Engl J Med* **328**: 1820. (A classical picture of this condition.)
Scheinberg IH, Jaffe ME & Sternlieb I (1987) The use of trientine in preventing the effects of interrupting pencillamine therapy in Wilson's disease. *N Engl J Med* **317**: 209.
Wilson SAK (1912) Progressive lenticular degeneration. A familial nervous disease associated with cirrhosis of liver. *Brain* **34**: 295.

CASE 119 Splenomegaly

Instruction

Examine this patient's abdomen.

Salient features

- Massive spleen. There may be associated anaemia.
- Start low while examining for the spleen and be gentle during palpation. Even if you are certain it is the spleen, you must go through the motions of ruling out a palpable kidney: do a bimanual palpation and check for ballottement; feel for the splenic notch; auscultate for splenic rub.

Proceed as follows:

- Look for enlarged lymph nodes and anaemia.
- Remember that the spleen must be at least two or three times its usual size before it can be felt.
- Remember that, normally, the spleen does not extend beyond the anterior axillary line and lies along the 9th, 10th and 11th ribs.

Diagnosis

This patient has massive splenomegaly (lesion), probably due to a myeloproliferative disorder (aetiology).

Questions

What is your diagnosis?

- Myeloproliferative disorder:
  Myelofibrosis, particularly in males.
  Chronic myeloid leukaemia, particularly in females.

How would you confirm your diagnosis?

Bone marrow examination.

Advanced-level Questions

In which other conditions is a massive spleen palpable?

- Malaria.
- Kala-azar.
- Gaucher's disease.

In which conditions is a moderately enlarged spleen (two to four finger-breadths or 4–8 cm) felt?

- Portal hypertension secondary to cirrhosis.
- Lymphoproliferative disorders such as Hodgkin's disease and chronic lymphatic leukaemia.

In which common conditions would the spleen be just palpable?

- Lymphoproliferative disorders.
- Portal hypertension secondary to cirrhosis.
- Infectious hepatitis.
- Glandular fever (infectious mononucleosis).
- Subacute endocarditis.
- Sarcoid, rheumatoid arthritis, collagen disease, idiopathic thrombocytopenia, congenital spherocytosis and polycythaemia rubra vera.

What do you know about the genetics of chronic myelocytic leukaemia?

The fusion of c-*abl* (normally present on chromosome 9) with *bcr* sequences on chromosome 22 is pathognomonic of the chronic phase of chronic myelocytic leukaemia (the Philadelphia chromosome). The p53 gene appears to be the culprit in cases of myeloid blast transformation and there are structural alterations of *RB1* or N-*ras* in less than 10% of the cases with myeloid blast crisis.

PCE Gaucher (1854–1918), Professor of Dermatology in France.
Sir David Weatherall, FRS, contemporary Regius Professor of Medicine, Oxford, who has the unique distinction of being both a molecular biologist and an astute clinician.
The 1902 Nobel Prize was awarded to Sir Donald Ross (1857–1932; born in Almora, India), University of Liverpool, for his work on malaria, in which he showed how it enters the organism and thereby laid the foundation for successful research on this disease and methods of combating it.

CASE 120 Felty's Syndrome

Instruction

Examine this patient's abdomen.

Salient features

- Mild to moderate splenomegaly.
- Rheumatoid arthritis.

Proceed as follows:

- Look for the following signs:
  Anaemia
  Vasculitis.
  Diffuse pigmentation.
  Leg ulcers.

Diagnosis

This patient has moderate splenomegaly with rheumatoid arthritis (lesions) due to Felty's syndrome.

Advanced level Questions

What is Felty's syndrome?

It is a rare complication of rheumatoid arthritis in which there is leucopenia with selective neutropenia and splenomegaly. The prognosis is poor because of recurrent Gram-positive infections.

Note. Splenectomy does not prevent sepsis.

What do you understand by the term 'hypersplenism'?

It implies removal of erythrocytes, granulocytes or platelets from the circulation by the spleen. Removal of the spleen is indicated when the underlying disorder cannot be corrected.

Criteria for hypersplenism include the following:
- Enlarged spleen.
- Destruction of one or more cell lines in the spleen.
- Normal bone marrow.

What are the indications for splenectomy?

- Hereditary spherocytosis in children.
- Autoimmune thrombocytopenia or haemolytic anaemia not controlled by steroids.
- To ameliorate hypersplenism in Gaucher's disease, thalassaemia, hairy cell leukaemia.
- Symptoms due to massive organomegaly.

What are the characteristic cells in a peripheral blood smear following splenectomy?

The presence of Howell–Jolly bodies (in all), siderocytes and spur cells (in 25% of patients).

What are the causes of asplenia?

Causes of asplenia include:
- Diminished function: sickle cell disease, thalassaemia, coeliac disease, SLE, lymphoma, leukaemia, amyloidosis.
- Surgical removal: hereditary spherocytosis, thalassaemia, lymphoma, idiopathic thrombocytopenia, traumatic rupture.

To which infections is the asplenic patient susceptible?

- *Streptococcus pneumoniae, Haemophilus* influenzae B, *Neisseria meningitidis* and malaria parasites cause significant risk.
- Less common causes include babesiasis, caused by tick-borne protozoa, and infection with *Capnocytophaga canimorus* following a dog bite.

What precautions would you advise an asplenic patient in the outpatient clinic?

- Vaccination.
  Pneumococcal vaccine – a single injection; booster doses at 5–10-
      year intervals.
  Hib vaccine – a single dose at the same time as pneumococcal
      immunization.
  Meningococcus groups A and C vaccine (although the majority of
      infections are due to group B strains for which there is no
      vaccine of proven efficacy).
- Antibiotic prophylaxis.
  Phenoxymethylpenicillin or amoxycillin.
- Foreign travel.
  Antimalarial chemoprophylaxis, other precautions (insect repellants,
      screens at night).

Augustus R Felty (1895–1964) was a physician at Hartford Hospital, Hartford,
Connecticut. He described this syndrome while he was working at the Johns
Hopkins Hospital, Baltimore.

Reference

Thorne C & Urowitz MB (1982) Long-term outcome in Felty's syndrome. *Ann
    Rheum Dis* **41**: 486.

CASE 121 Polycystic Kidneys

Instruction

Examine this patient's abdomen.

Salient features

- Arteriovenous fistulas in the arms or subclavian dialysis catheter
    (remember that polycystic kidneys constitute the third most common
    cause for chronic renal failure in the UK after glomerulonephritis
    and pyelonephritis).
- Palpable kidneys (confirm by bimanual palpation and ballottement;
    there is a resonant note on percussion due to overlying colon; the
    hand can get between the swelling and the costal margin).

Proceed as follows:

- Look for the following signs:
  Enlarged liver due to cystic disease.

Transplanted kidney may be palpable in either iliac fossa.

Third nerve palsy (berry aneurysms are associated with polycystic kidneys).

- Tell the examiner that you would like to investigate as follows:

  Check the blood pressure (hypertension develops in 75% of cases).

  Take a family history.

  Look for anaemia (due to chronic renal failure) or polycythaemia (due to increased erythropoiesis).

  Microscopic haematuria.

Remember that polycystic kidney disease is a misnomer as it is a systemic disorder affecting many organs.

Diagnosis

This patient has polycystic kidney disease (lesion and diagnosis) and is currently on dialysis as evidenced by the arteriovenous fistula in the arm (functional status).

Questions

How may polycystic disease present?

Haematuria, hypertension, urinary tract infection, pain in the lumbar region and uraemic symptoms.

Is the kidney involvement usually unilateral or bilateral?

The disease is universally bilateral; unilateral cases reported probably represent multicystic renal dysplasia.

Advanced-level Questions

What do you know about the prevalence of this disease?

Autosomal dominant polycystic kidney disease is one of the most common hereditary disorders, being ten times more common than sickle cell disease, 15 times more common than cystic fibrosis and 20 times more common than Huntington's disease. It has a worldwide distribution. In the white population the disease appears to occur in about 1 in 400 to 1 in 1000 people. Although the disease is rare in Africa and less common in American blacks than whites, the incidence of end-stage renal disease due to autosomal dominant polycystic kidney disease is similar in blacks and whites.

In which other conditions may bilateral renal cysts be observed in an ultrasonographic study?

Multiple simple cysts, autosomal recessive polycystic kidney disease in children, tuberous sclerosis and von Hippel–Lindau syndrome.

What are the criteria for diagnosis of polycystic kidney disease using ultrasonography?

The presence of at least two renal cysts (unilateral or bilateral) in individuals at risk and younger than 30 years may be regarded as sufficient to establish a diagnosis; among those aged 30–59 years the presence of at least two cysts in each kidney and among those aged 60 years and above at least four cysts in each kidney should be required.

How would you like to manage this patient?

- FBC, urea and electrolytes, serum creatinine, urine microscopy, urine culture.
- Ultrasonography of the kidneys to confirm the diagnosis.
- Family history should be ascertained (as the condition is autosomal dominant with nearly 100% penetrance).
- High resolution CT head scan or MRI as a screening test for intracranial aneurysms in those with a family history of intracranial aneurysms or subarachnoid haemorrhage.

In which other organs are cysts seen in this condition?

Liver (in 30% of cases), spleen, pancreas, lungs, ovaries, testes, epididymis, thyroid, uterus, broad ligament and bladder.

What are the neurological manifestations of this condition?

Subarachnoid haemorrhage from an intracranial berry aneurysm, causing death or neurological lesions in about 9% of patients.

What is the pathology?

Cysts develop in Bowman's capsule and at other levels in the nephron, displacing kidney tissue.

What cardiovascular manifestations have been reported in these patients?

- Mitral valve prolapse in 26%.

- Other lesions commonly seen are mitral, aortic and tricuspid valve regurgitation.

What do you know about Potter's classification of polycystic kidney disease?

There are three types:
- Type I – infantile polycystic disease of kidney.
- Type II – dysgenetic or hypogenetic cystic kidney, multicystic dysplastic kidney, unilateral multilocular cyst.
- Type III – adult polycystic disease of kidney with involvement of liver.

What are the renal manifestations of this disease?

- The main structural change is the formation of cysts. Cysts enlarge, lose their tubular connection and become isolated from the glomerulus, requiring transepithelial transport of solutes and fluids for further expansion. Cyst fluids have different compositions, some having high and others low sodium concentration.
- One of the earliest and most consistent functional abnormalities is a decrease in renal concentrating ability.
- There may be altered endocrine function as reflected by increased secretion of both renin (causing increased predilection to hypertension) and erythropoietin (resulting in better maintained haematocrit in renal failure, unlike in renal failure due to other causes; rarely can result in polycythaemia).

What are the causes of abdominal pain in this disease?

Infected cyst, haemorrage into cyst or diverticular perforation.

What are the complications of polycystic kidney disease?

Renal complications:
- Hypertension.
- Pain – back pain or abdominal pain.
- Gross or microscopic haematuria.
- Pyelonephritis.
- Proteinuria.
- Renal failure.

Extrarenal manifestations:
- Cystic: cysts in the liver, ovary, pancreas, spleen and central nervous system. Unlike renal cyst formation, liver cysts seem to be influenced by female hormones. Whilst men and women have the same frequency of liver cysts, massive liver cysts are almost exclusively found in women.

- Non-cystic:
    Cardiac valvular abnormalities – mitral valve prolapse, aortic valve abnormalities.
    Intracranial saccular aneurysm or berry aneurysm. Magnetic resonance angiography is the most reliable technique of non-invasive screening among such patients.
- Gastrointestinal – colonic diverticula.

What do you know about the genetic transmission of this disease?

The inheritance is autosomal dominant and in most families is linked to the α-haemoglobin gene complex and the phosphoglycerate kinase genes at the PKD1 locus on the short arm of chromosome 16. Patients not having the PKD1 locus have an older age at onset and later development of renal insufficiency. The second locus is on chromosome 4q13–q23. However, in 4% of families with the disorder it is caused by unknown mutations elsewhere in the genome.

What are the causes of death in these patients?

One-third of adult patients die from renal failure; another third die from the complications of hypertension (including heart disease, intracerebral haemorrhage and rupture of berry aneurysm). The remaining third die from unrelated causes.

Sir W Bowman (1816–1892), Surgeon at the Royal London Ophthalmic Hospital.
Jerome Kassirer, contemporary Renal Physician and Editor-in-Chief of the *New England Journal of Medicine*.
EL Potter (1901–), US pathologist. She also described Potter's syndrome with renal agenesis and characteristic of epicanthic folds, receding jaw and low set ears with less cartilage than usual.
OZ Dalgaard's study in 1957 clarified the autosomal dominant pattern of inheritance of the disease.

References

Gabow PA (1993) Autosomal dominant polycystic kidney disease. *N Engl J Med* **329**: 332.
Ravine D, Gibson RN, Walker RG, Sheffield LJ, Kincaid-Smith P & Danks DM (1994) Evaluation of ultrasonographic diagnostic criteria for autosomal dominant polycystic kidney disease 1. *Lancet* **343**: 824–827.
Wiebers DO & Torres VE (1992) Screening for unruptured intracranial aneurysms in autosomal dominant polycystic kidney disease. *N Engl J Med* **327**: 953–955.

CASE 122 Transplanted Kidney

Instruction

Examine this patient's abdomen.

Salient features

- Laparotomy scar (comment on the scar).
- Arteriovenous fistulas in arms.
- Transplanted kidney felt in either right or left iliac fossa.

Proceed as follows:

- Tell the examiner that you would like to look for other signs of uraemia (see page 544).
- Do know the differential diagnosis for masses in the right/left iliac fossa (see page 342).

Diagnosis

This patient has a transplanted kidney (lesion) probably due to diabetic nephropathy as evidenced by the sugar-free drinks by the bedside (aetiology).

Questions

Mention a few indications for renal transplantation.

End-stage renal diseases; the most common diseases that result in referral of patients for transplantation include:
- Diabetes mellitus with renal failure.
- Hypertensive renal disease.
- Glomerulonephritis.

Advanced-level Questions

Would you refer a patient for renal transplantation before instituting haemodialysis?

Referral for renal transplantation need not be delayed until the patient has begun dialysis. It is acceptable and, in fact, usually preferable to refer the patient to a renal transplant unit before dialysis is required. With judicious planning on the part of the general practitioner, renal physician and transplant surgical team, transplantation can be performed even before dialysis is even required.

In which age group is transplantation preferred to dialysis?

Infants and children have a high morbidity rate on long-term haemodialysis or peritoneal dialysis. Thus, renal transplantation from parents or siblings improves growth and allows a more normal lifestyle.

Is there any advantage to HLA-matching before transplantation?

Kidneys from living related donors who are HLA identical and also red blood cell ABO matched have a 90% survival rate at 1 year; less identical grafts tend to have a somewhat lower survival rate. Kidney transplants from matched cadaver donors survive nearly as long, especially if the receipient does not contain antibodies to donor antigens.

There is some evidence that HLA mismatching has a greater effect on living related than it does on cadaveric donor kidney transplantation. Recent evidence has shown that HLA-matched kidneys, particularly for DR, B and A antigens, are associated with long-term survival of the patient. Complete matching of DR, B and A loci is associated with the best chance of success. HLA-DR matching appears to have the greatest impact on survival, followed by B, and lastly the A loci.

Should repeated blood transfusions be avoided in a patient waiting for a renal transplant?

If the anaemia is well tolerated and is due to the renal failure *per se*, blood transfusion should be avoided as it carries a risk of HLA sensitization. Pretreatment of recipients with multiple blood transfusions from the *donor* tends to increase graft survival, in contrast to the deleterious effect on bone marrow engraftment.

What other factors are known to cause sensitization to HLA antigens?

Pregnancy, previously failed transplant.

What drugs are used for post-transplant immunosuppression?

Steroids, azathioprine and cyclosporin – used independently or in combination. Newer drugs include FK 506 and rapamycin.

What are the contraindications for kidney transplantation?

- A positive cross-match by cytotoxicity testing between recipient serum and donor cells is considered to be a contraindication for transplantation.

- Presence of HIV or other infectious agents on donor screening.

What are the complications of renal transplantation?

- Opportunistic infection, e.g. cytomegalovirus, *Pneumocystis*.
- Premature coronary artery disease.
- Hypertension – primarily to cyclosporin.
- Lymphomas and skin cancers.
- *De novo* glomerulonephritis in the transplanted kidney.
- Complications of steroid therapy, e.g. aseptic necrosis of bone.

What do you know about warm ischaemic time?

Shorter warm ischaemic time of the transplanted kidney is associated with longer survival of the recipient.

What is the survival rate following kidney transplant?

The 2-year kidney graft survival rate for living related donor transplantation is 85%, whereas in cadaveric donor transplantation it is about 70%.

What do you know about rejection of the transplanted kidney?

It may be acute or chronic and must be suspected when the graft is tender, the urine output is falling or the creatinine concentration is rising. It is a complex process in which both cell-mediated immunity and circulating antibodies play a role. Evaluation of a suspected rejection usually requires graft biopsy.

- Acute rejection is characterized by a lymphocytic interstitial infiltrate with destruction of epithelial cells. It usually responds to treatment which includes high-dose methyl prednisolone, antilymphocytic globulin and anti-T lymphocyte monoclonal antibody (OKT3) administration.
- Chronic rejection shows histological features of interstitial fibrosis, atrophy of tubules and proliferation of the arterial intima. There is no specific treatment and general management of chronic renal failure should be reinstituted.

Joseph E Murray (1919–), Professor of Surgery, Brigham and Women's Hospital and Harvard Medical School, was awarded the 1990 Nobel Prize for Medicine for his pioneering work on organ transplantation along with Thomas E Donnall (1920–) of the Fred Hutchinson Cancer Research Centre, Seattle, Washington, USA.

In 1966 Terasaki and coworkers reported the association between HLA matching and outcome in patients receiving cadaveric organs.

References

Sanfillipo F (1994) HLA matching in renal transplantation. *N Engl J Med* **331**: 803–805.

Teraski PI, Vredevoe DL, Mickey MR et al (1966) Serotyping for homotransplantation. VII. Selection of kidney donors for thirty-two recipients. *Ann N Y Acad Sci* **129**: 500–520.

CASE 123 Abdominal Aortic Aneurysm

Instruction

Examine this patient's abdomen.
This patient presented with low back pain; examine the abdomen.

Salient features

- Large expansile pulsation along the course of the abdominal aorta.
- Auscultate for bruit over the aneurysm and over the femoral pulses.
- Examine all peripheral pulses.

Proceed as follows:

- Tell the examiner that you would like to check the following:
  Urine for sugar.
  Blood pressure.
  Serum cholesterol.
  History of smoking.

Remember that:
- Popliteal artery aneurysms often coexist and, in fact, their presence should prompt the physician to look for an abdominal aortic aneurysm.
- Ninety per cent of the atherosclerotic abdominal aortic aneurysms are present below the origin of the renal arteries and can involve the aortic bifurcation.
- The infrarenal aorta is normally 2 cm in diameter; when it exceeds 4 cm an aneurysm is said to exist.

Diagnosis

This patient has a large pulsatile mass in the epigastrium (lesion) due to an aneurysm of the abdominal aorta (aetiology).

Questions

Which investigations would you do to confirm your diagnosis?

- Ultrasonography of the abdomen – a simple, cheap and accurate screening test.
- Large aneurysms require angiography.
- Magnetic resonance imaging is useful, particularly as it does not require administration of contrast.

Advanced-level Questions

How would you manage an abdominal aneurysm?

Aortic aneurysms more than 5 cm carry a high risk of rupture and hence should be referred to the vascular surgeon for surgery. Smaller aneurysms must be followed up; they enlarge at a rate of about 0.5 cm a year. In selected cases an endovascular prosthesis is preferred.

What is the prognosis of such aneurysms?

Mortality rate for a patient undergoing elective surgery is less than 5%, whereas that for a ruptured aneurysm is nearly 90%.

In 1951, C Dubost from Paris performed the first successful aortic resection for aneurysm.

Reference

Ernst CB (1993) Abdominal aortic aneurysm. *N Engl J Med* **328**: 1167.

CASE 124   Unilateral Palpable Kidney

Instruction

Examine this patient's abdomen.

Salient features

- One kidney is palpable (bimanually ballottable; there is a transverse band of colonic resonance on percussion and you will be able to insinuate your fingers between the mass and costal margin).

Proceed as follows:

- Look carefully for arteriovenous fistulas in the arms, haemodialysis catheters in the subclavian region.

Diagnosis

This patient has a unilateral palpable kidney (lesion) which may be due to either polycystic kidney disease or renal neoplasm (aetiology).

Questions

What are the common causes of a palpable kidney?

- Polycystic kidney disease.
- Renal carcinoma.
- Hydronephrosis.
- Renal cyst.
- Hypertrophy of the solitary functioning kidney.

What changes can occur in a kidney when the other is removed?

Long-term renal function remains stable in most patients with a reduction in renal mass of more than 50%. However, these patients are at increased risk for proteinuria, glomerulopathy and progressive renal failure. Hence it is important to monitor patients with remnant kidneys. Problems are most frequent in those in whom the amount of renal tissue removed is greatest and who have survived the longest.

Leon Fine, contemporary Professor and Chair of Medicine, University College Hospital, London.
Graeme Catto, contemporary Professor of Renal Medicine and Dean, Aberdeen Medical School.
HA Lee, Professor of Renal Medicine, Portsmouth, University of Southampton, who is also interested in metabolism.

References

Fine LG (1991) How little kidney tissue is enough? *N Engl J Med* **325**: 1097.
Novick AC, Gephardt G, Guz B, Steinmuller D & Tubbs RR (1991) Long term follow-up after partial removal of a solitary kidney. *N Engl J Med* **325**: 1058.

CASE 125 Abdominal Masses

Instruction

Examine this patient's abdomen.

Salient features

Patient 1 has an epigastric mass. Differential diagnosis:
- Carcinoma of the stomach: look for supraclavicular lymph nodes, hepatomegaly; comment on pallor and asthenia.
- Carcinoma of the pancreas: look for jaundice.
- Aneurysm of the abdominal aorta: look for pulsatile mass; check femoral and foot pulses; auscultate over the mass and the femoral pulses (see page 339).
- Retroperitoneal lymphadenopathy (lymphoma).

Patient 2 has a mass in the right iliac fossa. Differential diagnosis:
- Crohn's disease: look for mouth ulcers; tell the examiner that you would like to look for fistulas and take a history for chronic diarrhoea (see page 534).
- Carcinoma of the caecum: look for hard mass, lymph nodes.
- Look for lymph nodes elsewhere (see page 528); feel for liver and spleen; examine the drainage area of iliac lymph nodes (such as the leg, perianal area, external genitalia; do a rectal examination).
- Transplanted kidney: comment on the laparotomy scars, stigmata of renal failure and artificial arteriovenous fistulas.
- Appendicular abscess.
- Ileocaecal abscess, particularly in Asians.
- Ovarian tumours (must be mentioned as a differential diagnosis in female patients).

Less common causes of masses in the right iliac fossa:
- Amoebiasis.
- Carcinoid (ileal).
- Actinomycosis.
- Ectopic kidney.

Patient 3 has a mass in the left iliac fossa. Differential diagnosis:
- Diverticular abscess: look for tender, mobile mass.
- Carcinoma of the colon: look for hepatomegaly; tell the examiner that you would like to do a per rectal examination.
- Faecal mass (the mass may be moulded by pressure).
- Ovarian tumour (in females).

- Iliac lymph nodes: look for other lymph nodes, liver and spleen; examine the drainage areas.
- Transplanted kidney: comment on the laparotomy scar, look for signs of renal failure, arteriovenous fistulas (see page 564).

Note. The investigation of first choice in such patients is abdominal ultrasonography.

Robin Warren, Pathologist at Royal Perth Hospital in Western Australia, and Barry J. Marshall discovered that *Helicobacter pylori* causes peptic ulcer disease. In 1984, Marshall infected himself, by drinking a pure culture of *H. pylori*. After feeling fine for 5 days he experienced nausea and vomiting. Histology confirmed acute gastritis. In 1995 he received the Albert Lasker Clinical Medical Research Award. *H. pylori* has also been implicated in the causation of gastric cancer in Japanese people.

Reference

Warren JR & Marshall B (1983) Unidentified curved bacilli on gastric epithelium in active chronic gastritis. *Lancet* **i**: 1273–1275.

RHEUMATOLOGY

GENERAL GUIDELINES FOR EXAMINATION OF JOINTS

History

Ask the patient whether he or she has any pain, stiffness or difficulty in dressing or walking.

Examination

- *Look* at posture, gait and joint deformity.
- *Feel* for temperature, tenderness, joint fluid and crepitus of movement of the joints.
- *Move*: check passive and active movements of the joints; test stability of the joints.
- *Measure* muscle wasting and shortening of the limb.

EXAMINATION OF THE HANDS

1. Ask the patient, 'Are your hands painful?'

2. Inspect for joint deformity:
    - Swan-neck deformity (flexion at the distal interphalangeal joints and hyperextension of the proximal interphalangeal joints).
    - Boutonnière deformity (flexion of the proximal interphalangeal joints and hyperextension of the distal interphalangeal joint).
    - Z deformity of the thumb.
    - Ulnar deviation of the fingers.

3. Examine the nails:
    - Nail fold infarcts (rheumatoid arthritis).
    - Nail pitting, onycholysis, ridging, hyperkeratosis, discoloration (psoriasis).

4. Comment on the following:
   - Wasting of small muscles of the hand, in particular those on the dorsum of the hand.
   - Heberden's nodes, i.e. bony nodules at the distal interphalangeal joints (osteoarthroses).
   - Bouchard's nodes, i.e. bony nodules at the proximal interphalangeal joints (osteoarthroses).
   - Spindle-shaped deformity of the fingers.
   - Gouty tophi.

5. Examine the palms:
   - Wasting of the thenar or hypothenar eminence.
   - Thickening of the palmar fascia – Dupuytren's contracture (rheumatoid arthritis).
   - Palmar erythema (rheumatoid arthritis).
   - Tap over the flexor retinaculum to detect median nerve entrapment (Tinel's sign).

6. Get the patient to perform the following movements:
   - Unbuttoning of clothes.
   - Pincer movements.
   - Hand grip.
   - Abduction of the thumb.
   - Writing.

7. Test sensation of the index and little fingers.

8. Examine the elbows for the following signs:
   - Rheumatoid arthritis.
   - Gouty tophi.
   - Psoriatic plaques.

9. Tell the examiner that you would like to examine the other joints.

Note. When asked to examine the hands, consider the possibility of arthropathy, myopathy, neuropathy, a peripheral nerve lesion or acromegaly.

W Heberden, Sr (1710–1801), an English physician.
CJ Bouchard (1837–1915), a French physician.

EXAMINATION OF THE KNEES

- Ask the patient if the joints are sore.
- Expose both knees and lower thighs fully with the patient lying supine.

- Look for:
    Quadriceps wasting.
    Swelling of the joint.
- Feel:
    Temperature.
    Synovial thickening.
    Do the patellar tap (ballottement): fluid from the suprapatellar bursa
        is forced into the joint space by squeezing the lower part of the
        quadriceps and then the patella is pushed posteriorly with the
        fingers; this test indicates fluid in the synovial cavity.
- Movement:
    Test passive flexion and extension – make a note of the range of
        movements and feel for crepitus.
    Gently extend the knee and examine for fixed flexion deformity.
    Test the medial and lateral ligaments by steadying the thigh with the
        left hand and moving the leg with the right laterally and
        medially when the knee joint is slightly flexed – movement of
        more than 10 degrees is abnormal.
    Test the cruciate ligaments by steadying the foot with your elbow
        and moving the leg anteriorly and posteriorly with the other
        hand – laxity of more than 10 degrees is abnormal.
- Ask the patient to lie on his or her stomach and feel the popliteal fossa
    when the knee is extended.

EXAMINATION OF THE FEET

- Look:
    For skin rash, scars.
    At the nails for changes of psoriasis.
    At the forefoot for hallux valgus, clawing and crowding of the toes
        (rheumatoid arthritis).
    At the callus over the metatarsal heads which may occur in
        subluxation.
    At both the arches of the foot, in particular medial and longitudinal
        (flat foot, pes cavus).
- Palpate:
    Ankles for synovitis, effusion, passive movements at the subtalar
        joints (inversion and eversion) and talar joint (dorsiflexion and
        plantar flexion); remember that tenderness on movement is
        more important than the range of movement.
    Metatarsophalangeal joints for tenderness.
    Individual digits, for synovial thickening.
    Bottom of heel, for tenderness (plantar fasciitis), and Achilles
        tendon for nodules.

CASE 126 Rheumatoid Hands

Instruction

Examine this patient's hands.

Salient features

- Ask the patient for permission to examine her hands and then ask whether the hands are sore.

Proceed as follows:

- Comment on deformities such as the following:
    Subluxation at the metacarpophalangeal joint.
    Swan neck deformity.
    Boutonnière deformity (hyperextension at the terminal interphalangeal joint and flexion at the proximal interphalangeal joint).
    Z deformity of the thumb.
    Dorsal subluxation of the ulna at the carpal joint.
- Comment on the following signs:
    Nail-fold infarcts and vasculitic skin lesions.
    Palmar erythema.
    Wasting of the first dorsal interossei and other small muscles of the hand.
- Test grip and pincer movements. Quickly test for abductor pollicis brevis and interossei, and pinprick sensation over index and little fingers. The median nerve may be involved if there is associated carpal tunnel syndrome.
- Examine the elbow for rheumatoid nodules.
- Ask the patient to perform simple tasks involving hand function, such as unbuttoning her clothes, or writing.
- Tell the examiner that you would like to examine other joints.
- Highlight the following points:
    Whether terminal interphalangeal joints are spared or affected.
    Whether the arthritis is active (if the joints are inflamed) or inactive.

Diagnosis

This patient has swan neck deformity of the fingers (lesions) due to rheumatoid arthritis (aetiology) with marked active arthritis of the interphalangeal joints, and is unable to button her clothes (functional status).

Questions

What is the significance of rheumatoid arthritis?

The presence of nodules indicates seropositive and more aggressive arthritis.

Where else are nodules found?

Flexor and extensor tendons of the hand, sacrum, Achilles tendon, sclera, lungs and myocardium.

What are the skin lesions in rheumatoid arthritis?

Vasculitis, nail-fold infarcts.

What are the causes of anaemia in rheumatoid arthritis?

- Anaemia of chronic disease.
- Megaloblastic anaemia due to folate deficiency or associated pernicious anaemia.
- Felty's syndrome.
- Drugs: non-steroidal anti-inflammatory drugs (NSAIDs) causing iron deficiency anaemia; bone marrow suppression caused by gold.

What factors have been implicated in anaemia of chronic disease?

- Decreased production of red blood cells:
    Due to inadequate iron: impaired absorption and transport, failure to release iron stores.
    Due to decreased concentration or marrow resistance to erythropoietin.
    Ineffective erythropoiesis.
    Abnormal development of erythroid progenitor cells.
- Increased destruction of red cells

What is Felty's syndrome?

It is seen in some patients with severe rheumatoid arthritis and consists of splenomegaly, anaemia, leucopenia and thrombocytopenia (hypersplenism), and leg ulcers. Splenectomy ameliorates hypersplenism. Felty's syndrome is associated with positive rheumatoid factor.

What are the pulmonary manifestations of rheumatoid arthritis?

- Pleural effusion or pleurisy (seen in 25% of men with rheumatoid arthritis)
- Rheumatoid nodules.
- Fibrosing alveolitis.
- Caplan's syndrome (rheumatoid arthritis coexists with rounded fibrotic nodules 0.5–5 cm in diameter, mainly in the periphery of lung fields in coal-worker's pneumoconiosis).

What are the eye manifestations of rheumatoid arthritis?

- Episcleritis.
- Scleritis.
- Scleromalacia, scleromalacia perforans.
- Keratoconjunctivitis sicca.
- Sjögren's syndrome (see above).

What precautions are necessary before upper gastrointestinal endoscopy or general anaesthesia?

It is prudent to take a cervical spine radiograph to rule out atlanto-axial subluxation.

Which joints are commonly affected in rheumatoid arthritis?

Wrists, proximal interphalangeal joints and metacarpophalangeal joints of the hands, metatarsophalangeal joints and knees.

What is palindromic rheumatoid arthritis?

Palindromic onset is seen in some patients with recurrent episodes of joint stiffness and pain in individual joints lasting only a few hours or days. Hydroxychloroquine may be of value in preventing recurrences.

Advanced-level Questions

How would you treat the arthritis?

Prescribe NSAIDs (ibuprofen is the safest at conventional doses) including aspirin. If, after 1 month of NSAIDs, the symptoms persist with no sign of remission then a second-line drug should be added. Second-line drugs include hydroxychloroquine, sulphasalazine and pencillamine. Low-dose methotrexate and gold salts are used to prevent disease progression. Treatment with a monoclonal antibody to tumour necrosis factor produces significant but temporary improvement in the severity of arthritis, although more information about risks are required before it can be considered as viable treatment.

If the patient is known to experience gastric distress with NSAIDs, what precautions would you take while prescribing them?

Prophylaxis for NSAID-associated gastric distress may be attempted with concurrent administration of an H_2-receptor blocker (such as ranitidine), omeprazole or misoprostol. The latter is a prostaglandin analogue which has been shown to protect the gastric mucosa.

What are the neurological manifestations of rheumatoid arthritis?

- Peripheral neuropathy – glove-and-stocking sensory loss.
- Mononeuritis multiplex.
- Entrapment neuropathy, e.g. carpal tunnel syndrome.
- Cervical disease or atlanto-axial subluxation may cause cervical myelopathy.

What are the causes of proteinuria in patients with rheumatoid arthritis?

- Drug therapy: gold salts, penicillamine.
- Amyloidosis.

What is Sjögren's syndrome?

- The association of keratoconjunctivitis sicca (lack of lacrimal secretion) and xerostomia (dry mouth due to lack of salivary gland secretion) in association with a connective tissue disorder, usually rheumatoid arthritis. This syndrome may be associated with autoimmune thyroid disease, myasthenia gravis or autoimmune liver disease.
- The Schirmer filter paper test provides a crude measure of tear production. Filter paper is hooked over the lower eyelid and in normal people at least 15 mm is wet after 5 minutes, whereas in patients with keratoconjunctivitis sicca it is less than 5 mm.
- Anti-Ro (SSA) and anti-SS-B antibodies may be seen in this syndrome.
- Treatment is symptomatic with artificial tears (hypomellose drops or 1% methylcellulose), artificial saliva and NSAIDs for the arthritis.

What are the criteria for rheumatoid arthritis?

American Rheumatism Association criteria:
1. Morning stiffness for at least 1 hour for a duration of 6 weeks or more.

2. Swelling of at least three joints for 6 weeks or more.
3. Swelling of wrist, metacarpophalangeal or proximal interphalangeal joints for 6 weeks or more.
4. Symmetry of swollen joint areas for 6 weeks or more.
5. Subcutaneous nodules.
6. Positive rheumatoid factor.
7. Radiographic features typical of rheumatoid arthritis, i.e. erosions and periarticular osteopenia.

When four or more of the above criteria are met, there is 93% sensitivity and 90% specificity. It is important to note that the diagnosis of rheumatoid arthritis should not be made on the basis of these criteria alone if another systemic disease associated with arthritis is definitely present.

What are the poor prognostic factors?

- Systemic features: weight loss, extra-articular manifestations.
- Insidious onset.
- Rheumatoid nodules.
- Presence of rheumatoid factor more than 1 in 512.
- Persistent activity of the disease for over 12 months.
- Early bone erosions.

What are the factors leading to ulnar deviation of the hands?

- In the normal grip the fingers move to ulnar deviation.
- Weakening of radial sides of the joint capsule and the radial insertion of the interossei ligaments.
- The volar supports of the flexor tendon sheath are weakened by inflammation, allowing the tendon to bow in the direction of the ulna during gripping.
- Ulnar displacement of the extensor tendons in early deviation makes them slip, if the dorsal metacarpophalangeal joint is taut, and thereby exacerbates the development of ulnar deviation by acting as a bowstring.
- The joint capsules of metacarpophalangeal joints are weaker on radial sides than on ulnar sides.

AB Garrod coined the term rheumatoid arthritis in 1858.
HSC Sjögren, a Swedish ophthalmologist, described this condition in 1933.
A Caplan, a British physician, was an industrial officer in the Welsh coal mines.
In 1931 Philip S Hench (1896–1965) of the Mayo Clinic observed that arthritic pain temporarily decreased in pregnant women. He then studied the phenomena for the next 8 years that allergic conditions such as asthma, hay fever and food

sensitivity were also lessened in the presence of jaundice or pregnancy. He reasoned that a steroid hormone may be responsible, since hormone levels are high in the blood during pregnancy. Edward Kendall (1886–1972), Chief of the Division of Biochemistry, suggested the name 'corsone' on a piece of paper but Hench amended this to 'cortisone', and thus the steroid hormone was 'baptized'. The 1950 Nobel Prize for Medicine was jointly awarded to Kendall, Hench and Tadeus Reichstein (1897–) of Basel University, Switzerland, for their discoveries relating to the hormones of the adrenal cortex, their structure and biological effects.

References

Akil M & Amos RS (1995) Rheumatoid arthritis – II: Treatment. *Br Med J* **310**: 652–655.

Hench PS (1953) A reminiscence of certain events before, during and after the discovery of cortisone. *Minn Med* **36**: 705–710.

Porter DR & Sturrock RD (1993) Medical management of rheumatoid arthritis. *Br Med J* **307**: 425.

CASE 127 Ankylosing Spondylitis

Instruction

Examine this patient's back.
Examine this patient.

Salient features

- 'Question mark' posture (due to loss of lumbar lordosis, fixed kyphoscoliosis of the thoracic spine with compensatory extension of the cervical spine).
- Protuberant abdomen.

Proceed as follows:

- Ask the patient to look to either side – the whole body turns when the patient does this.
- Examine the cervical, thoracic and lumbar spines (remember that cervical spine involvement occurs later in the disease and results in pain and a grating sensation on movement of the neck).
- Measure the occiput-to-wall distance (inability to make contact when heel and back are against the wall indicates upper thoracic and cervical limitation).
- Perform Schober's test – this involves marking points 10 cm above and 5 cm below a line joining the 'dimple of Venus' on the sacral

promontory. An increase in the separation of less than 5 cm during full forward flexion indicates limited spinal mobility.

Note. Finger–floor distance is a simple indicator but is less reliable because good hip movement may compensate for back limitation.

- Examine for distal arthritis (occurs in up to 30% of patients and may precede the onset of the back symptoms). Small joints of the hand and feet are rarely affected.
- Measure chest expansion with a tape (less than 5 cm suggests costovertebral involvement).
- Tell the examiner that you would like to examine the following:
  Eyes for iritis, anterior uveitis (seen in 20% of patients).
  Heart for aortic regurgitation (seen in 4% of patients who have had the disease for over 15 years), cardiac conduction defects.
  Lungs for mild restrictive disease, apical fibrosis, apical cavities and secondary fungal infection.
  Central nervous system such as tetraplegia, etc.
  Foot for Achilles tendinitis and plantar fasciitis.

Remember:
- The four 'A's of ankylosing spondylitis: **a**pical fibrosis, **a**nterior uveitis, **a**ortic regurgitation, **A**chilles tendinitis.
- That psoriasis and Reiter's syndrome can also cause sacroiliitis.

Diagnosis

This patient has fixed kyphoscoliosis of the thoracic spine with loss of lumbar lordosis (lesion) due to ankylosing spondylitis (aetiology) on Schober's test; spinal movements are severely diminished (functional status).

Questions

What investigations would you like to do in this patient?

Anteroposterior view of sacroiliac joints and lateral radiographs of lumbar spine: the earliest changes are erosions and sclerosis of the sacroiliac joints. Later in the disease syndesmophytes may be found in the lumbosacral spine. In severe disease, involvement progresses up the spine, leading to a 'bamboo spine'. The New York criteria (1966) for the diagnosis of ankylosing spondylitis require a combination of clinical and radiographic features, but the diagnosis should be suspected on the basis of inactivity, spinal stiffness, and pain, with or without additional features.

In which other seronegative arthritic disorders is low back pain a feature?

Sacroiliitis is often seen in Reiter's syndrome, psoriatic arthritis, juvenile chronic arthritis and intestinal arthropathy.

How would you manage a patient with ankylosing spondylitis?

- Encourage exercise, particularly physical therapy to preserve back extension.
- NSAIDs, in particular indomethacin. Phenylbutazone is reserved for resistant cases.
- Surgical therapy, consisting of vertebral wedge osteotomy, is occasionally indicated.

Advanced-level Questions

What genetic counselling would you give this patient?

In HLA-B27-positive patients, the sibs have a 30% chance of developing this disease. Hence children of such patients who develop symptoms such as joint pains or sore eyes should be referred to a rheumatologist.

What is the natural history of the disease?

About 40% go on to develop severe spinal restriction; about 20% have significant disability; early peripheral joint disease, particularly of the hip, indicates a poor prognosis.

What is the risk in those with a 'bamboo' cervical spine when driving?

Increased susceptiblity to whiplash injury and restricted lateral vision.

What therapy may the patient have received in the past if the blood film shows a leukaemic picture?

In the past, patients were treated with irradiation of the spine. However, such patients tend to develop leukaemia several years after therapy.

Note. The term 'ankylosing spondylitis' derives from the Greek words, *ankylos* (bent or crooked) and *spondylos* (vertebra). Past names have included Marie–Strümpell disease and von Bechterew's disease.
The first clinical report of ankylosing spondylitis (1831) concerned a man from the Isle of Man. Vladimir von Bechterew of St Petersburg, Russia, described a series of cases between 1857 and 1927. Adolf Strümpell (1853–1926) of Erlangen, and Pierre Marie (1853–1940) of Paris, independently described this condition in 1897 and 1898 respectively.

HC Reiter (1881–1969), a German physician.

Achilles is a figure from Greek mythology who was a hero of the Trojan war. His mother dipped him into the river Styx, holding him by his heel, to make him invulnerable to the attack. He slew Hector in this war, but was himself slain, wounded in his vulnerable heel by Paris.

Reference

Keat A (1995) Spondyloarthropathies. *Br Med J* **310**: 1321–1324.

CASE 128 Psoriatic Arthritis

Instruction

Examine this patient's hands.

Salient features

- Distal interphalangeal joint involvement.

Proceed as follows:

- Tell the examiner that you would like to:

    Examine the nails, looking for pitting, onycholysis, discoloration, thickening (nails are involved in 80% of patients with psoriatic arthritis).

    Look for psoriatic plaques in the extensor aspects of elbows, scalp, submammary region, umbilicus and natal cleft; describe these as reddish plaques with well-defined edges and silvery white scales.

- Comment on the fingers, which are sausage shaped due to tenosynovitis.

Diagnosis

This patient has nail pitting, psoriatic plaques and distal interphalangeal arthropathy (lesion) due to psoriasis (aetiology) and has good hand function (functional status).

Advanced-level Questions

What are the patterns of joint involvement seen in psoriasis?

- Asymmetrical terminal joint involvement.
- Symmetrical joint involvement as seen in rheumatoid arthritis.

- Sacroiliitis: this differs from ankylosing spondylitis, most notably in that the syndesmophytes tend to arise from the lateral and anterior surfaces of the vertebral bodies and not at the margins of the bodies.
- Arthritis mutilans – complicated by the 'telescoping' of digits.

What are the radiological features of psoriatic arthritis?

- 'Fluffy' periostitis.
- Destruction of small joints.
- 'Pencil and cup' appearance, osteolysis and ankylosis in arthritis mutilans.
- Non-marginal syndesmophytes in spondylitis.

What is the prognosis?

Deforming and erosive arthritis is present in 40% of cases and 11% are disabled by their arthritis.

References

Editorial (1988) Prognosis of psoriatic arthritis. *Lancet* **ii**: 375.
Lambert JR & Wright V (1977) Psoriatic spondylitis: a clinical and radiological description of the spine in psoriatic arthritis. *Q J Med* **46**: 411.
Reed WB (1961) Psoriatic arthritis: a complete clinical study of 86 patients. *Acta Derm Venereol* **41**: 396–403.

CASE 129 Scleroderma

Instruction

Look at these hands.

Salient features

- Thickening and tightening of the skin over fingers, sclerodactyly (finger pulp atrophy), beaking of nails (pseudoclubbing), atrophic nails, telangiectasia (nail-fold capillaries).
- Raynaud's phenomenon.
- Subcutaneous calcification (fingers, elbows and extensor aspect of the forearms).
- Vitiligo or pigmentation.

Proceed as follows:

- Assess hand function: pincer movements, handgrip, unbuttoning of clothes, abduction of thumb and writing.
- Examine the following:
  The joints for arthalgia or arthritis.
  The face for microstomia, difficulty in opening the mouth, beak-like or pinched appearance of the nose, blotchy telangiectasia.
  The abdomen for liver (primary biliary cirrhosis).
- Tell the examiner that you would like to ask about the following:
  Dysphagia.
  Raynaud's phenomenon.
  Dry eyes.

Diagnosis

This patient has sclerodactyly, tightening of the skin over hands and face (lesion) due to scleroderma (aetiology). He has difficulty in buttoning his clothes and has marked dysphagia due to oesophageal involvement (functional status).

Questions

What other organ systems are involved?

- Skin: Raynaud's phenomenon; localized morphea, local or generalized oedema, hyperpigmentation, telangiectasia, subcutaneous calcification, ulceration, particularly at the fingertips. Ten-year survival rate is 71% with skin tightness limited to fingers but 21% with diffuse truncal skin involvement. Ilioprost, a prostacyclin analogue, helps heal digital ulceration. Penicillamine improves the skin and prolongs survival in patients with early, rapidly progressive, systemic sclerosis.
- Musculoskeletal system: arthritis, myositis, myopathy, bone ischaemia with resorption of the phalanges.
- Gastrointestinal tract: dysphagia, reflux oesophagitis, large or small bowel obstruction.
- Lung: fibrosis, atelectasis, pulmonary hypertension; pneumonia.
- Kidney: glomerulonephritis, malignant hypertension (poorest prognosis with renal involvement). Angiotensin converting enzyme (ACE) inhibitors dramatically improve renal crisis.
- Heart: myocardial fibrosis.

Remember: the prognosis is worse in those with renal disease and in males. Patients with skin and/or gut involvement without other organ disease have the best prognosis.

What are the variants of scleroderma?

CREST syndrome (see below), eosinophilic fasciitis, Thibierge–Weissen-
bach syndrome.

What is 'CREST' syndrome?

Calcinosis, **R**aynaud's phenomenon, **o**esophageal dysmotility, **s**clerodac-
tyly and **t**elangiectasia. It has a more favourable prognosis than systemic
sclerosis, and is associated with the anticentromere antibody.

Advanced-level Questions

What are the criteria for diagnosis of scleroderma?

- Major criterion is proximal scleroderma (affecting metacarpophalan-
  geals and metatarsophalangeals).
- Minor criteria are as follows:
  Sclerodactyly.
  Digital tip pitting or loss of substance of distal finger pads.
  Bi-basal pulmonary fibrosis.

At least the two major or two or more minor criteria are required.

What are the subsets of scleroderma?

- Limited cutaneous scleroderma: where the skin is affected only at the
  extremities.
- Diffuse cutaneous scleroderma: skin of trunk and extremities affected.
- Scleroderma sine scleroderma: skin not affected, patients present with
  pulmonary fibrosis, scleroderma renal crisis, cardiac failure or
  malabsorption and pseudo-obstruction. The presence of anticentromere, scleroderma-70 and antinuclear antibodies can be
  helpful.

What are the causes of anaemia in such a patient?

- Iron deficiency from chronic oesophagitis.
- Folate and vitamin B_{12} deficiency from malabsorption.
- Anaemia of chronic disease.
- Microangiopathic haemolytic anaemia.

What are the phases of skin changes in scleroderma?

- An early oedematous phase (with pitting oedema of hands and possibly forearms, legs and face).
- The dermal phase.
- An atrophic phase, followed by contracture.
- Other skin changes occur, e.g. depigmentation.

What do you know about the pathogenesis of these skin changes?

The endothelial damage resulting from a circulatory protein factor has been implicated as an early component of the 'inflammatory' phase of scleroderma and endothelial damage may result in the capillary and arteriolar abnormalities demonstrated, as well as local access of circulating proteins acting on fibroblast-enhancing collagen secretion.

How would you manage a patient with scleroderma?

- Educational and psychological support.
- Treat vascular abnormalities such as Raynaud's phenomenon.
- Symptomatic treatment, e.g. omeprazole for oesophagitis.
- Early phase of diffuse form: immunosuppressive drugs (cyclophosphamide, methotrexate, antithymocyte globulin).
- Later stages: antifibrotic drugs (penicillamine, interferon).

What is the role of prednisone in the treatment of scleroderma?

Prednisone has little or no role in the treatment of scleroderma.

What are the common fatal events in this disease?

In most cases, death results from cardiac, renal or respiratory failure.

The first reports of scleroderma were by WD Chowne of London in 1842, and James Startin, also from London, in 1846. The term 'sclerodermie' was suggested by E Gintrac (1791–1877) of Bordeaux; Italian physician GB Fantonetti introduced the term 'skleroderma' in 1836.
Maurice Raynaud commented on the presence of Raynaud's phenomenon in scleroderma in 1863.
Heirich Auspitz (1835–1886) reported, in 1863, on death due to renal failure in scleroderma; this was proved to be a more than chance association by H Moore and H Sheehan of Liverpool in 1952.
David A Isenberg is Professor of Rheumatology, University College London.
Carol Black is Professor of Rheumatology, Royal Free Hospital.

References

Isenberg D & Black C (1995) Raynaud's phenomenon, scleroderma and overlap syndromes. *Br Med J* **310**: 795–798.

Masi AT, Rodnam GP, Medsger TA et al (1980) Preliminary criteria for classification of systemic sclerosis. *Arthritis Rheum* **23**: 581–590.

CASE 130 Painful Knee Joint

Instruction

Examine this patient's leg.
Examine this patient's joints.
Examine this patient's knee joint.

Salient features

- Pain on movement of the joint (take care not to hurt the patient).
- Swelling of the joint (you must demonstrate fluid in the joint).
- Check both active and passive movements.
- Look for disuse atrophy of the muscles around the joint.

Proceed as follows:

- Tell the examiner that you would like to investigate as follows:
  Examine other joints.
  Take a history of trauma and fever.
  X-ray the knee (anteroposterior and lateral views).
  Analyse the joint fluid for cells, sugar, protein and culture.

Diagnosis

This patient has a painful knee joint with restricted movement (lesion and functional status) following trauma while playing rugby (aetiology).

Questions

What are the common causes of a painful knee joint?

- Rheumatoid arthritis.
- Osteoarthrosis.
- Trauma.
- Septic arthritis (will require emergency removal of the pus to prevent joint damage).

- Viral infection.
- Gout.
- Pseudogout.
- Haemophilia.

Advanced-level Questions

What is palindromic rheumatoid arthritis?

Palindromic onset of rheumatoid arthritis refers to acute recurrent arthritis, usually affecting one joint, with symptom-free intervals of days to months between attacks. This term was introduced by PS Hench (see page 352) and EF Rosenberg.

A patient with a painful knee joint and a unilateral facial nerve palsy is seen by you in the outpatient department. Six weeks before this she developed an annular rash after a camping trip in Europe. What is your diagnosis and what confirmatory test would you carry out?

The diagnosis is Lyme disease and the confirmatory test is an antibody titre against *Borrelia burgdorferi*. The disease was first recognized in Lyme, Connecticut, USA.

CASE 131 Osteoarthrosis

Instruction

Look at this patient's hands.
Examine this patient's joints.

Salient features

- Heberden's nodes (bony swellings) at the terminal interphalangeal joints.
- Squaring of the hands due to subluxation of the first metacarpopha-langeal joint.

Proceed as follows:

- Tell the examiner that you would like to examine the hips and knees as these joints are usually involved (feel the knee for crepitus: it may be red, warm and tender, and have an effusion).

Diagnosis

This elderly patient has Heberden's nodes and squaring of the hands with involvement of the interphalangeal joints of the hands (lesions) due to osteoarthrosis (aetiology) and is unable to button his clothes (functional status).

Questions

Which other joints are frequently involved?

Spine, in particular cervical and lumbar spines.

Mention the types and a few causes of osteoarthrosis.

- Primary.
- Secondary:
    Trauma – affects athletes, pneumatic drill workers, anyone doing work involving heavy lifting.
    Inflammatory arthropathies – rheumatoid arthritis, septic arthritis, gout.
    Neuropathic joints – in diabetes mellitus, syringomyelia, tabes dorsalis.
    Endocrine – acromegaly, hyperparathyroidism.
    Metabolic – chondrocalcinosis, haemochromatosis.

What are Heberden's nodes?

Bony swellings seen at the terminal interphalangeal joints in osteoarthrosis.

What are Bouchard's nodes?

Bony swellings at the proximal interphalangeal joints in osteoarthrosis.

Advanced-level Questions

What are the typical radiological features?

- Subchondral bone sclerosis and cysts.
- Osteophytes.

What will the synovial aspirate show?

Fewer than 100 white blood cells per millilitre.

What do you understand by the term 'nodal osteoarthrosis'?

Nodal osteoarthrosis is a primary generalized osteoarthrosis with characteristic features. It occurs predominantly in middle-aged women and is autosomal dominant. It characteristically affects the terminal interphalangeal joints with the development of Heberden's nodes. The arthritis may be acute and, although there may be marked deformity, there is little disability. It can also affect the carpometacarpal joints of the thumbs, spinal apophyseal joints, knees and hips.

How would you manage a patient with osteoarthrosis?

● Change in lifestyle: maintain optimal weight, encourage exercise, use appropriate footwear.
● Drugs: simple analgesics, rubifacients, NSAIDs for acute flare-ups, intra-articular corticosteroid injections for acute flare-ups or patients unfit for surgery.
● Surgery: arthroscopic removal of loose body, arthroscopic washout or radioisotope synovectomy for persistent synovitis, joint replacement for hip and knee.

William Heberden (1710–1801) was a London physician who described the nodes as 'little hard knobs' and this was first published posthumously in 1802.
JK Spender (1886), of Bath, introduced the term osteoarthritis. Archibald E Garrod from London, established the modern usage and clinical differentiation from rheumatoid arthritis in 1907.
In 1884, CJ Bouchard (1837–1915) described nodes adjacent to the proximal interphalangeal joints identical to those at the distal interphalangeal joints.

References

Hamerman D (1989) The biology of osteoarthritis. *N Engl J Med* **320**: 1322.
Jones A & Doherty M (1995) Osteoarthritis. *Br Med J* **310**: 457–460.
Moskowitz RW (1987) Primary osteoarthritis. Epidemiology, clinical aspects and general management. *Am J Med* **83**(suppl 5A): 5.

CASE 132 Gout

Instruction

Examine this patient's hands or examine the feet.

Salient features

- Chronic tophaceous deposit with asymmetrical joint involvement.

Proceed as follows:

- Tell the examiner that you would like to proceed as follows:
    Examine the helices of the ears, olecranon bursae and Achilles
        tendons for tophi.
    Examine the feet or hands.

Note. Uric acid crystals are negatively birefringent, needle shaped and
may be deposited in bursae and bone marrow. They are demonstrable in
synovial fluid within leukocytes and free in the fluid during attacks of
gouty arthritis. They react with nitric acid and ammonium hydroxide to
give a purple colour (murexide test).

Diagnosis

This patient has a painful great toe with swelling of the joint (lesion) due
to gout (aetiology) and is unable to walk because of the pain (functional
status).

Questions

What is the basic pathophysiology of gout?

Gout is a metabolic disorder of purine metabolism. It is characterized by
hyperuricaemia due to either overproduction (75%) or underexcretion
(25%) of uric acid.

What are the different clinical manifestations of gout?

- Asymptomatic hyperuricaemia.
- Acute arthritis.
- Chronic arthritis.
- Chronic tophaceous gout.

How would you treat an acute attack of gout?

Prescribe an NSAID such as indomethacin. Refractory gout may require steroids.

What factors may precipitate acute gouty arthritis?

Drugs (diuretics, aspirin), copious consumption of alcohol, dehydration, surgery, fasting food high in purines (sweetbreads, liver, kidney and sardines).

Advanced-level Questions

Under what circumstances would you treat hyperuricaemia?

Frequent attacks of acute arthritis, renal damage and consistently raised serum uric acid levels. Before attempting to lower serum uric acid levels it is prudent to use colchicine to prevent acute attacks.

What is the drug of choice for controlling hyperuricaemia?

Allopurinol (a xanthine oxidase inhibitor).

What drugs would you use if the patient was allergic to allopurinol?

Uricosuric drugs such as probenecid, sulphinpyrazone.

What is pseudogout?

Pseudogout is an acute arthritis resulting from the release of calcium pyrophosphate dihydrate crystals (deposited in the bone and cartilage) into the synovial fluid.

Gout has been recognized from as early as the 4th century BC. Two concepts have prevailed that it occurs mainly in sexually active mature men and that gastronomic and sexual excesses may precipitate acute attacks. Antonj van Leewenhoeck (1632–1723) described the microscopic appearance of urate crystals from gouty tophus. In 1847 Alfred Garrod, in London, identified uric acid in the serum of a gouty man.

James Wyngaarden, contemporary Professor of Medicine, Duke University, USA, whose chief interest is metabolic and genetic diseases.

CASE 133 Ehlers–Danlos Syndrome

Instruction

Do a general examination.
Examine this patient's joints.

Salient features

Skin:
- The skin over the neck, axillae and groin is smooth and elastic. It can be stretched and, when released, it returns immediately to its normal position. Late in the disease it becomes lax, wrinkled and hangs in folds.

Proceed as follows:

- Look at bony prominences for bruising, haematomas and gaping wounds. Wounds heal forming tissue-paper or papyraceous or 'cigarette-paper' scars. Haematomas heal forming pseudotumours or nodules.

Joints:
- Kyphoscoliosis.
- Hypermobility of joints.

Proceed as follows:

- Tell the examiner that you would like to examine the following:
   The hernial orifices.
   The heart for mitral valve prolapse and aortic regurgitation.
   The eyes for myopia, retinal detachment.

Note. The three basic clinical criteria are: (1) fragile skin; (2) bleeding diathesis; (3) hypermobile joints.

Diagnosis

This patient has hypermobile joints (lesion) due to Ehlers–Danlos syndrome (aetiology).

Advanced-level Questions

What are the gastrointestinal manifestations of this syndrome?

- Marked tendency to herniate.

- Achalasia cardia.
- Eventeration of the diaphragm.
- Megacolon.

What are the cardiovascular manifestations?

- Mitral valve prolapse.
- Aortic dissection.

What precautions would you take in managing skin wounds?

As the skin wounds tend to be gaping, they should be approximated with care; removable sutures are usually left in place for twice the usual time.

What do you know about Ehlers–Danlos syndrome?

It comprises a group of heterogeneous disorders that result from defects in collagen synthesis and vary genetically and clinically from one another. The molecular defects of the following are known:

- Type VI: the most common and autosomal recessive form of inheritance. There is a defect in the enzyme protein, viz. lysyl hydroxylase, which is necessary for hydroxylation of lysyl residues during collagen synthesis. Only collagen types 1 and 3 are affected, and collagen types 2, 4 and 6 are normal. The predominant clinical features are ocular fragility with rupture of the cornea and retinal detachment. Some of these patients respond to ascorbic acid.
- Type IV: due to a defect in the structural gene for collagen type 3 and thus inherited as an autosomal dominant trait. As type 3 collagen is present largely in blood vessels and intestines, the typical features of this syndrome include rupture of the large arteries and colon, reducing life expectancy considerably. This is the most severe form of Ehlers–Danlos syndrome.
- Type VII: a defect in the conversion of procollagen to collagen, due to the mutation that affects one of the two type 1 collagen genes. Although in the single mutant allele only 50% of type 1 collagen chains are affected, heterozygotes manifest the syndrome because these abnormal chains interfere with the formation of normal collagen helices.
- Type IX: due to a defect in copper metabolism with high levels of copper in the cells but low levels of serum copper and caeruloplasmin. Because the gene influencing copper metabolism is on the X chromosome, it is inherited as an X-linked recessive trait. This disease illustrates how copper metabolism can affect connective tissue.

Note. Patients with type I, II and IV disease are often investigated for bleeding diathesis before the correct diagnosis is made. Because of joint instability and laxity, many patients with types I, II, III, VI and VII disease are investigated for developmental delay before it is recognized that they have this syndrome.

In which other condition is there a defect in collagen metabolism?

Osteogenesis imperfecta.

Note. At least some 14 types of collagen have been discerned: types 1, 2 and 3 are the interstitial or fibrillar collagen whereas types 4, 5 and 6 are amorphous and are present in the interstitial tissue and basement membranes.

What are the criteria for diagnosis of joint hypermobility?

Beighton's nine-point scoring for joint hypermobility assigns two points for each of the following four paired manoeuvres:
- Hyperextension of the fifth metcarpophalangeal joint to 90 degrees.
- Apposition of the thumb to the volar aspect of the forearm.
- Hyperextension of the elbow beyond 10 degrees.
- Hyperextension of the knee to beyond 10 degrees.

One point is assigned for the ability to place the palms of the hands on the floor with the knees extended.

Is hypermobility advantageous to musicians?

Lax fingers and wrists are good for flutists and string players, but lax knees and spines are bad for tympanists and others who stand while they play.

Edvard Ehlers (1863–1937), a Danish dermatologist, and HA Danlos, a French dermatologist, described this condition independently in 1901 and 1908 respectively.
It is widely believed that the oustanding virtuosity of the violionist Niccolò Paganini (1782–1840) was due to remarkable flexibility of the joints of his left hand – he could span three octaves with little effort.
Robert James Gorlin (b. 1923) described Gorlin's sign, which is the ability to touch the tip of the nose with the tongue in Ehlers–Danlos syndrome.

References

Beighton P, Solomon L & Soskolne CL (1973) Articular mobility in an African population. *Ann Rheum Dis* **32**: 413–418.

Larsson LG, Baum J, Mudholkar GS & Kollia GD (1993) Benefits and disadvantages of joint hypermobility among musicians. *N Engl J Med* **329**: 1079.

Liechtenstein JR, Martin OR, Kohn L, Byers PH & McKusick VA (1973) Defect in conversion of procollagen to collagen in the form of Ehlers-Danlos syndrome. *Science* **182**: 298.

Smith RD (1982) Paganini's hand. *Arthritis Rheum* **25**: 1385–1356.

CASE 134 — Charcot's Joint

Instruction

Examine this patient's joints.
Examine the locomotor system in this patient.

Salient features

- Enlargement of the affected joint (compare with the other side).
- Instability of the joint, in particular hypermobility of the joint.
- May be warm, swollen and tender in the early stages.
- Enlargement and crepitus may be present in the later stages.

Proceed as follows:

- Check sensation in the affected limb.
- Tell the examiner that you would like to investigate as follows:
    Do a thorough neurological examination, looking for loss of proprioception and/or pain sensation.
    Examine the urine for sugar (looking for evidence of diabetes mellitus).
    Ask for lancinating pains, check posterior column signs and look for Argyll–Robertson pupil (tabes dorsalis).
    Check for dissociated sensory loss (syringomyelia).

Diagnosis

This patient has Charcot's joint (lesion) due to diabetes mellitus (aetiology) and has marked deformity of the joint with restricted movement (functional status).

Questions

What do you understand by the term Charcot's joint?

It is a chronic progressive degenerative arthropathy resulting from a disturbance in the sensory innervation of the affected joint. It is a neuropathic arthropathy which represents a complication of various disorders affecting the nervous system. It results in gross deformity, osteoarthrosis and new bone formation from repeated trauma.

Mention a few conditions responsible for the development of Charcot's joints.

- Diabetic neuropathy – affecting tarsal joints, tarsometatarsal, metatarsophalangeal joints.
- Tabes dorsalis – affecting knee, hip, ankle, lumbar and lower dorsal vertebrae.
- Syringomyelia – affecting shoulder, elbow, cervical vertebra.
- Myelomeningocoele – affecting ankle, tarsus.
- Miscellaneous: hereditary sensory neuropathies, peripheral nerve injury, congenital insensitivity to pain, leprosy.

Jean Martin Charcot (1825–1893) was a French neurologist. He was a Professor of Pathology in 1872 and Professor of Nervous Diseases in 1882. The other conditions that bear his name include the following: Charcot's fever (intermittent fever due to cholangitis), Charcot's triad (intention tremor, nystagmus and scanning speech in multiple sclerosis), Charcot-Leyden crystals (seen in the sputum of asthmatics), Charcot–Marie–Tooth disease (peroneal muscular atrophy), Charcot-Wilbrand syndrome (visual agnosia).

Reference

Sinha S, Munichoodappa CS & Kozak GP (1972) Neuroarthropathy (Charcot's joints) in diabetes mellitus: clinical study in 101 cases. *Medicine* **51**: 191–210.

CASE 135 Still's Disease

Instruction

Examine this patient's joints.
Look at this patient.

Salient features

- Micrognathia.
- Joints usually involved are upper cervical apophyseal joints, carpometacarpal joints and terminal interphalangeal joints.

- Maculopapular rash.
- Splenomegaly and lymph node enlargement.

Proceed as follows:

- Tell the examiner that you would like to take a history of fever in the initial stages of the disease.

Diagnosis

This patient has micrognathia, arthropathy of terminal interphalangeal joints and a past history of maculopapular rash (lesion) due to Still's disease (aetiology).

Advanced-level Questions

What do you know about juvenile chronic arthritis?

The diagnosis is made when a child aged less than 16 years has arthritis for at least 6 weeks with no other apparent cause. After 6 months of disease three major patterns are seen:

- Still's disease (10–20% of cases) is defined as arthritis associated with daily temperature spikes to 39.4 °C (103 °F) for at least 2 weeks with or without maculopapular rash.
- Polyarticular juvenile chronic arthritis (15–25%) in which five or more joints are affected. Early fusion of the mandible and cervical spine result in a receding chin and early fusion of the cervical spine.
- Pauciarticular juvenile chronic arthritis (60–75%) which affects four or less joints; iritis is common in girls, whereas sacroiliitis is common in boys.

What are the complications of juvenile chronic arthritis?

- Pain, lethargy, anorexia and irritability.
- Joint contractures.
- Anaemia.
- Chronic anterior uveitis.
- Growth disturbance.
- Amyloidosis.
- Joint failure.

How would you treat a patient with juvenile chronic arthritis?

- Education about the disease, counselling and social support.
- Physical and occupational therapy: monitoring and recording range of

movement of joints, exercises to increase range of movement and muscle bulk, hydrotherapy, splinting.

- NSAIDs: naproxen, ibuprofen, piroxicam, indomethacin, diclofenac.
- Intra-articular steroids: triamcinolone, methylprednisolone acetate.

What is the risk of treating young children with salicylates?

Reye's syndrome has been reported in children treated with aspirin for fever accompanying viral infections such as influenza. Children with juvenile chronic arthritis who are treated continuously for long periods have not been shown to have an increased incidence of this syndrome.

What are the poor prognostic factors?

- Chronic and polyarticular arthritis, particularly in patients with a systemic or pauciarticular onset.
- Polyarticular onset and a positive test for immunoglobulin rheumatoid factor.

Which drugs have been used in the treatment of resistant juvenile rheumatoid arthritis?

- Pencillamine.
- Hydroxychloroquine.
- Methotrexate (long-term therapy should be avoided as it is known to cause hepatic fibrosis).

Sir George Fredrick Still (1868–1941), a London physician, described 12 children (in 1897) who had a polyarthritis which he stated should be distinguished from rheumatoid arthritis, and a further six children with a disease indistinguishable from adult rheumatoid arthritis. The distinctive findings in the first group included splenomegaly, lymphadenopathy, frequent occurrence of pericarditis and a predilection for cervical spine involvement. He also noted that fever and growth retardation were prominent features. The rash, however, was first described by Eric GL Bywaters.
RDK Reye (1912–1977), an Australian histopathologist.

References

Southwood TR (1995) Arthritis in children. *Br Med J* **310**: 728–731.
Starko KM, Ray CG, Dominquez LB et al (1980) Reye's syndrome and salicylate use. *Pediatrics* **66**: 859.
Still GF (1897) On a form of chronic joint disease in childhood. *Med Chir Trans* **80**: 47.
White PH & Ansell BM (1992) Methotrexate for juvenile rheumatoid arthritis. *N Engl J Med* **326**: 1077.

ENDOCRINOLOGY

EXAMINATION OF THE THYROID

Instruction

Examine the thyroid.
Test this patient's thyroid status.
Look at this patient's neck.

Salient features

- Introduce yourself to the patient and, while shaking hands, note whether the palms are warm and sweaty.
- *Inspection of the neck*:
    Look for the JVP.
    Scars of surgery (often missed by candidates).
    Enlarged cervical lymph nodes.
    Goitre.
- *Palpation* (always begin by palpating from behind):
    Seat the patient comfortably.
    Comment first on exophthalmos.
    While palpating the gland, ensure that there is a glass of water to swallow.
    Palpate the thyroid and note the following:
        Size – specify the World Health Organization grade (see below).
        Mobility.
        Texture – simple or nodular (solitary or multiple)?
        Tenderness.
    Pemberton's sign (on raising the arms above the head, patients with retrosternal goitres may develop signs of compression, i.e. suffusion of the face, syncope or giddiness).
    Palpate cervical lymph nodes.
    Feel the carotid arteries.
    Palpate for tracheal deviation.
    Percuss for retrosternal extension.
    Auscultate over the gland for bruit, carotid bruits.

Test sternomastoid function (this muscle may be infiltrated in thyroid malignancy).
- Thyroid *function* should then be assessed:
1. Eye signs:
    Lid lag.
    Exophthalmos.
    Lid retraction (sclera visible above the cornea).
    Extraocular movements.
2. Hands:
    Pulse for tachycardia or atrial fibrillation.
    Tremor.
    Acropachy or clubbing.
    Palmar erythema (thyrotoxicosis).
    Supinator jerks (inverted in hypothyroidism).
    Proximal weakness in the upper arm.
3. Skin: look for pretibial myxoedema.
4. Elicit the ankle jerks.

If you are permitted to ask questions, enquire about shortness of breath, dysphagia, about iodine-containing medications and possible exposure to radiation.

Questions

How would you grade the size of the goitre?

WHO grading of goitre:
    Grade 0   No palpable or visible goitre.
    Grade 1   Palpable goitre.
        1A   Goitre detectable only on palpation.
        1B   Goitre palpable and visible with neck extended.
    Grade 2   Goitre visible with neck in normal position.
    Grade 3   Large goitre visible from a distance.

What is the significance of the thyroid bruit?

The thyroid bruit is almost pathognomonic of Graves' disease and occurs only rarely in patients with colloid goitres or other thyroid disorders.

In 1915 Kendall isolated a crystalline product named thyroxine and in 1927 Harrington and Barger synthesized thyroxine.
In 1952 Gross and Pitt-Rivers identified tri-iodothyronine.

References

Gross J & Pitt-Rivers R (1952) The identification of 3,5,3′ L-triiodothyronine in human plasma. *Lancet* **i**: 439.

Harrington CR & Barger G (1927) Chemistry of thyroxine. *Biochem J* **21**: 169.

Kendall EC (1915) The isolation in crystalline form of the compound containing iodine which occurs in the thyroid. *JAMA* **64**: 2042.

CASE 136 Graves' Disease

Instruction

Look at this patient.
Determine this patient's thyroid status.

Salient features

- Patient is fidgety and restless.

Proceed as follows:

Hands:

- While shaking hands with the patient note the warm sweaty palms.
- Look for tremor, thyroid acropachy, onycholysis (Plummer's nails), vitiligo and palmar erythema.
- Check pulse (for tachycardia or the irregularly irregular pulse of atrial fibrillation).

Eyes:

- Comment on proptosis (after looking at the eyes from behind and above).
- Check for lid lag.
- Check for scars of previous tarsorraphy.

Neck:

- Mention previous thyroidectomy scar if present.
- Examine the neck for goitre and auscultate over the gland.

Lower limbs:

- Examine the shins for pretibial myxoedema (bilateral pinkish, brown dermal plaques).
- Test for proximal myopathy.
- Tell the examiner that you would like to ask the patient about the following:
  Easy irritability.
  Weight loss with increased appetite.

Frequent defaecation.
Oligomenorrhoea.
Dislike for hot weather.
Family history of thyroid disease.

Diagnosis

This patient has tremor, proptosis and lid lag (lesions) due to autoimmune Graves' disease (aetiology), and is in fast atrial fibrillation and hyperthyroid (functional status).

Questions

How would you confirm the diagnosis in this patient?

Serum thyroxine (T_4), serum thyroid-stimulating hormone (TSH) levels and thyroid autoantibodies.

What are the causes of hyperthyroidism?

- Primary: Graves' disease, toxic nodule, multinodular goitre, Hashimato's thyroiditis, iodine-induced, excess thyroid hormone replacement, postpartum thyroiditis.
- Secondary: pituitary or excess TSH hypersecretion, hydatidiform moles, struma ovarii, factitious.

What are the components of Graves' disease?

Hyperthyroidism with goitre, eye changes and pretibial myxoedema – they run independent courses.

Advanced-level Questions

What happens to radioactive iodine uptake in Graves' disease?

Radioactive iodine uptake increases in Graves' disease.

Mention a few causes of hyperthyroidism with reduced iodine uptake.

- Thyroiditis.
- Malignancy of thyroid.
- Struma ovarii.

What drugs are used in the treatment of thyrotoxicosis?

- Carbimazole.
- Methimazole.
- Propylthiouracil.

What are the disadvantages of antithyroid drugs?

- High rates of relapse once treatment is discontinued.
- Occasionally complicated by troublesome hypersensitivity reaction and very rarely by life-threatening agranulocytosis and hepatitis.

What are the advantages and disadvantages of radioactive iodine, compared with partial thyroidectomy for thyrotoxicosis?

Both radioactive iodine therapy and surgical thyroidectomy are extremely effective and usually result in permanent cure. Patients will require lifelong thyroxine replacement. Thyroid surgery is expensive, inconvenient, occasionally complicated by injury to surrounding structures in the neck in less skilled hands, and complicated by the risks of anaesthesia.

Radioactive iodine, although safe, may not be acceptable to patients who are sensitive to the calamities of Chernobyl and Hiroshima.

Is there an increased frequency of cancer in patients with Graves' disease?

There is little evidence to suggest an increased frequency of thyroid cancer in patients with Graves' disease.

Does thyrotoxicosis affect the bone?

Yes, chronic thyrotoxicosis is associated with osteoporosis.

If a patient with thyrotoxicosis develops muscle weakness following oral carbohydrate or intravenous dextrose, which condition comes to mind?

Hypokalaemic periodic paralysis, which occurs particularly in Asian men. These attacks may last for 7–72 hours.

What is the effect of iodine on thyroid status?

It may cause transient hypothyroidism (Wolff–Chaikoff effect) or hyperthyroidism (Jod–Basedow phenomenon).

Robert James Graves (1796–1853) was a Dublin physician who described this condition. In 1835 he described three patients and wrote of one patient, 'It was now observed that the eyes assumed a singular appearance for the eyeballs were apparently enlarged, so that when she slept or tried to shut her eyes her lids were incapable of closing, when the eyes were open, the white sclerotic could be seen, to a breadth of several lines all around the cornea'.

References

Franklyn JA (1994) The management of hyperthyroidism. *N Engl J Med* **330**: 1731–1737.

Graves R (1835) *London Med Surg J* **7**(Part II): 516.

Ladenson PW (1991) Treatment for Graves' disease – letting the thyroid rest. *N Engl J Med* **324**: 989.

CASE 137 Exophthalmos

Instruction

Examine this patient's face.
Perform a general examination of this patient.

Salient features

- Prominent eyeballs.

Proceed as follows:

- Look at the patient's eyes from behind and above for proptosis.
- Comment on lid retraction (the sclera above the upper limbus of the cornea will be seen); this is Dalrymple's sign.
- Comment on the sclera visible between the lower eyelid and the lower limbus of the cornea (i.e. comment on the exophthalmos). Most patients have bilateral exophthalmos with unilateral prominence.
- Check for lid lag (ask the patient to follow your finger and then move it along the arc of a circle from a point above her head to a point below the nose – the movement of the lid lags behind that of the globe); this is von Graefe's sign. Voluntary staring can result in a false lid lag, and the patient must be suitably relaxed before eliciting this sign.
- Check for extraocular movements and comment on the cornea.
- Look for the following:
  Signs of thyrotoxicosis (fast pulse rate, tremor and sweating).
  Goitre (listen for a bruit).
  Post-thyroidectomy scar.

Diagnosis

This patient has marked exophthalmos with ophthalmoplegia (lesions) with signs of thyrotoxicosis (functional status) due to Graves' disease (aetiology).

Advanced-level Questions

What eye signs of thyroid disease do you know?

Werner's mnemonic, NO SPECS:
> No signs or symptoms.
> Only signs of upper lid retraction and stare, with or without lid lag and exophthalmos.

> Soft tissue involvement.
> Proptosis.
> Extraocular muscle involvement.
> Corneal involvement.
> Sight loss due to optic nerve involvement.

How would you investigate this patient?

- History and clinical examination for signs of thyrotoxicosis and thyroid enlargement and bruit.
- Serum T_4, triiodothyronine (T_3), TSH.
- Thyroid antibodies.

Mention the factors implicated in the phenomenon of lid lag.

- Sympathetic overstimulation, causing overaction of Müller's muscle.
- Myopathy of the inferior rectus causing overaction of superior rectus and levator muscles.
- Restrictive myopathy of the levator muscle.

What is euthyroid Graves' disease?

The patient will be clinically and biochemically euthyroid but will have manifestations of Graves' ophthalmopathy. A thyrotrophin releasing hormone (TRH) stimulation test will show a flat response curve.

What would you recommend if a patient with unilateral exophthalmos is clinically and biochemically euthyroid?

- Ophthalmological referral.
- Ultrasonography of the orbit.

- CT scan of the orbit.

How is proptosis quantified?

It is assessed using a Hertel's exophthalmometer. The upper limit of normal is subject to ethnic variation, and usually more than 20 mm is considered as proptosis.

How would you manage a patient with Graves' ophthalmopathy?

The single most important aspect is a close liaison between the physician and the ophthalmologist.

Severe Graves' disease and visual loss should be treated immediately with high doses of corticosteroids, orbital irradiation and plasma exchange as an adjunct and, if there is no improvement within 72–96 hours, orbital nerve decompression by surgical removal of the floor and medial wall of the orbit is necessary.

Moderate ophthalmopathy improves substantially in 2–3 years in most patients. In the interim the patient is treated symptomatically:
- Pain and grittiness is treated with methylcellulose eye drops by day and a lubricating eye ointment at night.
- Exposure keratitis may be relieved by lateral tarsorraphy, surgery of the lower eyelid.
- Diplopia may be relieved by prisms or surgery of the extraocular muscles.
- Static or worsening ophthalmopathy is an indication for steroids, orbital decompression or orbital irradiation.
- Patients should be advised to stop smoking.

Mild ophthalmopathy should be rectified by cosmetic eyelid surgery. It is important to remember that patients can be distressed by their appearance. During the early acute phase patients will have considerable symptomatic relief from the following measures:
- Elevating the head at night.
- Diuretics to reduce oedema.
- Tinted glasses for protection from the sun, wind and foreign bodies.

Does the treatment for hyperthyroidism affect Graves' ophthalmopathy?

Yes. Ophthalmopathy caused by Graves' disease may first appear or worsen during or after treatment for hyperthyroidism; iodine-131 is more likely to cause this than antithyroid drugs or surgery. Hypothyroidism should be avoided.

Mention the less important eponyms related to thyroid eye disease.

These include:
- Infrequent blinking – Stellwag's sign.
- Tremor of closed eyelids – Rosenbach's sign.
- Difficulty in everting upper eyelid – Gifford's sign.
- Absence of wrinkling of forehead on sudden upward gaze – Joffroy's sign.
- Impaired convergence of the eyes –Möbius' sign.
- Weakness of at least one of the extraocular muscles – Ballet's sign.
- Paralysis of extraocular muscles – Jendrassik's sign.
- Poor fixation on lateral gaze – Suker's sign.
- Dilatation of pupil with weak adrenaline solution – Loewi's sign.
- Jerky pupillary contraction to consensual light – Cowen's sign.
- Increased pigmentation of the margins of eyelids – Jellinek's sign.
- Upper lid resistance on downward traction – Grove's sign.
- Abnormal fullness of the eyelid – Enroth's sign.
- Unequal pupillary dilatation – Knie's sign.
- When the eyeball is turned downwards, there is arrest of the descent of the lid, spasm and continued descent – Boston's sign.
- When the clinician places his or her hand on a level with the patient's eyes and then lifts it higher, the patient's upper lids spring up more quickly than the eyeball – Kocher's sign.

J Dalrymple (1804–1852), an English ophthalmologist.
Exophthalmos associated with goitre and non-organic heart disease was first described by English physician, Caleb Hillard Parry (1775–1822) in a paper published posthumously in 1825. He graduated in medicine from Edinburgh and practised in Bath. He described hyperthyroidism before Graves' disease.
In 1977 Solomon et al presented the evidence that three independent autoimmune diseases tended to occur concomitantly in the same euthyroid Graves' ophthalmopathy: idiopathic hyperthyroidism, Hashimato's thyroiditis and Graves' ophthalmopathy.
Anthony Toft, an endocrinologist, is President of the Royal College of Physicians of Edinburgh.

References

Bahn RS & Heufelder AE (1993) Pathogenesis of Graves' ophthalmopathy. *N Engl J Med* **329**: 1468–1475.
Fleck BW & Toft AD (1990) Graves' ophthalmopathy. *Br Med J* **300**: 1352.
Parry CH (1825) *Elements Path Ther* **2**: 11.
Prummel MF, Mouritis Mph, Blank L, Berghout A, Koornneef L & Wiersinga WM (1993) Randomised double-blind trial of prednisone versus radiotherapy in Grave's ophthalmopathy. *Lancet* **342**: 949–953.
Werners SC (1977) Classification of the eye changes of Graves' disease. *J Clin Endocrinol Metab* **44**: 203–204.

CASE 138   Hypothyroidism

Instruction

Look at this patient's neck.
Look at this patient.
Do a general examination.

Salient features

- Coarse, dry skin (look for yellowish tint of carotenaemia – 'peaches and cream' complexion).
- 'Dirty elbows and knees' sign.
- Puffy lower eyelids.
- Loss of outer third of eyebrows, xanthelasma.
- Slow pulse.

Proceed as follows:

- Examine the neck for goitre and the scar of previous thyroidectomy.
- Check the ankle jerks, looking for delayed relaxation.
- Tell the examiner that you would like to check for the following:
    Proximal muscle weakness.
    Cerebellar signs.
    Carpal tunnel syndrome.
- Tell the examiner that you would like to take a history of the following:
    Cold intolerance.
    Change in the voice (hoarse, husky).
    Lethargy, undue tiredness.
    Constipation.
    Moderate weight gain in spite of loss of appetite.
    Menorrhagia.
    Radio-iodine therapy for previous Graves' disease (the patient may have associated eye signs of Graves' disease).

Diagnosis

This patient has delayed ankle jerks, puffy lower eyelids, slow pulse and hoarse husky voice (lesions) indicating that he has hypothyroidism (functional status); the cause needs to be determined (aetiology).

Questions

How is delayed relaxation best elicited in the ankle?

Get the patient to kneel on a chair with his hands holding the back of the chair and then elicit the jerks on either side.

What are the causes of goitre?

- Idiopathic (majority).
- Hashimato's thyroiditis.
- Graves' disease.
- Iodine deficiency (simple goitre).
- Puberty, pregnancy, subacute thyroiditis, goitrogens (lithium, phenyl-butazone).

What is the thyroid status in Hashimato's disease?

Hypothyroidism (usually).

What is the single best clinical indicator for hypothyroidism?

Delayed ankle jerks.

What is the best laboratory indicator for hypothyroidism?

Serum TSH levels.

How would you investigate a simple goitre?

Estimation of serum T_3, T_4, TSH and thyroid antibodies.

What is the cause for delayed relaxation in hypothyroidism?

The exact cause is not known. It is probably due to decreased muscle metabolism.

How would you manage this patient with hypothyroidism?

Oral thyroxine replacement therapy for life. The therapeutic dose varies between 100 and 200 μg per day taken as a single dose. Dose adjustments are made once in 3 weeks. The dose is adjusted depending on the clinical response and suppression of raised serum TSH levels.

What is the hazard in treating the elderly?

Rapid T_4 replacement may precipitate angina and myocardial infarction. The starting dose in the elderly is 50 µg per day.

What are the cardiovascular manifestations of hypothyroidism?

- Bradycardia.
- Mild hypertension.
- Pericarditis and pericardial effusion.
- High low-density lipoprotein, low high-density lipoprotein levels, hypercholesterolaemia.
- Diminished cardiac output and cardiac failure.
- Coronary artery disease.
- ECG changes: low-voltage T and P waves, prolongation of QT interval.

What are the neurological manifestations of hypothyroidism?

- Delayed deep tendon reflexes (Woltman's sign).
- Carpal tunnel syndrome, peripheral neuropathy.
- Myxoedema madness.
- Myxoedema coma.
- Pseudodementia.
- Deafness to high tones (Trotter's syndrome). In Pendred's syndrome, babies are born with a goitre, deafness and mental retardation.
- Cerebellar syndrome.
- Hoffmann's syndrome, i.e. muscle aches with myotonia in myxoedema. In infants, muscle involvement may result in Kocher–Debré–Sémélaigne syndrome or 'infant Hercules'.

What other conditions are associated with Hashimato's thyroiditis?

- Addison's disease.
- Diabetes mellitus.
- Graves' disease.
- Hypoparathyroidism.
- Premature ovarian failure.
- Pernicious anaemia.
- Rheumatoid arthritis.
- Sjögren's syndrome.
- Ulcerative colitis.
- SLE.
- Haemolytic anaemia.

What do you understand by the term 'sick euthyroid syndrome'?

In severe acute non-thyroidal illness or following surgery, changes in pituitary–thyroid function result in altered thyroid indices but, despite this, patients remain euthyroid. On recovery from the illness, the indices of thyroid function return to normal. The changes in thyroidal indices include:

- Decrease in extrathyroidal conversion of thyroxine T_4 to tri-iodothyronine (T_3), the active form of the thyroid hormone.
- A decrease in thyrotrophin secretion, which causes decreased thyroidal secretion and, in time, decreases in serum T_4 concentrations and further decreases in serum T_3 concentrations – the latter due to both decreased secretion of T_3 by the thyroid and diminished availability of T_4 for peripheral conversion to T_3.
- Decreased production or diminished affinity for thyroidal hormones of one or more major serum thyroid hormone-binding proteins – thyroxine-binding globulin, transthyretin and albumin. These decreases can result in decreased serum total thyroxine levels but not in free T_4 or T_3. Serum concentrations of reverse T_3 (which is inactive) are increased because its deiodination is impaired.

The complete clinical description of myxoedema was first given by Gull in 1873, but it was Ord in 1878 who coined the word myxoedema when, at autopsy, he found extensive deposits of mucin in the skin of the feet. WW Gull (1816–1890), FRS, graduated from Guy's Hospital in London and was created a Baronet when he treated the then Prince of Wales, who had typhoid. He was a good teacher and said that 'Savages explain, science investigates'.

Emil Theodor Kocher (1841–1917), Swiss Professor of Surgery in Berne, was awarded the Nobel Prize in 1909 for his work on the physiology, pathology and surgery of the thyroid gland. He was the first to excise the thyroid gland for goitre and described myxoedema following thyroidectomy – 'cachexia strumipriva'. His name is associated with: (1) Kocher forceps; (2) Kocher's transverse cervical incision for thyroidectomy; (3) Kocher's operation for the wrist; (4) Kocher's oblique right subcostal incision for gallbladder surgery; (5) Kocher manoeuvre for reduction of a dislocated shoulder; and (6) Kocher syndrome describing splenomegaly and lymphadenopathy with thyrotoxicosis.

R Debré and G Sémélaigne were both French physicians.

H Hashimato (1881–1934), a Japanese surgeon.

Johann Hoffmann (1857–1919), a German neurologist.

References

Ber A (1954) The sign of 'dirty' knees and elbows. *Acta Endocrinol* (Copenh) **16**: 305.

Debré R & Sémélaigne G (1935) Syndrome of diffuse muscular hypertrophy in infants causing athletic appearance. Its connection with congenital myxoedema. *Am J Dis Child* **50**: 1351.

Gull WW (1873) On a cretinoid state supervening in adult life in women. *Trans Clin Soc London* **7**: 180–185.

Jellinek EH & Kelly RE (1960) Cerebellar syndrome in myxoedema. *Lancet* **ii**: 225.

Ord WM (1878) On myxoedema, a term proposed to be applied to an essential condition in the 'cretinoid' affection occasionally observed in middle-aged women. *Med Chir Trans* **61**: 57.

Trotter WR (1960) The association of deafness with thyroid dysfunction. *Br Med Bull* **16**: 92.

Utiger RD (1995) Altered thyroid function in nonthyroidal illness and surgery. *N Engl J Med* **333**: 1562–1563.

CASE 139 Pretibial Myxoedema

Instruction

Look at this patient's legs.

Salient features

- Red thickened swellings above the lateral malleoli – peau d'orange appearance – which progresses to thickened non-pitting oedema of the feet.

Proceed as follows:

- Examine the following:
  The hands for acropachy, palmar erythema and warm, sweaty palms.
  The neck for goitre and thyroidectomy scar.
  The eyes for exophthalmos.
  The pulse for tachycardia and atrial fibrillation.
- Tell the examiner that you would like to know whether or not the patient has had any treatment, in particular radioactive iodine.

Remember pretibial myxoedema dermopathy is a late manifestation of Graves' disease and its onset is usually followed by the diagnosis of hyperthyroidsim and ophthalmopathy.

Diagnosis

This patient has pretibial myxoedema (lesion) with ophthalmopathy and signs of thyrotoxicosis (functional status) which is due to Graves' disease.

Questions

What investigations would you do?

Serum T_4, T_3 and TSH.

How are these lesions treated?

- Intralesional steroids or fluorinated corticosteroids applied under polythene occlusion.
- Plasmapheresis.
- Cytotoxic therapy.
- Octreotide.

NB: Surgical excision should be avoided because surgical scars may aggravate the dermopathy and precipitate recurrence.

Advanced-level Questions

What are the types of pretibial myxoedema?

Three major classes of thyroid dermopathy have been identified:
- Non-pitting oedema accompanied by hyperkeratosis, pigmentation and pinkish, brownish red or yellowish discoloration of the skin. Plaque formation and nodularity are characteristically absent in this group.
- Plaque form consisting of raised, discrete or confluent plaques.
- Nodular form, characterized by nodule formation.

Less common types:
- Elephantiasic form.
- Polypoid form.

NB: Almost all patient tend to have ophthalmopathy, which is usually severe.

What is the histology of pretibial myxoedema?

- Characteristic features include fraying and oedematous appearance on routine staining with haematoxylin and eosin, and increase of alcian blue–periodic acid–Schiff-positive mucinous material, with resultant connective tissue fibre separation.
- Review of pathology reports does not show any distinguishing microscopic characteristics for various clinical forms of this dermopathy.

Mention a few symptoms that would indicate hyperthyroidism.

Excessive sweating, preference for cold weather, increased appetite and weight loss, nervousness, tiredness and palpitations, increased bowel movement.

How can hyperthyroidism present in the elderly?

Thyrotoxicosis can present in the elderly with atrial fibrillation, and such patients may lack other common signs of thyrotoxicosis; this is known as apathetic hyperthyroidism.

Reference

Fatourechi V, Pajouhi M & Fransway AF (1994) Dermopathy of Graves disease (pretibial myxoedema). *Medicine* **73**: 1–7.

CASE 140 Multinodular Goitre

Instruction

Examine this patient's neck.

Salient features

- Middle-aged or elderly patient.
- Multinodular goitre.
- Atrial fibrillation.
- Signs of thyrotoxicosis (see page 377).

Diagnosis

This patient has a multinodular goitre (lesion) and is hyperthyroid with atrial fibrillation (functional status).

Questions

What is the natural history of thyrotoxicosis in nodular goitre?

It is permanent and there are no spontaneous remissions; therefore, antithyroid drugs to decrease thyroid hormone secretion is not appropriate long-term therapy.

How would you investigate a nodular goitre?

- *Ultrasonography* of the thyroid gland indicates whether goitre is *cystic* or *solid.*
- If solid, perform an isotope scan to indicate hot or cold nodule.
- If hot nodule, T_3, T_4, TSH.
- If cold nodule, fine-needle aspiration.

How would you treat such a patient?

- Beta-blockers to control thyrotoxicosis.
- Warfarin in atrial fibrillation to prevent embolic complications.
- Radioiodine for hyperthyroidism.
- Surgery if the patient refuses radioiodine and for large multinodular goitres.

Advanced-level Questions

How do you differentiate between Graves' disease and toxic nodular goitre?

Graves' disease	Toxic nodular goitre
Younger age group	Older individuals
Diffuse goitre	Nodular enlargement of the gland
Eye signs common	Rare
Atrial fibrillation is uncommon	Atrial fibrillation is common (about 40% of the patients)
Other autoimmune diseases are common	Uncommon

What factors influence the decision to proceed to radiotherapy?

Patient's age, sex, diagnosis, severity of hyperthyroidism, presence of other medical conditions, access to radioiodine (I-131), and patient and doctor preference.

What are the contraindications to radioiodine therapy?

- Breastfeeding and pregnancy.
- Situations where it is clear that the safety of other persons cannot be guaranteed.
- Patients who are incontinent who are unwilling to have a urinary catheter.
- Allergy to iodine.

What are the indications for radioiodine therapy in hyperthyroidism?

- Hyperthyroidism due to Graves' disease with moderate goitre (40–50 g), with no significant eye signs and first presentation.

- Toxic multinodular goitre in older persons complicated by heart failure or atrial fibrillation.
- Toxid adenoma, usually with mild hyperthyroidism.
- Ophthalmopathy with thyroid dysfunction with stable eye disease.
- Ablation therapy in those with severe manifestations such as heart failure, atrial fibrillation or psychosis.

What advice would you give to patients who are administered radioiodine?

- Depending on the dose, they should avoid journeys on public transport, stay off work, avoid places of entertainment or close contact with other people for up to 12 days and avoid non-essential close personal contact with children and pregnant women for up to 27 days.
- Patients should be warned that in the first fortnight after administration of therapy they may experience palpitations or other exacerbations of symptoms, particularly when not euthyroid before treatment.
- The importance of regular follow-up should be emphasized and the need to report the recurrence of thyrotoxic symptoms or the development of hypothyroidism.
- Patients should be informed that atrial fibrillation often reverts to normal rhythm and that digitalis may then be discontinued.
- Patients should be reminded to avoid pregnancy for 4 months after radioiodine therapy.

CASE 141 Cushing's Syndrome

Instruction

Examine this patient.
Look at this patient's face.

Salient features

- Moon-like facies, acne, hirsutism and plethora (due to telangiectasia).

Proceed as follows:

- Examine the following:
  The mouth for superimposed thrush.
  The interscapular area for 'buffalo hump'.
  Increased fat pads and bulge above supraclavicular fossae (more specific for Cushing's syndrome).
  The abdomen for thinning of skin and purple striae (also seen over

the shoulders and thighs) – said to be present on almost all patients.

The limbs for bruising, wasting of the limbs, weakness of the muscles of the shoulders and hips – get the patient to squat (proximal myopathy).

- Tell the examiner you would like to:

Ask the patient whether she is taking steroids.

Ask the patient whether she has back pain and then examine the spine, looking for evidence of osteoporosis and collapse of vertebra, kyphoscoliosis.

Test the urine for glucose.

Measure the blood pressure.

Check visual fields (for pituitary tumour).

Examine the fundus for optic atrophy, papilloedema, signs of hypertensive or diabetic retinopathy.

Note. Hirsutism is not common in Cushing's syndrome caused by exogenous steroids because they suppress adrenal androgen secretion.

Also comment on signs of asthma, rheumatoid arthritis, SLE, fibrosing alveolitis (as these are conditions that are treated with long-term steroids).

Diagnosis

This patient has moon-like facies, acne and supraclavicular pads of fat (lesions), which are features of Cushing's syndrome caused by long-term steroid therapy (aetiology) for asthma. The patient is now steroid dependent and is disabled by proximal myopathy and kyphoscoliosis due to osteoporosis (functional status).

Questions

Mention some causes of Cushing's syndrome.

- Steroids, including adrenocorticotrophic hormone (ACTH).
- Pituitary adenoma (Cushing's disease).
- Adrenal adenoma.
- Adrenal carcinoma.
- Ectopic ACTH (usually by small cell carcinoma of the lung).

What is the difference between Cushing's disease and Cushing's syndrome?

Cushing's disease is increased production by the adrenals secondary to excess pituitary ACTH, whereas Cushing's syndrome is caused by excess steroid from any cause.

How would you investigate such a patient?

Tests to *confirm the diagnosis*
- 24-hour urinary free cortisol: this is the most direct and reliable practical index of cortisol secretion. The reason is that plasma concentrations of corticotrophins and cortisol fall and rise episodically, in normal subjects, in Cushing's syndrome and in ectopic ACTH syndrome.
- Overnight dexamethasone test.
- Plasma cortisol.

Tests to *determine the site of hormone production*:
- Low- and high-dose dexamethasone test: low-dose dexamethasone fails to suppress urinary steroid secretion in Cushing's disease whereas high-dose dexamethasone (2 mg Q6H for 2 days) suppresses at least 50% of urinary steroid secretion.
- CXR for carcinoma of the bronchus.
- Plain radiograph of the abdomen for adrenal calcification.
- Ultrasonography of the abdomen for adrenal tumours.
- If Cushing's disease is suspected:
  > Plasma ACTH, radiography of pituitary, MRI gadolinium enhancement, and bilateral measurement of corticotrophin in the inferior petrosal sinus.
  > Corticotrophin-releasing hormone (CRH) test (helpful in distinguishing pituitary-led Cushing's disease from ectopic corticotrophin secretion).

How would you manage Cushing's syndrome?

- Cushing's disease: trans-sphenoidal microadenomectomy, pituitary irradiation, total bilateral adrenalectomy.
- Adrenal tumour: surgical resection, mitotane therapy, resection of recurrent tumour.
- Ectopic ACTH: surgical resection of tumour.
- Taper corticosteroid therapy.

Advanced-level Questions

What is pseudo-Cushing's syndrome?

In chronic alcoholics and patients with depression there may be increased urinary excretion of steroids, absent diurnal variation of plasma steroids and a positive overnight dexamethasone test. All these investigations return to normal on discontinuation of alcohol or improvement of emotional status.

Harvey Williams Cushing (1869–1939) was Professor of Surgery at Harvard. He was awarded the Pulitzer Prize for his biography of Osler.

Christopher Edwards, contemporary Principal, Imperial College, London; his chief interest is metabolism of steroids.

References

Cushing H (1932) The basophil adenomas of the pituitary body and their clinical manifestation. *Bull Johns Hopkins Hosp* **1**: 137.

Orth DN (1995) Cushing's syndrome. *N Engl J Med* **332**: 791–803.

CASE 142 — Addison's Disease

Instruction

Look at this patient, who presented with weakness, loss of appetite and weight loss.

Salient features

- The striking abnormality is hyperpigmentation.

Proceed as follows:

- Examine for hyperpigmentation:
  The hand: compare the creases with your own.
  The mouth and lips for pigmentation.
  Areas not usually covered by clothing: nipples, areas irritated by belts, straps, collars or rings.
- Look for vitiligo.
- Tell the examiner that you would like to investigate as follows:
  Ask if the patient has been sitting in the sun.
  Examine the blood pressure, in particular for postural hypotension.
  Ask questions regarding fatigue, weakness, apathy, anorexia, nausea, vomiting, weight loss and abdominal pain.
  Look for sparse axillary and pubic hair.
  Examine the abdomen for adrenal scar (if the scar is pigmented, think of Nelson's syndrome and examine field defects).
- If you suspect Addison's disease tell the examiner that you would like to do a short tetracosactrin test (synacthen test).

Diagnosis

This patient has postural hypotension, marked hyperpigmentation and sparse axillary hair (lesion) due to autoimmune Addison's disease (aetiology). The patient has marked hypoadrenalism (functional status).

Questions

What is the size of the heart in Addison's deficiency?

The heart is small.

Mention some causes of hyperpigmentation.

- Suntan.
- Race.
- Uraemia.
- Haemochromatosis.
- Primary biliary cirrhosis.
- Ectopic ACTH.
- Porphyria cutanea tarda.
- Nelson's syndrome.
- Malabsorption syndromes.

Mention some causes of Addison's disease.

- 80% idiopathic.
- Tuberculosis.
- Metastasis.
- HIV infection.

Which conditions may be associated with Addison's disease?

Graves' disease, Hashimato's thyroiditis, primary ovarian failure, pernicious anaemia, polyglandular syndromes.

Advanced-level Questions

What are the components of Schmidt's syndrome?

Addison's disease and hypoparathyroidism.

What do you know about polyglandular syndromes?

They are autoimmune in nature and are of two types:
- Type I: chronic mucocutaneous candidiasis, hypoparathyroidism and Addison's disease.
- Type II: consists of Addison's disease, insulin-dependent diabetes and

thyroid disease (hyperthyroidism or hypothyroidism). This syndrome is also known as 'autoimmune polyendocrinopathy–candidiasis–ectodermal dysplasia'.

What are the features of Allgrove's syndrome?

Adrenal insensitivity to ACTH (resulting in cortisol deficiency), achalasia, alacrima and neurological disease.

How would you investigate this patient?

- FBC (for lymphocytosis, eosinophilia).
- Electrolytes (for hyponatraemia, hyperkalaemia, hyperchloraemic acidosis, hypercalcaemia).
- Blood glucose, looking for hypoglycaemia.
- Short tetracosactrin (synacthen) test; if positive, follow up with a prolonged ACTH stimulation test.
- ACTH and cortisol levels.
- Adrenal autoantibodies.
- CXR for TB.
- Plain radiograph of the abdomen for adrenal calcification.
- CT scan of the adrenals.

How would you manage this patient if the underlying aetiology is autoimmune?

- Replacement steroids: prednisolone 5 mg *mane* and 2.5 mg *nocte*; adjust dose depending on serum levels and clinical well-being.
- Fludrocortisone 0.025–0.15 mg daily; adjust dose depending on postural hypotension.
- Give steroid card and Medic Alert bracelet.
- Stress the importance of regular therapy, and increase the dose in the event of stress such as dental extraction or urinary tract infection. It is also important to tell the patient that this therapy is lifelong and that an ampoule of hydrocortisone should be kept at home.
- Follow up every 6 months.

Note. In addisonian crisis, intravenous fluids and hydrocortisone should be administered (after drawing a blood sample for cortisol determination).

Thomas Addison (1793–1860) qualified from Edinburgh and worked at Guy's Hospital, London. He wrote *The Constitutional and Local Effects of the Disease of the Suprarenal Capsules*. Armand Trosseau in Paris labelled the disease 'maladie d'Addison'. Addison also first described morphea.

John F Kennedy, past president of the USA, reportedly had Addison's disease and was on replacement corticosteroid therapy.

References

Addison T (1855) Disease of the suprarenal capsules. *London Med Gaz* **43**: 517.
    (The original description of this disease.)
Vita JA, Silverberg SJ, Goland RS et al (1985) Clinical clues to the causes of
    Addison's disease. *Am J Med* **78**: 461.

CASE 143 Acromegaly

Instruction

Examine this patient's face.
This patient complains of excessive sweating; examine him.
Examine this patient's hands.

Salient features

Hands:
- On shaking hands there is excessive sweating.
- Large hands with broad palms, spatulate fingers; there is an increase in
  the 'volume' of the hands.

Proceed as follows:

- Look for evidence of carpal tunnel syndrome (tap over the flexor
  retinaculum for Tinel's sign).
Face:
- Prominent supraorbital ridges.
- Large nose and lips.
- Protrusion of the lower jaw (prognathism); ask the patient to clench his
  teeth and note the malocclusion and splaying of the teeth (i.e.
  interdental separation).

Proceed as follows:

- Ask the patient to show his tongue and look for macroglossia and for
  impressions of the teeth on the edges of the tongue (see page 577).
- Test for bitemporal hemianopia (see page 126) and optic atrophy.
- Tell the examiner that you would like to examine the following:
      Neck for goitre.
      Axillae for skin tags (molluscum fibrosum), acanthosis nigricans
          (black velvety papillomas).
      Chest for cardiomegaly, gynaecomastia and galactorrhoea.
      Abdomen for hepatosplenomegaly.

Joints for arthropathy, i.e. osteoarthrosis, chondrocalcinosis.
Spine for kyphosis.
Blood pressure for hypertension (present in 15% of cases).
Urine for sugar (impaired glucose tolerance).
Old photographs of the patient for comparison.

Diagnosis

This patient has a protruding lower jaw, splaying of teeth and large spade-like hands (lesions) which are features of acromegaly due to a pituitary tumour (aetiology).

Questions

Would you like to ask the patient a few questions?

Ask about any increase in size of shoes, gloves and hat, and whether the wedding ring is tight to wear.

Advanced-level Questions

Mention some causes of macroglossia.

- Acromegaly.
- Amyloidosis.
- Hypothyroidism.
- Down's syndrome.

How can this condition present?

One-third of patients notice a change in their features, one-third are noticed to have a change in their features by their GPs and the remaining third have symptoms such as excessive sweating and visual difficulties.

What are the complications of acromegaly?

- Cardiomegaly and heart failure.
- Hypertension.
- Impaired glucose tolerance.
- Hypopituitarism.
- Carpal tunnel syndrome.
- Arthritis of the hip, knee and spine.
- Spinal stenosis resulting in cord compression.
- Visual field defects.

What are the indicators of disease activity?

- Symptoms such as headache, increase in size of ring, shoe or dentures.
- Excessive sweating.
- Skin tags.
- Glycosuria.
- Hypertension.
- Increased loss of visual fields.

How would you investigate this patient?

Biochemical tests: .
- Non-suppressibility of growth hormone levels to less than 2 ng ml^{-1} after oral administration of 100 g glucose.
- Plasma insulin-like growth factor levels (allows assessment of the efficacy of initial therapy and in the post-therapeutic period).
- Also serum T_4, prolactin, testosterone; evaluate pituitary function – static and dynamic tests.
- Calcium levels (to exclude multiple endocrine neoplasia (MEN) type 1 syndrome).

Radiography:
- Pituitary fossa (enlarged sella).
- Sinuses.
- Chest (cardiomegaly).
- Hand (terminal phalangeal 'tufting').
- Foot (terminal phalangeal 'tufting', lateral view shows increased thickness of the heel pad).
- CT scan (MRI scan is more reliable).

Other investigations:
- Formal perimetry.
- Obtain old photos.
- New photos of face, torso, hands on the chest.
- ECG.
- Triple stimulation test – if hypopituitarism is suspected.

What therapeutic options are available?

- Neurosurgical intervention – typically trans-sphenoidal – is the primary therapeutic choice for almost all patients. Diaphoresis and carpal tunnel syndrome often improve within 1 day of surgery. Although growth hormone levels fall immediately, insulin-like growth factor levels fall gradually.
- Radiation therapy is a primary treatment option for a few patients who have acromegaly but are not surgical candidates.

- Octreotide and bromocriptine are valuable as adjunctive therapy.

Remember the aim of treatment should be symptomatic control and a growth hormone concentration of less than 5 mU l^{-1}.

Mention four common causes of death in such patients.

- Cardiac failure.
- Tumour expansion (mass effect and haemorrhages).
- Effects of hypertension.
- Degenerative vascular disease.

Mention other conditions with excess growth hormone secretion.

- Multiple endocrine neoplasia type 1 (parathyroid hyperplasia, pituitary tumours and gut tumours).
- McCune–Albright syndrome (polyostotic fibrous dysplasia, sexual precocity and café-au-lait spots).
- Carney complex, which consists of multicentric tumours in many organs of autosomal dominant aetiology (including cardiac myxomas, myxomas in breast, testes, pigmented skin lesions and pigmented nodular hyperplasia).

In 1886 Pierre Marie (1853–1940) used the term acromegaly in describing two patients and reviewed eight previously published papers describing patients with presumed acromegaly. He described Charcot–Marie–Tooth disease.

In 1887 Minkowski deduced that acromegaly is related to pituitary tumour.

In 1891 the New Syndenham Society published a translation of Marie's original paper and a review by Souza-Leite of 48 patients.

Fuller Albright, Professor of Endocrinology at Massachussetts General Hospital and Harvard Medical School, whose chief interest was calcium metabolism.

References

Acromegaly Therapy Consensus Development Panel (1994) Consensus Statement: benefits versus risks of medical therapy for acromegaly. *Am J Med* **97**: 468.

Ezzat S, Forester MJ, Berchtold P, Redelmeier DA, Boerlin V & Harris AG (1994) Acromegaly: clinical and biochemical features in 500 patients. *Medicine* **73**: 233.

Marie P (1886) Sur deux cas d'acromegalie. Hypertrophie singulière non-congénitale des extrémités supérieures, inférieures et céphaliques. *Rev Med* **6**: 297–333.

Marie P & de Souza-Leite JD (1891) *Essays on Acromegaly*. London: New Sydenham Society.

Melmed S (1990) Acromegaly. *N Engl J Med* **322**: 967–975.

Minkowski O (1887) Uber einen Fall von Akromegalie. *Berl Klin Wochenschr* **24**: 371–374.

CASE 144 Hypopituitarism (Simmonds' Disease)

Instruction

Look at this patient.

Salient features

- Patient is pale; the skin is soft.
- Paucity of axillary and pubic hair.
- Atrophy of breast (in females).

Proceed as follows:

- Tell the examiner that you would like to investigate as follows:
    Examine the blood pressure for postural hypotension.
    Check visual fields: bitemporal hemianopia may be present.
    Examine the fundus for optic atrophy.
    Examine the external genitalia for hypogonadism (small testes).
    Take a history:
        In a male, of the frequency of shaving, impotence.
        In a female, of postpartum haemorrhage, amenorrhoea.

Diagnosis

This patient has pale soft skin and absence of axillary hair with atrophied breasts (lesion) due to hypopituitarism (functional status) secondary to postpartum necrosis (aetiology).

Questions

Mention a few causes of hypopituitarism.

- Iatrogenic – from surgical removal of the pituitary or irradiation.
- Chromophobe adenoma (particularly in males).
- Postpartum pituitary necrosis (in females) – known as Sheehan's syndrome.

Rare causes:
- Craniopharyngioma.
- Metastatic tumours, granulomas (TB, sarcoid, haemochromatosis, histiocytosis X).

How would you assess such a patient?

- FBC for normochromic normocytic anaemia.
- Urea and electrolytes for hyponatraemia due to dilution. Hyperkalaemia does not usually occur because aldosterone production is not affected.
- Measurement of pituitary hormone levels (ACTH, TSH, luteinising hormone (LH), growth hormone, prolactin).
- Measurement of target organ secretion (T_4, T_3, serum cortisol, testosterone, oestrogen and progesterone levels).
- Pituitary stimulation tests:
  Thyrotrophin-releasing hormone (TRH) stimulation tests.
  Tetracosactrin (synacthen) tests.
  Insulin hypoglycaemia test.
  Luteinizing hormone releasing hormone (LHRH) tests.
- Skull radiography.
- MRI provides the best image of parasellar lesions. The posterior pituitary usually has a high-intensity signal on sagittal MRI that is absent in central diabetes insipidus.
- Assessment of visual fields (formal perimetry).

In what order do the hormone secretions generally fail?

In general growth hormone, follicle-stimulating hormone (FSH) and LH secretions become deficient early, followed by TSH and ACTH. Last of all, antidiuretic hormone (ADH) secretions diminish and fail.

How would you treat such patients?

The mainstay of therapy is lifetime replacement of deficient end-organ deficiencies (thyroid, adrenal and gonads).

Advanced-level Questions

What is the Houssay phenomenon?

Houssay showed that diabetes of pancreatectomized dogs improved after hypophysectomy. A diminishing requirement of insulin by diabetics may be a sign of hypopituitarism with diminished secretion of growth hormone and ACTH (and thus corticosteroids). Similarly, diabetes due to acromegaly may improve with pituitary surgery or octreotide therapy.

Morris Simmonds of Hamburg described this condition in 1914.
Bernado Alberto Houssay (1889–1971), an Argentinian physiologist in Buenos Aires, was awarded the Nobel Prize for his discovery of the part played by the hormone of the anterior pituitary lobe in the metabolism of sugar. The other half of the Nobel Prize was awarded to Carl and Gerty Cori of St Louis, Missouri, USA, who were awarded the prize for their discovery of the course of the catalytic conversion of glycogen.

CASE 145   Gynaecomastia

Instruction

Look at this patient's chest.

Salient features

- Unilateral or bilateral enlargement of the breasts in a male patient.

Proceed as follows:

- Palpate to confirm the presence of glandular tissue.
- Tell the examiner that you would like to investigate as follows:
    Look for stigmata of cirrhosis of the liver.
    Take a drug history – oestrogens, digoxin, spironolactone, cimetidine, diazepam, alkylating agents, methyldopa, clomiphene.

Diagnosis

This patient has gynaecomastia (lesion) due to spironolactone therapy (aetiology), which is cosmetically distressing to the patient (functional status).

Questions

Mention the physiological causes of gynaecomastia.

- Newborn.
- Adolescence.
- Ageing.

Mention a few pathological causes.

- Chronic liver disease.
- Thyrotoxicosis.
- Klinefelter syndrome.
- Viral orchitis.
- Renal failure.
- Neoplasms (bronchogenic carcinoma, testicular carcinoma).
- Drugs associated with gynaecomastia include:
    Antibiotics: isoniazid, ketoconazole, metronidazole, miconazole.
    Cardiovascular drugs: atenolol, captopril, digoxin, enalapril, methyldopa, nifedipine, spironolactone, verapamil.
    Antiulcer drugs: cimetidine, ranitidine, omeprazole.
    Psychoactive drugs: diazepam, tricyclic antidepressants.

Advanced-level Questions

How would you investigate such a patient?

- CXR for metastatic or bronchogenic carcinoma.
- Plasma β-human chorionic gonadotrophin – detectable levels implicate a testicular tumour or lung or liver neoplasm.
- Plasma testosterone and luteinizing hormone in the diagnosis of hypogonadism.
- Serum oestradiol (usually normal).
- Other: serum prolactin, serum thyroxine and TSH, and chromosomal analysis for Klinefelter's syndrome.

What are the causes of a feminizing state?

- Absolute increase in oestrogen formation by tumours.
- Increased availability of oestrogen precusors, e.g. as a result of cirrhosis.
- Increased extraglandular oestrogen synthesis.
- Relative increase in ratio of oestrogen to androgen, e.g. as a result of testicular failure.
- Drugs.

Ancient Egyptian sculptures and paintings suggest that the pharaoh Tutankhamen (1357–1339 BC) had gynaecomastia.

Reference

Braunstein GD (1993) Gynaecomastia. *N Engl J Med* **328**: 490.

CASE 146 Carpopedal Spasm (Post-Thyroidectomy Hypoparathyroidism)

Instruction

Look at this patient's hands.

Salient features

- Spasm of the hands – fingers are extended, except at the metacarpophalangeal joints, and the thumb is strongly adducted.

Proceed as follows:

- Look at the feet for spasm and then investigate as follows:
    Tap over the facial nerve (in front of the tragus of the ear) – there is contraction of the lips and facial muscles (Chvostek's sign or Chvostek–Weiss sign).
    Look into the mouth for candidiasis (may be seen in primary hypoparathyroidism) and defective teeth.
    Finger nails may be thin and brittle.
    Check for thyroidectomy scar.
    Look for cataracts.
- Tell the examiner that you would like to perform the following tests:
    Do a skull radiograph (looking for basal ganglia calcification).
    Check serum calcium and magnesium levels.
    ECG for prolonged QT intervals and T-wave abnormalities.
    Slit-lamp examination for early posterior lenticular cataract formation.

Diagnosis

This patient has carpopedal spasm (lesion) due to hypoparathyroidism as a complication of thyroidectomy (aetiology).

Questions

What is Trousseau's sign?

The cuff is inflated just above the systolic pressure for 3 minutes and this will cause the hand to go into spasm.

Advanced-level Questions

Mention any drugs that you would use cautiously in hypoparathyroidism.

Frusemide, as it may enhance hypocalcaemia, and phenothiazine drugs, because they may precipitate extrapyramidal symptoms.

How would you manage an acute attack of hypoparathyroid tetany?

- Maintain airway.
- Slow intravenous calcium gluconate and oral calcium.
- Vitamin D preparations.
- Magnesium (if associated hypomagnesaemia).

What are the causes of hypoparathyroidism?

- Damage during thyroid or neck surgery.
- Idiopathic.
- Destruction of the parathyroid gland due to the following:
  Radioactive iodine therapy.
  External neck irradiation.
  Haemochromatosis and Wilson's deficiency.
  Metastatic disease from the breast, lung, lymphoproliferative disorder.
- Dysembryogenesis (DiGeorge's syndrome).
- Polyglandular autoimmune syndrome (PGA type 1) which is also known as autoimmune polyendocrinopathy–candidiasis–ectodermal dystrophy (APECD) (see page 396).

What are the biochemical features of hypoparathyroidism?

Typically it consists of low serum calcium, high serum phosphate and normal alkaline phosphatase levels and reduced urine calcium excretion.

What do you know about pseudohypoparathyroidism?

It is a condition characterized by end-organ resistance to parathyroid hormone. The biochemistry is similar to that of idiopathic hypoparathyroidism except that patients with pseudohypoparathyroidism do not respond to injected parathyroid hormone. These patients are moon faced, short statured and mentally retarded and may have short fourth or fifth metacarpals. Patients without hypocalcaemia but who have these phenotypic abnormalities are said to have 'pseudopseudohypoparathyroidism'.

What are the main physiological effects of parathyroid hormone?

It results in a net increase of ionized calcium in the plasma as a result of:
- Increased bone osteoclastic activity resulting in increased delivery of calcium and phosphorous to the extracellular compartment.
- Enhanced renal tubular absorption of calcium.
- Inhibits the absorption of phosphate and bicarbonate by the renal tubule.
- Stimulates the synthesis of 1,25-dihydrocholecalciferol (vitamin D) by the kidney.

Frantisek Chvostek (1835–1884) was Professor of Medicine in Vienna, Austria.
Nathan Weiss (1851–1883), an Austrian physician.
Armand Trousseau (1801–1867), a Parisian physician, was the first to refer to adrenal insufficiency as Addison's disease.

References

Davis RH, Fourman P & Smith JWG (1960) Problems of parathyroid insufficiency after thyroidectomy. *Lancet* **ii**: 1432.
Juan D (1979) Hypocalcaemia: differential diagnosis and mechanisms. *Arch Intern Med* **139**: 1166.

 CASE 147 Carcinoid Syndrome

Instruction

Look at this patient who was told by her GP that she has a 'nervous bowel'.

Salient features

- Flushed face ('fire-engine' face).
- Telangiectasia.

Proceed as follows:

- Tell the examiner that you would like to:
    Listen to the chest for wheeze (bronchial carcinoid).
    Listen to the heart (right-sided murmurs in intestinal, gastric, hepatic and ovarian carcinoid, left-sided murmurs in bronchial carcinoid).
    Look for hepatomegaly (nodular and firm due to metastases, may be pulsatile due to tricuspid regurgitation).
    Confirm a history of chronic intermittent diarrhoea.

Diagnosis

This patient has facial flushing and tricuspid regurgitation (lesion) due to carcinoid syndrome (aetiology) and is in cardiac failure (functional status).

Advanced-level Questions

What are the cardiac lesions seen in metastatic carcinoid from the liver?

- Right-sided valvular lesions, including tricuspid stenosis or regurgitation, and pulmonary stenosis or regurgitation. (Note bronchial carcinoids metastasize to the left side of the heart.)
- Endocardial fibrosis.

How is the diagnosis confirmed?

- Raised urinary levels of 5-HIAA (hydroxyindoleacetic acid).

How are these tumours treated?

- Emergency treatment includes prednisolone.
- Severe diarrhoea: hydration, diphenoxylate with atropine, cyproheptadine or methysergide.
- Octreotide (a somatostatin analogue) is associated with a significant reduction in 5-HIAA concentration.
- Surgery is useful for localized carcinoid.
- Chemotherapy in advanced disease (fluorouracil, streptozocin, dacarbazine).

Reference

Sjoerdsma A, Weissbach H & Udenfriend S (1956) A clinical, physiologic and biochemical study of patients with malignant carcinoid (argentaffinoma). *Am J Med* **20**: 520–532.

CASE 148 Obesity

Instruction

Look at this patient.

Salient features

- Patient has excessive adipose tissue.

Proceed as follows:

- Tell the examiner that you would like to:
    Measure the height and body-weight (to determine body–mass index).
    Check blood pressure.
    Assess urine sugar.
    Check serum lipids.
    Examine the joints to exclude osteoarthrosis.
    Assess pulmonary function (sleep apnoea).
    Determine family history of obesity.
    Exclude secondary causes (hypothyroidism, Cushing's syndrome).

Diagnosis

This patient has gross obesity (lesion) of genetic origin, complicated by hypertension and osteoarthrosis.

Advanced-level Questions

Is obesity of genetic origin?

Although many obese individuals are blamed for being obese – by their friends, physicians, family and by themselves – increasingly it has been shown that genetic influences have a substantial influence on body–mass index. The *ob* gene is an adipocyte-specific gene that encodes leptin, a protein that regulates body-weight. Animals with mutations in the *ob* gene are obese and lose weight when given leptin. In humans, serum leptin concentrations correlate with the percentage of body fat, suggesting that most obese people are insensitive to endogenous leptin (leptin resistance).

What is body–mass index?

It is a measure to determine the presence of excessive adipose tissue and is calculated by dividing the body-weight in kilograms by the height in metres squared. The normal spread of the body–mass index is from 20 to 25 kg m^{-2}.

What is morbid obesity?

It is relative weight greater than 200% and is associated with a tenfold increase in the mortality rate.

Mention some adverse health consequences of obesity.

They have a greater risk for diabetes mellitus, stroke, coronary artery disease, premature mortality, thromboembolism, gallstones, reflux oesophagitis, sleep apnoea, polycythaemia, and cancer of the colon, rectum, prostate, uterus, breast and ovary.

What patterns of obesity correlate with premature coronary artery disease?

Central obesity (abdomen and flank) and when there is excessive visceral fat within the abdominal cavity rather than subcutaneous fat around the abdomen.

How would you manage such patients?

- Multidisciplinary approach to weight loss: hypocaloric diets, exercise, social support.
- Drugs: fenfluramine, phenteramine.
- Surgery: vertical banded gastroplasty, gastric bypass operations.

What are the mechanisms of obesity?

- Insensitivity to leptin, presumably in the hypothalamus.
- Neuropeptide Y-induced hyperphagia.
- Deficiency of production or action of anorexigenic hypothalamic neuropeptides.
- Increased secretion of insulin and glucocorticoid.

Mention some syndromes where obesity is a prominent feature.

Cushing's syndrome (see page 392), Laurence–Moon–Biedl syndrome (see page 304), pickwickian syndrome (see page 606), Alstrom's syndrome, Prader–Willi syndrome.

References

Lindpainter K (1995) Finding an obesity gene: a tale of mice and men. *N Engl J Med* **332**: 679.

Rohner-Jeanrenaud F & Jeanrenaud B (1996) Obesity, leptin and the brain. *N Engl J Med* **324**: 325.

Zhang Y, Proenca R, Maffei M, Barone M, Leopald L & Friedman JM (1994) Positional cloning of the mouse *obese* gene and its human analogue. *Nature* **372**: 425–432.

DERMATOLOGY

CASE 149 — Maculopapular Rash

Instruction

Would you like to perform a general examination of this patient?
Look at this patient.

Salient features

- Reddish, blotchy maculopapular rash over the trunk (check the chest, back and axillae) and limbs.

Proceed as follows:

- Palpate the surface of the rash to confirm your inspectory findings.
- Check the mucous membranes of the mouth.
- Tell the examiner that you would like to ask the patient some questions:
    Ask whether or not the rash itches.
    Ask where the rash started and ask the patient to describe its evolution.
    Take a drug history.
    Examine for lymph nodes (glandular fever) – some examiners may expect you to examine the lymph nodes as a part of the general examination. If lymph nodes are palpable, then examine all groups (cervical, supraclavicular, axillary and inguinal).

Note. Avoid waffling descriptions such as 'skin rash'.

Diagnosis

This patient has a maculopapular rash (lesion) due to ampicillin ingestion (aetiology), which usually resolves on discontinuing the drug (functional status).

Questions

What is your differential diagnosis?

- Drug-induced rash (e.g. ampicillin, cephalosporins).
- Glandular fever.

What is your differential diagnosis when the rash is associated with lymphadenopathy?

- Glandular fever.
- Lymphoproliferative disorders such as Hodgkin's disease.
- HIV infection.

CASE 150 Purpura

Instruction

Examine this patient's skin.

Salient features

- Small circumscribed bleeding into the skin – purpura or larger lesions – bruises or ecchymoses.

Proceed as follows:

Look for an underlying cause:
> Comment on the patient's age – consider senile purpura.
> Comment on the distribution – Henoch-Schönlein purpura is seen over the buttocks and lower limbs (see page 422).

- Look for the following signs:
> Rheumatoid arthritis where purpura is drug induced (steroids, gold).
> Anaemia (leukaemia, marrow aplasia or infiltration).
> Chronic liver disease.
> Ulcers in the mouth (severe neutropenia).
> Bleeding gums, corkscrew hair and perifollicular haemorrhages of scurvy (particularly in the elderly).
> Stigmata of Ehlers–Danlos syndrome.
> Bleeding from multiple venepuncture sites (disseminated intravascular coagulation).

- Tell the examiner that you would like to investigate as follows:
> Take a drug history – steroids, anticoagulants, carbimazole, phenylbutazone, chloramphenicol.
> Examine for spleen, liver and lymph nodes.

Diagnosis

This patient has purpura (lesion) which is due to ingestion of steroids (aetiology) and is cosmetically unacceptable to the patient (functional status).

Questions

What are the common causes of purpura?

- Senile purpura, due to senile changes in the vessel walls.
- Purpura induced by steroids or anticoagulants.
- Thrombocytopenia due to leukaemia and marrow aplasia.

What are causes of bruising?

- Thrombocytopenia: idiopathic thrombocytopenic purpura, marrow replacement by leukaemia or secondary infiltration.
- Vascular defects: senile purpura, steroid-induced purpura, Henoch–Schönlein purpura, scurvy, von Willebrand's disease, uraemia.
- Coagulation defects: haemophilia, anticoagulants, Christmas disease.
- Drugs: thiazides, sulphonamides, phenylbutazone, sulphonylureas, sulindac, barbiturates.

Advanced-level Question

What do you know about Moschcowitz's syndrome?

Moschcowitz syndrome or thrombotic thrombocytopenic purpura is an acute disorder characterized by thrombocytopenic purpura, microangiopathic haemolytic anaemia, transient and fluctuating neurological features, fever and renal impairment.

E Moschcowitz (1879–1964), New York physician.
In 1951 William Harrington, then a trainee in haematology at the Barnes Hospital in St Louis, Missouri, had severe thrombocytopenia immediately after voluntarily receiving plasma from a patient with the disease, establishing beyond doubt that a plasma factor causes the destruction of platelets in chronic idiopathic thrombocytopenic purpura.

CASE 151 Psoriasis

Instruction

Look at this patient.
Do a general examination.

Salient features

- Well-demarcated salmon pink plaques with silvery white scales over extensor surfaces, scalp, naval and natal cleft. They often tend to have a pink or red line in the intergluteal fold.

Proceed as follows:

- Look at the nails for pitting and onycholysis (separation of the nail plate from the bed).
- Tell the examiner that you would like to take a history of:
  Joint pains (see page 356 for psoriatic arthropathy).
  Symptoms (itching, pain, flexural intertrigo, limitation of manual dexterity), cosmetic problems or both.

Diagnosis

This patient has silvery white scales and nail pitting (lesion) due to psoriasis (aetiology), with considerable itching (functional status).

Questions

How common is this condition?

It affects 1–2% of the population of the UK.

What are the typical features of psoriatic plaques?

Distinguishing features include:
- Silvery colour of the scaling.
- The moist red surface on removal of the scales (Bulkeley's membrane).
- Capillary bleeding on abrasion of this membrane.

Advanced-level Questions

How is the severity of involvement usually estimated?

- The patient's own perception of the disability.
- Objective assessment of disability.

It is usually estimated by using the Psoriasis Area and Severity Index which takes into consideration the area of involvement, thickness, redness and scaling. The maximal score on this index is 72, with mild, moderate and severe having scores of <10, 10–50 and >50 respectively.

What are the types of psoriasis?

Depending on the natural history:
- Type 1: young patients with a strong family history have a more aggressive disorder.
- Type 2: older patients with no family history have a more indolent course.

Depending on the nature of skin lesion:
- Chronic plaque psoriasis.
- Guttate psoriasis.
- Pustular psoriasis – localized or generalized.
- Erythrodermic psoriasis.

What do you know about the genetics of psoriasis?

Polygenic inheritance is likely, although it has been located to the distal end of the long arm of chromosome 17 in several kindreds.

What do you know about the pathology of plaque psoriasis?

- Hyperproliferation of the epidermis.
- Inflammation of the epidermis and dermis.

What do you understand by the term Koebner's phenomenon.

Injury or irritation of psoriatic skin tends to provoke lesions of psoriasis in the site in some patients – this is known as the Koebner's phenomenon.

Mention a few exacerbating factors?

- Drugs: beta-blockers, ACE inhibitors, lithium, indomethacin, anti-malarials, alcohol.
- Psychological factors
- Infection: β-haemolytic streptococci, HIV virus (pre-existing psoriasis may become more refractory to therapy and plaque psoriasis may change to the guttate form in patients with HIV positivity).
- Injury to the skin: mechanical injury, sunburn.

How would you manage a patient with psoriasis?

- Educate the patient that there is no cure and that only suppression of the disease is possible.
- Indications for treatment include symptoms (itching, pain, flexural intertrigo, limitation of manual dexterity), cosmetic problems or both.
- Initial treatment is topical when less than 20% of the body is involved.
    Topical therapy includes:
    Emollients (soft yellow paraffin or aqueous cream).
    Keratolytic agents (salicylic acid).
    Coal tar is usually used in combination with ultraviolet B phototherapy (PUVA B).
    Anthralin (often used according to the Ingram regimen – a daily coal tar bath, ultraviolet B phototherapy and 24-hour application of an anthralin paste containing salicylic acid).
    Topical steroids.
    Calcipotriol (vitamin D_3) is known to act locally to increase extracellular calcium concentrations, which leads to increased keratinocyte differentiation and decreased proliferation and scaling. It is an excellent alternative to steroids.
- Systemic therapy:
    Phototherapy (ultraviolet B radiation).
    Photochemotherapy (methotrexate with ultraviolet A therapy).
    Methotrexate.
    Etretinate (vitamin A derivative), retinoids.
    Systemic steroids.
    Cyclosporin.
- Novel approach:
    Anti-CD4 monoclonal antibody.

What are the indications for systemic treatment?

- Failure of topical therapy.
- Repeated hospital admissions for topical treatment.
- Extensive plaque psoriasis in the elderly.
- Generalized pustular or erythrodermic psoriasis.
- Severe psoriatic arthropathy.

What underlying condition would you suspect when psoriasiform lesions are seen on the nose, ears, fingers and toes?

Such lesions are paraneoplastic eruptions associated with squamous cell carcinoma of the oropharynx, tracheobronchial tree and oesophagus – this is known as Bazex syndrome.

B Russell, in 1950, proposed that psoriasis be known by the eponym Willan–Plumbe syndrome. The first clear descriptions were by Willan (1808) and Plumbe (1824).

References

Greaves MW & Weinstein GD (1995) Treatment of psoriasis. *N Engl J Med* **332**: 581.
Russell B (1950) Lepra, psoriasis, or the Willan–Plumbe syndrome. *Br J Dermatol Syphilis* **62**: 359–361.

CASE 152 Bullous Eruption

Instruction

Look at this patient.

Salient features

- Bullous eruption.

Proceed as follows:

- Comment on the distribution: knee, thighs, forearms and umbilicus in the elderly (pemphigoid).
- Look in the mouth for ulceration; if the blisters break easily, leaving denuded skin, it is more likely to be pemphigus.
- Tell the examiner that a biopsy of the skin is essential to confirm the diagnosis.

Diagnosis

This patient has a bullous eruption (lesion) due to sulphonamides (aetiology) which is widespread with involvement of mucous membrane (functional status).

Questions

What do you understand by the term 'bulla'?

It is a circumscribed elevation of the skin, larger than 0.5 cm, and containing fluid.

How would you confirm the diagnosis?

A biopsy of a fresh blister (less than 12 hours old) with a portion of perilesional skin for histology and immunofluorescent studies.

Advanced-level Questions

Mention a few blistering conditions.

- Common: friction, insect bites, drugs, burns, impetigo, contact dermatitis.
- Uncommon:
    Autoimmune bullous diseases (pemphigoid, pemphigus vulgaris, dermatitis herpetiformis, immunoglobulin-A-mediated diseases, bullous erythema multiforme, epidermolysis bullosa acquisita).
    Porphyria cutanea tarda.
    Paraneoplastic pemphigus.

How would you manage a patient with pemphigus vulgaris?

Barrier nursing, antibiotics, intravenous fluids, large doses of systemic steroids, usually with immunosuppressive drugs – azathioprine, cyclophosphamide or methotrexate – which act as steroid-sparing agents. Other drugs used include dapsone, nicotinamide, gold and cyclosporin.

What are the forms of pemphigus?

There are two main forms; both occur commonly in middle age. These include:
- Pemphigus vulgaris and its variant pemphigus vegetans. The vulgaris form begins in the mouth in over 50% of cases.
- Pemphigus foliaceus and its variant pemphigus erythematosus. These are more superficially blistering conditons. The foliaceus form may be drug induced, e.g. penicillamine toxicity, or is associated with autoimmune disease.

What are the characteristics of pemphigus vulgaris?

Pemphigus vulgaris is characterized by bullae in the epidermis. It is often preceded by bullae in the mucous membrane. Superficial separation of the skin after pressure, trauma or on rubbing the thumb laterally on the surface of uninvolved skin may cause easy separation of the epidermis (Nikolsky's sign). Biopsy shows disruption of epidermal intercellular connections called acanthocytolysis. Immunofluorescence shows intercellular deposition of immunoglobulin G in the epidermis.

What are the characteristics of bullous pemphigoid?

It is a relatively benign condition with remissions and exacerbations. Characteristically, tense blisters are present in the flexural areas, typically in the elderly. The bullae are subepidermal and immunoelectron microscopy shows that deposits of immunoglobulin G and complement 3 (C3) are found in the lamina lucida of the basement membrane.

What do you know about herpes gestationis?

It is a self-limiting disease with the initial appearance of bullae in the periumbilical region, usually in the fifth or sixth month of pregnancy. It may recur in subsequent pregnancies. Menses and oestrogen are known to precipitate flare-ups. The blisters are subepidermal with C3 in the basement membrane and serum complement-fixing immunoglobulin antibody. Corticosteroids, usually systemic, are the treatment of choice.

How would you manage generalized forms of autoimmune bullous disease?

- Systemic steroid therapy is usually chosen first to treat patients with generalized forms of any autoimmune bullous disease except those mediated by immunoglobulin A. Topical steroids have little, if any, value in the treatment of such patients, although they are sometimes effective in patients with localized disease.
- Other immunosuppressive drugs: many patients with moderate to severe pemphigus, bullous pemphigoid, cicatricial pemphigoid or epidermolysis bullosa acquisita require a second immunosuppressive drug (such as azathioprine or cyclophosphamide), either for its corticosteroid-sparing effect or to achieve complete remission. The specific choice is a matter of personal experience, concern over the relative toxic effects, and possible contraindications. Some patients have been treated successfully with prednisone and cyclosporin, but the latter alone is not beneficial. Low-dose methotrexate plus prednisone may benefit patients with pemphigus or bullous pemphigoid.
- Dapsone and related drugs: dapsone is the drug of choice for patients with dermatitis herpetiformis or linear immunoglobulin A dermatosis who are not allergic to sulphonamides. It inhibits the chemotaxis of neutrophils, reducing their accumulation in the upper dermis and thus diminishing tissue inflammation. The response is rapid, with most lesions resolving within 48–72 hours. Alternatives to dapsone include sulphapyridine, sulfoxone sodium and sulphamethoxypyridazine. Dapsone is effective as monotherapy in only a minority of patients with bullous pemphigoid.

- Chrysotherapy: systemic gold is rarely used as an alternative or adjunct to prednisone therapy in patients with pemphigus because it is efficacious in only a subgroup of patients and carries the potential risk of side-effects on prolonged administration.
- Plasmapheresis: is used in patients with severe pemphigus unresponsive to conventional therapy and high titres of pemphigus autoantibodies. Plasmapheresis may also be beneficial in patients with bullous pemphigoid even in the absence of detectable autoantibodies, although its mechanism of action in such patients is not known.
- Gluten-free diets in dermatitis herpetiformis.
- Other therapies: extracorporeal absorption of antibodies for pemphigus, combination tetracycline and nicotinamide in bullous pemphigoid, colchicine in immunoglobulin A dermatosis.

PV Nikolsky (b. 1858), Professor of Dermatology, first in Warsaw and later in Rostov.

Reference

Fine JD (1995) Management of acquired bullous diseases. *N Engl J Med* **333**:1475–1483.

CASE 153 Henoch–Schönlein Purpura

Instruction

Look at this patient's legs.

Salient features

- Purpuric rash over the legs and buttocks.

Proceed as follows:

- Tell the examiner that you would like to examine the rest of the body – including arms, body, scalp and behind the ears – for distribution of rash.
- Examine the mouth to confirm or rule out involvement of mucous membranes.
- Tell the examiner that you would like to investigate as follows:
  Ask the patient about the following:
  Joint pains (knees and ankles are commonly involved).
  Abdominal pain.

The rash – its onset and evolution.
Recent drug ingestion.
Examine the urine for haematuria.

Diagnosis

This patient has purpuric rash over the legs and buttocks with renal involvement (lesions) due to Henoch–Schönlein purpura (aetiology). I would like to know his 24-hour urine output and levels of urea and electrolytes to determine renal function (functional status).

Advanced-level Questions

What do you know about Henoch–Schönlein purpura?

Henoch–Schönlein or anaphylactoid purpura is a distinct, self-limiting vasculitis which occurs in children and young adults. It is a disorder characterized by non-thrombocytopenic purpura, arthralgia, abdominal pain and glomerular nephritis. It is due to circulating immunoglobulin (Ig) A-containing immune complexes. It usually lasts between 1 and 6 weeks and subsides without sequelae if renal involvement is mild. The presence of IgG indicates a worse prognosis. Adults are more likely to develop renal involvement.

What investigations would you like to do?

● Examine the urine for haematuria and proteinuria.
● Antinuclear factor.
● Venereal Disease Research Laboratory test.
● Skin biopsy to detect arteriolar and capillary vasculitis.

What is the differential diagnosis?

● Drug-induced purpura.
● SLE.
● Gonococcal arthralgia.
● Keratoderma blenorrhagicum.
● Secondary syphilis.

How would you classify vasculitis clinically?

● Purpuric disorders: Henoch–Schönlein purpura, leukocytic vasculitis.
● Microscopic polyarteritis: polyarteritis nodosa.

- Aortic type: Takayasu disease, polyarteritis nodosa (in the latter, the subclavian artery is spared).
- Pulmonary type: Wegener's granulomatosus, Churg–Strauss syndrome.

This disorder was first reported in the English literature by Willan in 1808.

Eduard Heinrich Henoch (1820–1910) qualified in Berlin, where he ran the neurology department; he studied under Schönlein and eventually became a paediatrician. In 1874 he reported the coexistence of purpura and gastrointestinal haemorrhage.

Johannes Lucas Schönlein (1793–1864) was initially Professor of Medicine in Würzburg but, because of his liberal views, he was dismissed; he eventually became Professor of Medicine, first in Zurich and then in Berlin. In 1837 he reported the coexistence of purpura and arthritis.

Anthony Fauci, contemporary Director of the National Institute of Allergy and Infectious Diseases and Director of AIDS Research, NIH, Bethesda, whose chief interests include immunological disorders including AIDS.

References

Anonymous (1991) Case records of the Massachusetts General Hospital. Case 35–1991. *N Engl J Med* **325**: 643–651.

Goldstein AR, White RH, Akuse R & Chantler C (1992) Long-term follow up of childhood Henoch–Schönlein nephritis. *Lancet* **339**: 280.

CASE 154 Ichthyosis

Instruction

Look at this patient.
Examine this patient's skin.
Perform a general examination on this patient.

Salient features

- Rough, dry skin with fish-like scales.

Proceed as follows:

- Examine the palms for dry skin and hyperkeratotic creases.
- Tell the examiner that you would like to investigate as follows:
    Take a family history of the disorder.
    Ask whether or not it is of recent onset (underlying malignancy).

Note. Although ichthyosis is said not to be increased in frequency in HIV/AIDS, it may be more severe when associated with this condition.

Diagnosis

This patient has rough, dry skin with fish-like scales (lesion) due to ichthyosis (aetiology), which causes severe itching and may be cosmetically unacceptable (functional status).

Advanced-level Questions

What do you know about ichthyosis?

Ichthyosis can be classified as follows:
1. *Inherited* ichthyosis is present from birth or childhood and may be apparent only in winter.
   - Ichthyosis vulgaris: present from childhood; autosomal dominant; spares flexural areas; associated with atopy.
   - X-linked ichthyosis: present from birth; over the trunk; associated with corneal opacities.
   - Lamellar ichthyosis: autosomal recessive; present from birth; seen over the body, palms and soles; associated with ectropion.
   - Epidermolytic hyperkeratosis: autosomal dominant; present since birth; predominant flexural involvement.
2. *Metabolic* ichthyosis:
   - Refsum's disease – a metabolic disorder of lipid metabolism.
3. *Malignancy* – as a cutaneous marker:
   - Hodgkin's disease.
   - Multiple myeloma.
   - Breast cancer.

How would you manage such patients?

Regular use of emollients and moisturizing creams. Creams containing urea are useful.

S Refsum, a Norwegian physician.

CASE 155 — Hereditary Haemorrhagic Telangiectasia (Rendu–Osler–Weber Disease)

Instruction

Examine the patient's face.
Perform a general examination.
Look at this patient's face.

Salient features

- Punctiform lesions and dilated small vessels present on the face, in particular around the mouth.
- The patient may be pale (due to iron deficiency anaemia).

Proceed as follows:

- Look into the patient's mouth and inspect the tongue and palate for telangiectasia.
- Examine the nail beds, arms, trunk for telangiectasia.
- Tell the examiner that you would like to ask the patient the following questions:
    Does it run in the family (autosomal dominant)?
    Is there a history of gastrointestinal bleeding?
    Is there a history of epistaxis?
    Is there a history of dyspnoea, fatigue, cyanosis or polycythaemia? (pulmonary arteriovenous malformations).
    Is there a history of headaches, subarachnoid haemorrhage? (cerebral arteriovenous malformations).
- Tell the examiner that you would like to examine:
    The chest for bruits (pulmonary arteriovenous malformations with a predilection for lower lobes).
    For signs of cardiac failure caused by left-to-right shunting and hepatic bruits (both due to hepatic arteriovenous malformations).

Diagnosis

This patient has multiple telangiectasia around the mouth and on the tongue and lips (lesion), probably hereditary in nature (aetiology). The patient is severely anaemic, probably as a result of upper gastrointestinal bleeding, and is currently receiving a blood transfusion (functional status).

Questions

What do you understand by the term 'telangiectasia'?

Telangiectasia is a cluster of dilated capillaries and venules.

Mention a few conditions in which telangiectasia are seen.

- Of the face:
    Those who work outdoors in a temperate or cold climate (e.g. farmers).
    In mitral stenosis.
    Myxoedema.
    Transitory phenomenon during pregnancy.
- Other sites:
    Secondary to irradiation.
    Scleroderma (CREST syndrome).
    Dermatomyositis.
    SLE.
    Acne rosacea.
    Lupus pernio.
    Polycythaemia.
    Necrobiosis lipoidica diabeticorum.

Advanced-level Questions

What do you know about the genetics of hereditary telangiectasia?

Advances in molecular genetics have shown that this condition is actually a group of autosomal dominant disorders with genetic linkages established to chromosome 9q33–q34 in some families and to chromosome 12q in others. In one form of the condition (at chromosome 9q3) the gene encodes the protein endoglin (which is the most abundant protein on endothelial cells), which binds to transforming growth factor β.

What do you know about the pathology of the condition?

In the skin:
- The small telangiectasias are focal dilatations of postcapillary venules with prominent stress fibres in the pericytes along the luminal border.
- In fully developed telengiectasia, there is marked dilatation of the venules, which are also convoluted. They extend along the entire

dermis, with excessive layers of smooth muscle devoid of elastic fibres. These often are directly connected to dilated arterioles.
- Mononuclear cells, predominantly lymphocytes, accumulate in the perivascular space.

In the lungs, liver and brain: arteriovenous malformations lack capillaries and consist of direct connections between arteries and veins.

What are the clinical criteria for diagnosing hereditary haemorrhagic telangiectasia?

The presence of any two of the following:
- Recurrent epistaxis.
- Telangiectasia at a site other than in the nasal mucosa.
- Evidence of autosomal dominant inheritance.
- Visceral involvement.

What are the complications of hereditary telangiectasia?

- Epistaxis (usually begins by the age of 10 years and age 21 in most; it becomes more severe in later decades in about two-thirds of affected patients).
- Gastrointestinal haemorrhage (usually does not manifest until the fifth or sixth decade). Arteriovenous malformations, angiodysplasias and telangiectasias are present in the stomach, duodenum, small bowel, colon and liver.
- Iron deficiency anaemia.
- Haemoptysis, cyanosis, clubbing, cerebral abscess and embolic stroke due to pulmonary arteriovenous malformations.
- Headache and subarachnoid haemorrhage.

How would you manage such patients?

- Anaemia: ferrous sulphate, multiple blood transfusions.
- Epistaxis: oestrogen, cauterization, septal dermatoplasty, laser ablation and transcatheter embolotherapy of arteries leading to the nasal mucosa.
- Cutaneous telangiectasia: cosmetic therapy with topical agents, laser ablation.
- Pulmonary arteriovenous malformations: embolotherapy, surgical resection or ligation of arterial supply.
- Gastrointestinal telangiectasia: blood transfusions, photocoagulation, oestrogen–progestogen therapy.
- Brain and spinal cord arteriovenous malformations: embolotherapy, neurosurgery, stereotactic surgery.
- Active bleeding: epsilon aminocaproic acid.

This condition was described by HJLM Rendu, a French physician, in 1896, by Sir William Osler in 1901 and by F Parkes Weber, a London physician, in 1936.

References

Guttmacher AE, Marchuk DA & White RI Jr (1995) Hereditary haemorrhagic telangiectasia. *N Engl J Med* **333**: 918–924.

McDonald MT, Papenberg KA, Ghosh S et al (1994) A disease locus for hereditary haemorrhagic telangiectasia maps to chromosome 9q33-34. *Nat Genet* **6**: 197–204.

Phillips MD (1994) Stopping bleeding in hereditary telangiectasia. *N Engl J Med* **330**: 1822.

Saba HI, Morelli GA & Logrono LA (1994) Treatment of bleeding in hereditary hemorrhagic telangiectasia with aminocaproic acid. *N Engl J Med* **330**: 1789.

Shovlin CL, Hughes JMB, Tuddenham EGD et al (1994) A gene for hereditary haemorrhagic telangiectasia maps to chromosome 9q3. *Nat Genet* **6**: 205–209.

CASE 156 — Herpes Labialis

Instruction

Look at this patient's mouth.

Salient features

• Small vesicles with an erythematous base on the lips and around the mouth.

Proceed as follows:

• Look for vesicles in the mouth (gingiva, tongue, soft and hard palate) and pharynx.

Diagnosis

This patient has small vesicles around the mouth (lesion) due to herpes labialis (aetiology), which is causing severe itching (functional status).

Questions

What usually causes a 'cold sore'?

Herpes simplex virus (HSV) type I: in children it causes asymptomatic gingivostomatitis; in adults there may be severe stomatitis with mouth ulcers, local lymph node enlargement and systemic features.

What do you know about HSV-II?

HSV-II causes genital infection, called vulvovaginitis. Women with genital herpes ought to have cervical screening as a link is suspected with carcinoma of the cervix.

Advanced-level Questions

What are the complications of herpes infections?

- Erythema multiforme.
- Disseminated infection in the immunocompromised individual.
- Herpes keratitis, scarring and visual impairment.
- Herpes simplex encephalitis (propensity for the temporal lobe).
- Herpetic whitlow (infection of the finger).
- Herpes gladiatorum (infection of the skin, described among wrestlers).
- Visceral infections, especially in viraemia in HIV (oesophagitis, pneumonitis, hepatitis).
- Neonatal HSV infection (neonates less than 6 weeks of age); usually visceral and/or central nervous system infection.
- Herpes simplex meningitis.

How would you confirm your clinical diagnosis?

- Scrapings of the base of the lesions stained with either Wright, Giemsa (Tzanck preparation) or Papanicolaou's stain will demonstrate characteristic giant cells or intranuclear inclusions of herpes infection (does not differentiate from zoster infection).
- Isolation of virus in tissue culture.
- Demonstration of HSV antigens in scrapings from lesions.

How would you treat herpes labialis?

Acyclovir cream applied locally.

What drugs are available for herpes simplex infections?

- Mucocutaneous herpes: topical acyclovir, foscarnet.
- Eye infections: idoxuridine, trifluorothymidine, and topical vidarabine.
- Encephalitis: intravenous acyclovir.
- Neonatal infections: high-dose intravenous vidarabine and acyclovir.

In a patient suspected of herpes encephalitis, which test allows early detection?

HSV DNA polymerase chain reaction (PCR) in the cerebrospinal fluid.

CASE 157 Herpes Zoster Syndrome (Shingles)

Instruction

Look at this patient.

Salient features

- Vesicular rash along a dermatome (usually affects thoracic and lumbar dermatomes).
- Enlargement of a draining lymph node.

Proceed as follows:

- Tell the examiner that you would like to ask about the following:

   Pain, particularly in the ophthalmic branch of the trigeminal nerve, and in the lower thoracic dermatomes (postherpetic neuralgia occurs in about 50% of patients with zoster over the age of 60 years).

   Past history of chickenpox.

   Presence of an underlying immunocompromised state (e.g. recurrent zoster indicates a poorer prognosis in patients with established AIDS). Zoster occurs at least seven times more frequently in homosexual men with HIV infection than in HIV-negative controls.

- Remember that the virus affects both the posterior horn of the spinal cord and the skin supplied by sensory fibres that pass through the diseased root ganglion.

Diagnosis

This patient has a vesicular rash along the 6th thoracic dermatome (lesion) due to herpes zoster (aetiology), and has severe local pain (functional status).

Advanced-level Questions

In which layer of the skin are the vesicles formed?

They are formed in the prickle-cell layer of the epidermis as a result of the 'balloon degeneration' of cells and serous exudation from the corium.

How does this condition present?

Pain in the distribution of the dermatome; malaise; fever, followed a few days later by a rash in the same distribution as the pain. Starts as macules then forms vesicles and then pustules.

Which nerve is affected when the lesions are present on the tip of the nose?

The ophthalmic division of the trigeminal nerve.

How would you confirm the diagnosis?

The diagnosis is usually clinical. It is confirmed by rising viral titres and isolation of the virus from the blister.

How would you manage such a patient?

- Topical idoxuridine 5% solution if caught in the first 36 hours of the eruption.
- Pain relief, including amitriptyline in severe cases.
- Intravenous acyclovir in the immunocompromised individual.
- Interferon appears to be effective in limiting zoster in patients with cancer.

Is varicella-zoster immune globulin (VZIG) useful in preventing zoster eruptions?

There are no known means of effectively preventing zoster eruptions; however, results on the effectiveness of the recently developed live attenuated varicella vaccine are awaited. Although there is considerable controversy, with arguments for and against universal vaccination, the American Academcy of Pediatrics has recently adopted a position in support of universal vaccination of healthy non-immune children and adults.

What are the complications of herpes zoster?

- Corneal ulcerations.
- Gangrene of the affected area.
- Phrenic nerve palsy.
- Meningoencephalitis.
- Ramsay Hunt syndrome.
- Postherpetic neuralgia.
- Disseminated zoster including pneumonia.

What are the features of herpes zoster in patients with HIV infection?

It is usually unidermatomal and uneventful. However, it may be multidermatomal, disseminated recurrent, or chronically persistent as a hyperkeratotic nodular lesion.

How does the varicella zoster virus affect the central nervous system in patients with AIDS?

In acquired immune deficiency syndrome the virus may cause the following:
- Multifocal encephalitis.
- Ventriculitis.
- Acute haemorrhagic meningomyeloradiculitis.
- Focal necrotizing myelitis.
- Vasculitis of the leptomeningeal arteries.

J Ramsay Hunt (1874–1937), a US neurologist.

References

American Academy of Pediatrics Committee on Infectious Diseases (1995). Recommendations of the use of live attenuated varicella vaccine. *Pediatrics* **95**: 791–796.
Gilden DH (1994) Herpes zoster with postherpetic neuralgia – persisting pain and frustration. *N Engl J Med* **330**: 932.
Gray F, Belec L, Lecs MC et al (1994) Varicella-zoster virus infection of the central nervous system in the acquired immune deficiency syndrome. *Brain* **117**: 987.
Wood MJ (1994) A randomised trial of acyclovir for 7 days or 21 days with and without prednisolone for treatment of acute herpes zoster. *N Engl J Med* **330**: 896.

CASE 158 Lichen Planus

Instruction

Look at this patient's skin.

Salient features

- Papular, purplish, flat-topped eruption with fine white streaks (Wickham's striae) over the anterior wrists and forearms, sacral region, legs and penis.

Proceed as follows:

- Look into the mouth for a lace-like pattern of white lines and papules. (Remember that oral lichen planus must be differentiated from leukoplakia.)
- Examine the scalp for cicatricial alopecia.
- Examine the nails for longitudinal ridging, pterygium formation from the cuticle, 20-nail dystrophy with roughened nail surface and brittle free nail edge, total nail loss.
- Comment on eruptions which are present along linear scratch marks (Koebner's phenomenon).
- Tell the examiner that you would like to take a history of:
  Drug ingestion (gold, organic mercurials, chloroquine, mepacrine, methyldopa, quinine, chlorpropamide, tolbutamide).
  Occupational history (whether the patient is in contact with colour film developer).

Note. The three cardinal features of lichen planus are the typical skin lesions, histopathological features of T-cell infiltration of the dermis in a band pattern, and IgG and C3 immunofluorescence at the basement membrane of the dermis.

Diagnosis

This patient has violaceous, flat-topped eruptions (lesion) due to lichen planus (aetiology) with several scratch marks indicating moderately severe pruritus (functional status).

Advanced-level Questions

Mention a few conditions that present as white lesions in the mouth.

- Leukoplakia.
- Candidiasis.
- Aphthous stomatitis.
- Squamous papilloma.
- Verruca vulgaris.
- Secondary syphilis.

Mention a few conditions in which ulcers can be found in the mouth.

- Erosive lichen planus.
- Pemphigus vulgaris.
- Recurrent aphthous ulcers.
- Behçet's disease.

- Stevens–Johnson syndrome.
- Recurrent herpes simplex.

What is the prognosis in lichen planus?

Lichen planus is a benign condition which lasts for months to years. It may be recurrent. Oral lesions may be persistent.

How would you manage these lesions?

- Local measures: local steroid creams or intralesional steroids.
- General measures: PUVA, isotretinoin, dapsone.

LF Wickham (1860–1913), a French dermatologist.
H Koebner (1838–1904), a German dermatologist.

CASE 159 Vitiligo

Instruction
Look at this patient.

Salient features
- Hypopigmented patches which are distributed symmetrically; sometimes the border may be hyperpigmented. The distribution often includes wrists, axillae, perioral, periorbital and anogenital skin.

Proceed as follows:
- Look at the scalp for alopecia.
- Tell the examiner that you would like to ask:
     Whether or not it runs in the family.
     About other autoimmune disorders (hypothyroidism, Addison's disease).

Note. Scratching when the disease is active may induce lesions along the scratch marks; this is termed isomorphic response or Koebner's phenomenon.

Diagnosis
This patient has vitiligo (lesion) which is of autoimmune origin (aetiology) and can be cosmetically distressing to the patient (functional status).

Advanced-level Questions

Mention some associated conditions.

Organ-specific autoimmune conditions:
- Thyroid disease – Graves' disease, myxoedema, Hashimato's disease.
- Pernicious anaemia.
- Diabetes mellitus.
- Alopecia areata.
- Addison's disease.

Which fungal condition can be mistaken for vitiligo?

Pityriasis versicolor (caused by the fungus *Malassezia furfur*).

How would you manage such patients?

- Cosmetics are useful for concealing disfiguring patches.
- When less than 20% of the skin is involved, topical methoxsalen with long-wavelength ultraviolet A (UVA) is used, followed by thorough washing and application of an SPF 15 sunscreen.
- When more than 20% of the skin is affected, oral methoxsalen with UVA.
- New lesions of vitiligo may benefit from topical steroids.
- Newer therapies include epidermal autografts and cultured epidermis combined with PUVA.

Note. On the whole, treatment of vitiligo remains unsatisfactory.

Mention a few conditions in which hypopigmentation is common.

- Hypopituitarism.
- Albinism.
- Phenylketonuria.
- Leprosy.
- Burns.
- Radiodermatitis.
- Piebaldism (an autosomal dominant condition manifested by a white forelock).
- Ash leaf spots (tuberous sclerosis).

What is the histology of vitiligo?

Characteristically there is partial or complete loss of pigment-producing melanocytes in the epidermis. In contrast, some forms of albinism have melanocytes but no melanin pigment is produced because of lack of or a defect in the tyrosinase enzyme.

Why are melanocytes progressively lost in this condition?

The various theories of pathogenesis include:
- Autoimmune destruction due to circulating antibodies against the melanocytes and impaired cell-mediated immunity.
- Self-destruction by toxic intermediates of melanin production.
- Neurohumoral factors.

Reference

Hertz KC, Gazze LA, Kirkpatrick CH & Katz SI (1977) Autoimmune vitiligo, detection of antibodies to melanin-producing cells. *N Engl J Med* **297**: 634.

**CASE
160** **Raynaud's Phenomenon**

Instruction

Examine this patient's hands.

Salient features

- Hands may be painful – ask the patient.
- The hands and fingers are cyanosed and cold, or may be warm and red or blue. The thumbs are rarely affected.

Proceed as follows:

- Examine the hands carefully for signs of scleroderma (tightening of skin, telangiectasia).
- Examine the face for tightening of skin around the mouth (scleroderma), butterfly rash (SLE).
- Tell the examiner that you would like to ask the patient about the following:
    The different phases of Raynaud's phenomenon (in idiopathic Raynaud's disease the cold dead-white hands (ischaemia) become blue (stasis) and finally red (reactive hyperaemia) and painful.
    Sensory changes secondary to vasospasm (numbness, stiffness, aching pain).

Occupation (polishing tools, vibrating tools).

Dysphagia (CREST syndrome).

Butterfly rash, arthralgia, xerostomia (SLE, collagen vascular disorder).

Use of electrically heated gloves.

- Tell the examiner that you would like to examine upper limb pulses and blood pressure in both upper limbs (useful in the detection of cervical rib).

Diagnosis

This patient has cold, blue hands (lesion) due to Raynaud's phenomenon (aetiology) and is unable to continue her occupation, which requires using a vibratory hand drill (functional status).

Advanced-level Questions

What are the causes of Raynaud's phenomenon?

- Immunological and connective tissue disorders:
  Scleroderma.
  SLE.
  Dermatomyositis.
  Rheumatoid arthritis.
  Mixed connective tissue disorders.
- Obliterative arterial disease:
  Atherosclerosis.
  Thoracic outlet syndrome, cervical rib.
- Occupational:
  Vibration, causing white fingers.
  Cold injury, e.g. from handling frozen commodities.
  Vinyl chloride.
- Drugs:
  Beta-blockers.
  Bromocriptine.
  Sulphasalazine.
  Ergot alkaloids.
  Combination of bleomycin and vincristine (as for testicular cancer).
- Miscellaneous:
  Cold agglutinins.
  Cryoglobulins.
  Idiopathic.

What investigations would you do to look for autoimmune rheumatic disease in a patient with Raynaud's phenomenon?

- FBC, ESR.
- Total immunoglobulin and electrophoresis strip.
- Urine analysis.
- Nail-fold capillaroscopy.
- Chest radiography.
- Renal and liver function tests.
- Test for antinuclear antibody.
- Hand radiography.

What drugs have been used to treat Raynaud's syndrome?

Nifedipine, nitrates, stanazolol, inositol nicotinate, naftidrofuryl oxalate, prostaglandin 12, thymoxamine, guanethidine, prazosin.

What is the role of surgery in treating Raynaud's disease?

In patients resistant to medical therapy with severe, frequent attacks, and if trophic changes have occurred interfering with work, dorsal sympathectomy may be indicated.

Do you know of any other vasospastic conditions?

- White finger syndrome.
- Livedo reticularis.
- Erythromelalgia.
- Chilblains.

Maurice Raynaud (1834–1881) described the sign in 1862. He was a physician at Hôpital Lariboisière, Paris.

References

Grigg MH & Wolfe JHN (1991) ABC of vascular diseases: Raynaud's syndrome and similar conditions. *Br Med J* **303**: 913.

Isenberg D & Black C (1995) Raynaud's phenomenon, scleroderma and overlap syndromes. *Br Med J* **310**: 795–798.

Raynaud M (1888) On local and symmetrical gangrene of the extremities. In: Barlow T (translator) *Selected Monographs*, vol. 121. London: New Sydenham Society.

CASE 161 Systemic Lupus Erythematosus

Instruction

Examine this patient's face (usually young females).

Salient features

- Butterfly rash – follicular plugging, scales, telangiectasia and scarring affecting the bridge of the nose and cheeks (the patient may be cushingoid due to steroids).

Proceed as follows:

- Examine the following:
    - Conjuctiva for anaemia (often Coombs' test positive).
    - Mouth ulcers (seen in one-third of cases).
    - Scalp for alopecia.
    - Sun-exposed areas and elbows for vasculitic rash, subcutaneous nodules.
    - Nails for splinter haemorrhages, nail-fold capillaries and periungal infarcts.
    - Hands for palmar erythema, Raynaud's phenomenon, arthritis.
    - Knees for vasculitic rash.
    - Feet for secondary oedema (secondary to nephrotic syndrome).
- Tell the examiner that you would like to examine the urine for proteinuria.

Note. SLE principally affects skin, joints, kidney and serosal membranes.

Diagnosis

This patient has a butterfly rash of the face with telangiectasia (lesion) due to systemic lupus erythematosus (aetiology) and has renal failure probably due to lupus nephritis as evidenced by the haemodialysis catheter (functional status).

Advanced-level Questions

What is the histology of the skin rash in SLE?

- Liquefactive degeneration of the basal layer of the epidermis together with oedema at the dermoepidermal junction. Immunofluorescence

microscopy shows deposition of immunoglobulin and complement
along the dermoepidermal junction.
- Oedema of the dermis accompanied by infiltrates of perivascular
  mononuclear cells.
- Vasculitis with fibrinoid necrosis of the vessels.

What are the skin manifestations of SLE?

Butterfly rash, periungal erythema, nail-fold telangiectasia, alopecia,
livedo reticularis, hyperpigmentation, urticaria, purpura, scarring eruption
of discoid lupus.

What are the criteria for diagnosis of SLE?

Any four of the following 11 criteria are required to make a diagnosis:
- Malar rash.
- Discoid rash.
- Photosensitivity.
- Oral ulcers.
- Arthritis – non-erosive arthritis.
- Serositis – pleuritis, pericarditis.
- Renal involvement – proteinuria, cellular casts (nephritis is more
  common in patients with anti-native DNA).
- Neurological involvement – seizures, psychosis.
- Haematological involvement – haemolytic anaemias, leucopenia,
  thrombocytopenia.
- Antinuclear antibody – seen in over 95% of patients.
- Immunological disorder – positive LE cell, anti-DNA antibody, false-
  positive syphilitic serology.

Note. American Rheumatic Association (ARA) criteria are intended to
provide a degree of diagnostic certainty primarily for research purposes. It
is often possible to be reasonably confident about a diagnosis of SLE on
less strict clinical grounds. A diagnosis of SLE is usually made when
patients have three or four typical manifestations, such as a characteristic
skin rash, thrombocytopenia, serositis or nephritis and antinuclear
antibodies. Polyarthritis and dermatitis are the most common manifestations. It should be noted that antibodies to double-stranded DNA and the
so-called Smith antigen (Sm) are virtually diagnostic of SLE.

What do you know about SLE in older patients?

The initial presentation of idiopathic SLE usually occurs between the first
and fourth decades of life. However, about 10% of cases may first occur in

patients over 60 years of age. Patients with SLE after the age of 50 years less often present with malar rash, arthritis and nephritis.

Diagnosis of SLE in older patients must be one of exclusion. The frequency of low titres on antinuclear antibody tests increases with advancing age, and a positive test may be associated with malignant disease or chronic infection.

What do you know about drug-induced lupus erythematosus?

- Procainamide is responsible for the majority of the cases. Other causes include hydralazine, isoniazid.
- Drugs causing lupus-like syndrome do not seem to aggravate primary SLE.
- Although multiple organs are affected, nephritis and central nervous system features are not ordinarily present.
- Antihistone antibodies are characteristic of drug-induced lupus, but are not specific for this syndrome; anti-native DNA is almost never detected.
- Clinical manifestations and many laboratory features return to normal after the offending drug is withdrawn.

How useful is the detection of antinuclear antibodies in the diagnosis of SLE?

The detection of antinuclear antibodies (ANAs) is a sensitive screening test for SLE. Since ANAs occur in 95% of the patients, it is hard to be certain of the diagnosis in their absence. The degree of positivity is diagnostically important. Serum dilutions below which normal serum may be positive for these antibodies vary in different laboratories. Titres that are less than two times higher than the normal limit in any laboratory ought to be viewed sceptically. The positive predictive value of the test increases with higher titres.

What are the patterns of lupus nephritis?

The World Health Organization's morphological classification of lupus nephritis describes five patterns:
- Normal by light, electron and immunofluoroscence microscopy (rare).
- Mesangial lupus glomerulonephritis.
- Focal proliferative glomerulonephritis.
- Diffuse proliferative glomerulonephritis.
- Membranous glomerulonephritis.

Note. None of these patterns is specific for lupus.

How would you manage a patient with SLE?

- Avoidance of sunlight provocation. In Britain patients should avoid being outside from 11am to 3pm from March to September and should wear protective clothing, including hats; patients should holiday in temperate latitudes or during the winter. In addition, sun block creams such as titanium dioxide (rather than barrier cream) are essential.
- Avoidance of drug provocation – penicillin, sulphonamides.
- Encourage the patient to join the Lupus Society.
- Educate the patient that no therapy is curative and that medical treatment is largely empirical, selected on the basis of specific manifestations (see table below).

Disease manifestations	Treatment
Serological abnormalities and minor cytopenia unaccompanied by symptoms	No treatment
Rash and mild systemic symptoms	Antimalarial drugs
Mild or moderate arthritis, fever, pleuropericarditis	NSAIDs or low-dose prednisolone
Malaise, weight loss and lymphadenopathy	Low-dose steroids
High fever, active inflammatory glomerulonephritis, severe thrombocytopenia, severe haemolytic anaemia and most neurological disturbances	High-dose prednisolone (> 60 mg per day for 4–6 weeks)
Rapidly progressive renal disease	Intravenous administration of bolus doses of 1000 mg methylprednisolone
Lupus nephritis with high histological activity score	Oral or intravenous cyclophosphamide with high dose steroids
Thromboembolism with antiphospholipid antibody	Long-term anticoagulation
Severe disease	Experimental treatments*

* Experimental treatments include apharesis, intravenous γ-globulin, cyclosporin, immunoadsorption, photochemotherapy, nodal irradiation and various monoclonal antibodies.

What are the common causes of death in SLE?

The most common causes of death are renal failure and intercurrent infections followed by diffuse central nervous system disease.

RRA Coombs (b. 1921), Professor of Immunology at Cambridge, is reported to have said 'red blood cells were primarily designed by God as tools for the immunologist and only secondarily as carriers of haemoglobin.'

Ferdinand von Hebra (1816–1880) from Vienna described an eruption that occurs 'mainly on the face, on the cheeks and nose in a distribution not dissimilar to a butterfly' in 1845.

Pierre Louis Alphée Cazenave (1795–1877) from Paris first used the term lupus érythémateux in 1851.

Sir William Osler (1849–1919) first described the systemic manifestations of systemic lupus erythematosus under the name exudative erythema between 1895 and 1904.

References

Cervaera R and the The European Working Party on SLE (1993). Systemic lupus erythematosus: clinical and immunologic patterns of disease expression in a cohort of 1000 patients. *Medicine* **72**: 113.

Hay EM & Snaith ML (1995) Systemic lupus erythematosus and lupus-like syndromes. *Br Med J* **310**: 1257–1261.

Mills JA (1994) Systemic lupus erythematosus. *N Engl J Med* **330**: 187.

Tan EM, Cohen AS, Fries JF et al (1982) The 1982 criteria for classification of SLE. *Arthritis Rheum* **25**: 1271.

CASE 162 Phlebitis Migrans

Instruction

Look at this patient's leg: he has had similar such lesions at different sites at intervals.

Salient features

• Inflamed superficial leg veins.

Proceed as follows:

• Ask the patient about local trauma (including intravenous infusions).
• Tell the examiner that you would like to investigate for the underlying malignancy, usually carcinoma of the pancreas or stomach (Trousseau's sign).

Diagnosis

This patient has migratory phlebitis (lesion) and I would like to investigate for an underlying pancreatic or gastric malignancy (aetiology).

Advanced-level Questions

In which other condition is superficial phlebitis a prominent sign?

Thromboangiitis obliterans.

Is superficial thrombophlebitis associated with deep vein thrombosis?

It may be associated with occult deep vein thrombosis in about 20% of cases, although pulmonary emboli are rare.

Is phlebitis more frequently associated with plastic venous catheters or with steel intravenous needles?

It is more likely to be associated with plastic catheters, but this may be due to its remaining in the vein for longer periods.

How is superficial phlebitis treated?

- Local heat, elevation of the leg, and NSAIDs.
- When very extensive or in proximity to the saphenofemoral junction, ligation and division of the the saphenous vein at the saphenofemoral junction (as pulmonary embolism may result if the phlebitis of the saphenous vein extends into the deep vein).
- Septic thrombophlebitis, which is usually due to *Staphylococcus aureus*, requires excision of the involved vein up to its junction with an uninvolved vein in order to control infection.

What other dermatoses complicate pancreatic disease?

- Panniculitis.
- 'Bronze' pigmentation of haemochromatosis.
- 'Necrolytic migratory erythema' of glucagonoma syndrome.
- Cutaneous haemorrhage of acute pancreatitis – 'bruising' of the left flank (Grey Turner's sign) or umbilicus (Cullen's sign).

Armand Trousseau (1801–1867), physician at the Hôtel-Dieu in Paris, noted the sign as his death warrant, confirming his suspicion of an underlying malignancy.
G Grey Turner (1877–1951), Professor of Surgery, Hammersmith Hospital, London.
TS Cullen (1868–1953), Canadian born, Professor of Gynaecology, Johns Hopkins Hospital, Baltimore, USA.

References

Prandoni P, Lensing AWA, Büller HR et al (1992) Deep vein thrombosis and the incidence of subsequent symptomatic cancer. *N Engl J Med* **327**: 1128–1133.

Silverstein RL & Nachman RL (1994) Cancer and clotting –Trousseau's warning. *N Engl J Med* **327**: 1163-1164.

Trousseau A (1872) Phlegmasia albia dolens. In: *Lectures on clinical medicine, delivered at the Hôtel-Dieu, Paris*, pp. 281–295. London: New Wydenham Society.

CASE 163 Erythema Multiforme

Instruction

Perform a general examination.

Salient features

- Target-shaped lesions, usually over the limbs. A classical target lesion consists of three concentric zones of colour change.
- Pleomorphic eruption with macules, papules and bullae.

Proceed as follows:

- Look at the mucous membranes of the mouth and eyes (Stevens–Johnson syndrome).
- Tell the examiner that you would like to proceed as follows:
  Examine the external genitalia for ulcers.
  Take a history of preceding sore throat or cold.
  Take a drug history (barbiturates, sulphonamides).

Note. Erythema multiforme is a cell-mediated hypersensitivity reaction to many different immunological insults, including drugs and infectious agents such as viruses (most notably herpes simplex). In its so-called 'minor' form, it is manifested by heterogeneous cutaneous eruption, at times bullous.

Diagnosis

This patient has target-shaped lesions (lesion) due to sulphonamides (aetiology) which usually resolve on discontinuing the drug (functional status).

Questions

What is the underlying aetiology?

- Infections (herpes simplex, mycoplasma, streptococcal).
- Drug hypersensitivity (sulphonamides, penicillin, barbiturates, salicylates, antimalarials).
- Collagen vascular disorder (SLE, dermatomyositis, periarteritis nodosa).
- Malignancy (carcinomas and lymphomas).
- Multiple myeloma.
- Idiopathic – in 50% of cases no cause may be found.

Advanced-level Questions

How would you investigate this patient?

- Viral titres, in particular for herpes simplex type 1.
- Complement fixation test for mycoplasma.
- Antistreptolysin O (ASO) titres.

If the above are negative:
- Serum(s) antibodies.
- Protein electrophoresis, urine for Bence-Jones proteins.

What is the histology of erythema multiforme?

- Early lesions: superficial perivascular lymphocytic infiltrate with oedema of the dermis, accompanied by degeneration and necrosis of keratinocytes and margination of lymphocytes at the dermoepidermal junction.
- Late lesions: upward migration of lymphocytes into the epidermis, discrete and confluent portions of the epidermis necrose resulting in blister formation and subsequently erosions (due to sloughing of the epidermis).
- Target lesions: characterized by central necrosis surrounded by perivenular inflammation.

What do you understand by the term 'Stevens – Johnson syndrome'?

Stevens–Johnson syndrome, also referred to as erythema multiforme major, is characterized by fever and mucous membrane involvement (usually oral cavity, eye and genital) in addition to the eruptions of erythema multiforme.

How would you manage a patient with erythema multiforme and Stevens – Johnson syndrome?

- Symptomatic treatment with antipyretics, intravenous fluids and antibiotics.
- Systemic corticosteroids, although the role of steroids is controversial.
- Other immunosuppressive drugs used in recurrent erythema multiforme and Stevens–Johnson syndrome include levamisole, azathioprine, dapsone, thalidomide, high-dose intravenous immunoglobulin and cyclosporin.
- Acyclovir is recommended by some authors as a therapeutic trial in any patient with severe recurrent erythema multiforme, even if no preceding herpes simplex infection has been documented.
- Other therapeutic options:
    Localized care including use of antibiotic creams, ointments, sterile dressing, special beds containing beads, amnion dressings on denuded skin.
    Ophthalmological care includes use of artificial tears and topical vitamin A.
    Extensive denudation of the skin is best treated in a burns unit.

Erythema multiforme is a self-limiting condition, but Stevens–Johnson syndrome may be fatal.

FC Johnson (1894–1934) and AM Stevens (1884–1945), both American paediatricians, described this condition in 1922 in a paper entitled 'A new eruptive fever with tonsillitis and ophthalmia'.
H Bence-Jones (1814–1873), English physician, St George's Hospital, London.

Reference

Stevens AM & Johnson FC (1922) A new eruptive fever associated with stomatitis and ophthalmia: report of two cases in children. *Am J Dis Child* **24**: 526–533.

CASE 164 Erythema Ab Igne

Instruction

Examine this patient's legs.
Examine this patient's abdomen.

Salient features

- Reticular erythematous or pigmented rash, usually on the forelegs (or abdomen), known as 'Granny's tartan'.

Proceed as follows:

- Look for features of hypothyroidism (pulse, ankle jerks).
- Tell the examiner that you would like to proceed as follows:
  Ask the patient whether she exposed the affected area to heat.
  Measure T_4 and thyroid-stimulating hormone (TSH) levels.

Note. If the rash is present over the anterior abdominal wall or lumbar region, it is very likely that there is an intra-abdominal malignancy.

Diagnosis

This patient has a reticular pigmented rash (lesion) on the abdomen due to local heat from a hot-water bag (aetiology); I would like to exclude an underlying intra-abdominal malignancy.

Advanced-level Questions

How may erythema ab igne be complicated?

Epitheliomas may develop in keratoses, which form in later stages of this condition.

What other reticulated rashes do you know?

- Livedo reticularis, seen in the following conditions:
  Polyarteritis nodosa.
  SLE.
  Occult malignant neoplasm.
  Atherosclerotic microemboli to the skin.
  Physiological in young women (it is most apparent on the thighs of young females playing outdoor sports on a cold day).
- Cutaneous marmota seen in children.

Mention some skin abnormalities related to heat or cold.

- Erythema ab igne.
- Livedo reticularis (due to cold in young women).
- Raynaud's phenomenon.
- Chilblains.

CASE 165   Hirsutism

Instruction

Examine this patient.

Salient features

- Excessive hair growth, particularly over the face and upper and lower limbs.

Proceed as follows:

- Tell the examiner that you would like to:
  Take a menstrual history.
  Check the blood pressure and urine for sugar.
  Comment on cushingoid features, if any.
  Look for signs of virilization (receding hairline, breast atrophy, clitoromegaly).

Questions

What do you understand by the term hirsutism?

Hirsutism is the male pattern of hair growth in women and consists of excessive *terminal* hair (androgen-sensitive hair). It is abnormal, particularly on the chin, sternum, upper abdomen and upper back in women. Terminal hair may normally occur on the arms, legs, upper lips, linea alba and periareolar area in women. The degree of hirsutism can be assessed by the Ferriman–Gallwey Score, a simple, semiquantitative method of recording distribution and severity of excess body hair.

Why do you want to take a menstrual history?

If menstruation is normal, it indicates that there is no increase in testosterone production. However, if menstruation is abnormal, the commonest cause is polycystic ovary disease (POCD or Stein–Leventhal syndrome), which is the underlying cause in 92% of the women with hirsutism (the popular belief that most cases of hirsutism are idiopathic is untrue).

Advanced-level Questions

What other causes of hirsutism can you tell us?

- Cushing's syndrome.
- Adrenal or ovarian tumours.
- Acromegaly.
- Drugs:
    Those that increase *vellus* growth: phenytoin, minoxidil, diazoxide, cyclosporin.
    Those that increase *terminal* hair growth: androgens.
- Familial.

What is the relationship between body-weight and hirsutism?

Hirsute women are more likely to be obese than non-hirsute women. Thus, weight loss must be a priority in treating overweight women with hirsutism.

What is the role of testosterone in hirsutism?

Testosterone is the most potent androgen and is derived directly from ovarian secretion (60%) and from peripheral conversion of androstenedione (40%). About 65% of testosterone is strongly bound to sex hormone-binding globulin (SHBG) and 33% is weakly bound to albumin. The remaining 2% is free testosterone and can enter target cells to exert its androgenic effect. In the skin it is converted to dihydrotestosterone (DHT) which stimulates the hair follicle. Other androgens include androstenedione (secreted in equal amounts by adrenals and ovaries) and dehydroepiandrosterone (derived exclusively from the adrenals).

What is the pathophysiology of POCD?

It is due to an abnormality of pulsatile secretion of the gonadotrophin-releasing hormone (GnRH) causing increased luteinizing hormone (LH) and follicle-stimulating hormone (FSH) secretion. This results in hyperplasia of the ovarian thecal cell leading to multiple follicular cysts and excessive androgen synthesis and anovulation. (Remember that POCD is the association of hyperandrogenism with chronic anovulation in women without specific underlying diseases of adrenals or pituitary glands.)

How would you investigate a patient with suspected POCD?

- Ovarian ultrasonography is the most accurate investigation; typically it shows thickened capsules, multiple 3–5-mm cysts and a hyperechogenic stroma.
- Biochemistry:
    Total testosterone levels may be normal, but free androgens are raised.

Sex hormone-binding globulin (SHBG) level is low.

LH:FSH ratio is raised, usually greater than 2:1, but FSH level is low or normal.

Mild hyperprolactinaemia is common and rarely exceeds $1500 \, \text{mU} \, \text{l}^{-1}$.

Is glucose metabolism affected in POCD?

POCD is associated with hyperinsulinaemia and insulin resistance, and consequently may have impaired glucose tolerance. The site of insulin resistance in these patients is skeletal muscle and fatty tissue but not hepatic resistance (the latter being a feature of non-insulin-dependent diabetes mellitus). It is believed that full expression of polycystic ovary disease requires the interaction of insulin abnormality with an underlying disorder of androgen biosysthesis, and that an abnormality of insulin alone is unlikely to cause hyperandrogenism.

How would you treat hirsutism?

- Treatment is directed towards the underlying cause of hyperandrogenism.
- Mild hyperandrogenism which is idiopathic or mild POCD: oral contraceptives.
- Severe hirsutism: antiandrogens (spironolactone, cyproterone acetate, flutamide), finasteride (5 α-reductase inhibitor) prevent the cutaneous conversion of testosterone to active dihydrotestosterone, GnRH analogues (leuprolide, nafarelin).
- Local treatment: shaving, epilation, waxing, electrolysis or bleaching.

IF Stein (1887–), a US gynaecologist.
ML Leventhal (1901–1971), a US obstetrician.

References

Adams, J, Polson DW & Franks S (1986) Prevalence of polycystic ovaries in women with anovulation and idiopathic hirsutism. *Br Med J* **293**: 355.

Conway GS & Jacobs HS (1990) Hirsutism. *Br Med J* **301**: 619.

Ferriman D & Gallwey JD (1961) Clinical assessment of body hair growth in women. *J Clin Endocrinol Metab* **21**: 1440–1447.

Franks S (1995) Polycystic ovary syndrome. *N Engl J Med* **333**: 853–861.

MacKenna TJ (1994) Screening for sinister causes of hirsutism. *N Engl J Med* **331**: 1015.

Stein IF & Leventhal ML (1935) Amenorrhea associated with bilateral polycystic ovaries. *Am J Obstet Gynecol* **29**: 181–191.

CASE 166 Acanthosis Nigricans

Instruction

Perform a general examination.

Salient features

- Black, velvety overgrowth seen in the axillae, neck, umbilicus, nipples, groins or facial skin.

Proceed as follows:

- Look for the following signs:
  Tripe palms (roughness of the palmar and plantar skin).
  Filiform growths around the face and mouth, and over the tongue.
- Tell the examiner that you would like to investigate for underlying malignancy, in particular adenocarcinoma of the stomach and for endocrine disorders (diabetes, Cushing's syndrome, acromegaly).

Diagnosis

This patient has a velvety black overgrowth in the axillae (lesion) and I would like to exclude an underlying adenocarcinoma, particularly of the stomach (aetiology).

Advanced-level Questions

What is the histology of acanthosis nigricans?

- Undulating epidermis with numerous sharp peaks and valleys.
- Variable amount of hyperplasia, hyperkeratosis and slight pigmentation of the basal cell layer (but no melanocytic hyperplasia).

With which conditions is acanthosis nigricans associated?

Benign conditions:
    Diabetes associated with marked insulin resistance.
    Cushing's syndrome.
    Acromegaly.
    Stein–Leventhal syndrome.
Malignant conditions (due to abnormal production of epidermal growth factors):
    Adenocarcinomas, lymphomas.

What is the relationship between the course of the skin lesion and the underlying malignancy?

The acanthosis nigricans may precede the neoplasm by more than 5 years. In about two-thirds of cases the course parallels that of the tumour, including remission with cure.

Mention some cutaneous manifestations of visceral malignancy.

- Dermatomyositis.
- Migratory thrombophlebitis.
- Ichthyosis.
- Paget's disease of the nipple.
- Tylosis.

Acanthosis is hyperplasia of the stratum spinosum of the epidermis.

References

Curth HO (1976) Classification of acanthosis nigricans. *Int J Dermatol* **15**: 592.
Ellis DL, Kafka SP, Chow JC et al (1987) Melanoma growth factors, acanthosis nigricans, the sign of Leser–Trélat, and multiple acrochordons. A possible role for alpha-transforming growth factors in cutaneous neoplastic syndromes. *N Engl J Med* **317**: 1582.

CASE 167 Lipoatrophy

Instruction

Look at this patient.
Look here (the examiner pointing at the patient's thighs).

Salient features

- Atrophy of the subcutaneous fat leading to disfiguring excavations and depressed areas.

Proceed as follows:

- Tell the examiner that you would like to know whether:
    The patient is taking insulin for diabetes.
    The patient has a past history of renal disease (mesangiocapillary glomerulonephritis).

Diagnosis

This patient has atrophy of subcutaneous fat or lipoatrophy (lesion) due to local injection of subcutaneous insulin (aetiology).

Advanced-level Questions

With which conditions is lipoatrophy associated?

- Mesangiocapillary glomerulonephritis.
- Localized scleroderma.
- Morphea.
- Chronic relapsing panniculitis.

What advice would you give this patient on insulin?

The insulin should be changed to a more purified form. The purified form should be injected directly into the atrophic area, which often results in the restoration of the local contours.

What is the mechanism of lipoatrophy atrophy?

This complication results from an immune reaction.

Can lipohypertrophy occur with insulin injections?

Yes, as a consequence of the pharmacological effects of insulin being deposited in the same location repeatedly. Rotation of injection sites can prevent this complication. It can occur with purified insulins and responds best to liposuction.

The 1923 Nobel Prize in Medicine was awarded for the discovery of insulin to a Canadian surgeon, Sir Fredrick G Banting (1891–1941) and Scottish physiologist, John JR Macleod (1876–1935) working in Toronto. Banting shared his monetary prize with Charles Best whereas Macleod shared his prize with JJ Collip (the latter purified insulin to the point that it could be used in humans). Macleod corrected Banting's deficiencies on carbohydrate metabolism and provided him with laboratory support including the services of a graduate student in physiology viz., Charles Best.

CASE 168 Lupus Pernio

Instruction

Look at this patient's face.

Salient features

- Reddish blue or violaceous plaques on the nose, cheeks, ears and fingers, with telangiectasia over and around the plaques.

Proceed as follows:

- Tell the examiner that you would like to do radiography for hilar adenopathy.

Diagnosis

This patient has violaceous plaques on his face (lesion) due to sarcoidosis (aetiology) which is cosmetically disfiguring (functional status).

Advanced-level Questions

What is the differential diagnosis of such a lesion?

- Rhinophyma.
- Lupus vulgaris.
- Leprosy.

What are the cutaneous manifestations of sarcoid?

- Erythema nodosum.
- Micropapular sarcoid.
- Scar infiltration.
- Sarcoid plaques of limbs, shoulders, buttocks and thighs.

How may sarcoid present?

- Acute sarcoidosis usually presents in the third decade, characterized by erythema nodosum, parotid enlargement and hilar lymphadenopathy.
- Chronic sarcoidosis usually presents in the fifth decade with an insidious onset characterized by fatigue, dyspnoea, arthralgia and lupus pernio. Bone cysts are another feature.

How would you investigate such a patient?

- FBC and ESR (leukopenia, eosinophilia and raised ESR).
- CXR (there are three stages of sarcoidosis depending on radiographic findings and include Stage I where there is bilateral hilar adenopathy alone, Stage II where there is both hilar adenopathy and lung parenchymal involvement and Stage III with parenchymal involvement alone).
- Slit-lamp examination of the eyes.
- Kviem's test (the antigen is cultured in human spleen and thus, increasingly, it is recommended that this test should not be performed because of the risk of transmitting viral infections).
- Mantoux test (skin anergy is present in 70%).
- Serum angiotensin-converting enzyme levels (raised in 40–80% with active disease, although this finding is neither sensitive nor specific enough to have diagnostic significance).
- Lung function tests (usually restrictive changes with decreased lung volumes and diffusing capacity; occasionally airflow obstruction).
- Serum calcium levels (hypercalcaemia in 10% of patients).
- Gallium-67 scan.
- Bronchoalveolar lavage (usually characterized by an increase in lymphocytes and a high CD4:CD8 ratio).
- Histological confirmation: transbronchial lung biopsy; biopsy of lymph node, skin, liver, gums and minor salivary glands (presence of non-caseating granulomas with typical manifestations is generally required for diagnosis of sarcoidosis).

What is the prognosis and treatment of sarcoidosis?

- Acute sarcoidosis usually regresses spontaneously within 2 years and does not recur; it may not require treatment.
- Chronic sarcoidosis may require systemic corticosteroids in order to prevent serious disability and even death from respiratory failure.

What are the specific indications for systemic steroids in sarcoidosis?

- Progressive deterioration in lung function, particularly transfer factor and vital capacity. Serial evaluation should be performed every 2 months initially, gradually increasing the intervals between follow-up to about 4–5 months; patients should be followed for at least 2 years after steroids are stopped.
- CNS involvement.
- Hypercalcaemia.
- Severe ocular disease.

- Hepatitis.
- Cutaneous lesions.
- Constitutional symptoms.
- Symptomatic pulmonary lesions.

What are the ocular manifestations of sarcoidosis?

- Anterior uveitis, seen in about 5% of all cases:
    Acute.
    Chronic – mutton fat keratic precipitates, iris nodules.
- Retinal vasculitis, neovascularization.
- Vitreous opacities.
- Choroidal granulomata.
- Optic nerve granuloma.

What is Löfgren's syndrome?

Erythema nodosum and hilar adenopathy in a patient with sarcoidosis.

What is the source of the raised angiotensin converting enzyme level in sarcoidosis?

It is derived from the cell membranes of epithelioid cells in the sarcoid granuloma and its synthesis is controlled by epithelioid cells.

MA Kviem (b. 1892), a Norwegian pathologist.
CPM Boeck (1845–1917), Professor of Medicine and dermatologist in Oslo, Norway, first described the disease as 'mutliple benign sarcoid'.
S Löfgren, a Swedish physician.
D Geraint James, contemporary Professor of Medicine, Royal Free Hospital, London; his chief interest is sarcoidosis. His wife, Dame Sheila Sherlock, is a renowned hepatologist.
C Mantoux (1877–1947), a French physician from Cannes, who showed that his intradermal test was more sensitive than the older Pirquet subcutaneous tests using tuberculin.

References

James DG & Jones Williams W (1984) *Sarcoidosis and other Graulomatous Disorders*. Philadelphia: WB Saunders.
Spalton DJ & Saunders MD (1981) Fundus changes in histologically confirmed sarcoidosis. *Br J Ophthalmol* **65**: 348–358.

CASE 169 Xanthelasma

Instruction

Examine this patient's eyes.

Salient features

- Xanthelasmata (flat yellow nodules or plaques) seen on eyelids and around both eyes, particularly on the inner canthus.

Proceed as follows:

- Look for the following signs:
    Corneal arcus.
    Jaundice, generalized pigmentation, scratch marks (primary biliary cirrhosis).
    Tendon xanthomata.
    Palmar xanthomata.
- Tell the examiner that you would like to check the following:
    Urine sugar.
    Blood pressure.
    Pulse and ankle jerks (hypothyroidism).

Remember that blood lipids can often be normal.

Diagnosis

This patient has xanthelasmata on the eyelids (lesions) and I would like to test serum lipids to exclude an underlying lipid disorder (aetiology).

Advanced-level Questions

In which conditions are xanthelasmata seen?

Those in which there is an increase in serum cholesterol:
- Type IIb hyperlipidaemia – increased cholesterol and triglycerides.
- Type IIa hyperlipidaemia – increased cholesterol only.
- Type III hyperlipidaemia – equal increase in cholesterol and triglycerides.

Mention a few secondary causes of hyperlipidaemia.

Diabetes mellitus, hypothyroidism, nephrotic syndrome, cholestatic jaundice, excess alcohol intake, oral contraceptives.

How would you manage a patient with hyperlipidaemia?

- Lifestyle advice.
- Dietary modification (usually adequate for those whose cholesterol level is in the range 6.5–8 mmol l^{-1}).
- Avoidance of alcohol, smoking, oestrogens and thiazides.
- Exercise.
- Control of hypertension and diabetes.
- Lipid-lowering drugs.

Mention a few lipid-lowering drugs.

- Ion exchange resin: cholestyramine.
- Fibrates: bezafibrate, gemfibrozil.
- Sitostanol-ester margarine (a plant sterol that reduces serum cholesterol concentration by inhibiting cholesterol absorption).
- Hydroxymethylglutaryl (HMG) coenzyme A (CoA) reductase inhibitors: simvastatin, pravastatin, lovastatin. These drugs block the endogenous synthesis of cholesterol and reduce levels of low-density lipoprotein cholesterol.
- Nicotinic acid derivatives: nicotinic acid, probucol.

Are HMG CoA reductase inhibitors useful in patients with hypercholesterolaemia and coronary heart disease?

Yes, the Scandinavian Simvastatin Survival Study (the 4S trial) demonstrated a survival benefit from lowering cholesterol with simvastatin in patients with coronary disease.

What is the role of HMG CoA reductase inhibitors in patients with hypercholesterolaemia and no signs of coronary heart disease?

A recent study from Scotland showed that treatment with pravastatin significantly reduced the incidence of myocardial infarction (30% reduction) and death from cardiovascular causes (33% reduction) without adversely affecting the risk of death from non-cardiovascular causes in men with moderate hypercholesterolaemia and without a history of myocardial infarction. This has been confirmed by the 'CARE' trial.

James Scott, contemporary Professor and Chairman of the Department of Medicine at Hammersmith Hospital, London, is a physician, biochemist and molecular biologist. He has made a considerable contribution to lipid and cardiovascular research.

References

Miettinen TA, Puska P, Gylling H, Vanhanen H & Vartainen E (1995) Reduction of serum cholesterol with sitostanol-ester margarine in a mildly hypercholesterolaemic population. *N Engl J Med* **333**: 1308-1312.

Scandinavian Simvastatin Survival Study Group (1994) Randomised trial of cholesterol lowering in 4444 patients with coronary heart disease: The Scandinavian Simvastatin Survival Study (4S). *Lancet* **344**: 1383-1389.

Shepherd J, Cobbe SM, Ford I et al (1995) Prevention of coronary heart disease with pravastatin in men with hypercholesterolaemia. *N Engl J Med* **333**: 1301-1307.

CASE 170 **Necrobiosis Lipoidica Diabeticorum**

Instruction

Look at this patient's legs.
Examine this patient's back.

Salient features

- Usually seen in females (two to four times more frequently than in men).
- Sharply demarcated oval plaques seen on the shin, arms or back.
- The plaques have a shiny surface with yellow waxy centres and brownish red margins with surrounding telangiectasia.

Proceed as follows:

- Tell the examiner that you would like to check the urine for sugar.

Diagnosis

This patient has plaques with yellow waxy centres on the shins (lesions) due to diabetes mellitus (aetiology) which are cosmetically disfiguring (functional status).

Advanced-level Questions

What is the histology of these lesions?

Collagen degeneration surrounded by epithelioid and giant cells.

What may complicate it?

Ulceration of the plaque.

What treatment is available for such lesions?

- Good diabetic control.
- Whirlpool therapy, occlusive dressings, aspirin, pentoxifylline.
- Local steroids.
- Excision and skin grafting.

What other skin lesions are usually seen on the shins?

- Erythema nodosum (see page 492).
- Pretibial myxoedema (see page 388).
- Diabetic dermopathy.
- Erythema ab igne (see page 448).
- Livedo reticularis.

What are the other skin lesions seen in diabetes?

- Granuloma annulare.
- Chronic pyogenic infections and carbuncles (indicating poor control).
- Eruptive xanthomata (from hypertriglyceridaemia associated with poor glycaemic control) (see page 446).
- Xanthelasmata (see page 459).
- Lipoatrophy and lipohypertrophy (see page 455).
- Leg ulcers and gangrene.
- Acanthosis nigricans (see page 453).
- Peripheral anhydriosis (due to autonomic neuropathy).
- Vulval candidiasis.

Reference

Templeton SF & Caughman SW (1993) Necrobiosis lipoidica diabeticorum. *N Engl J Med* **329**: 320 (A classical photograph of the lesion; candidates are encouraged to refer to this photograph.)

CASE 171 Radiotherapy Marks

Instruction

Look at this patient's chest.

Salient features

Patient 1:
- Telangiectasia over the chest wall.
- There may be a unilateral mastectomy.

Diagnosis

This patient has telangiectasia and a unilateral mastectomy (lesion), indicating that she has had radiotherapy (aetiology) for breast cancer in the past.

Patient 2:
- India-ink marks over the chest.
- Localized erythema in the same region.

Diagnosis

This patient has India-ink marks over the chest with localized erythema (lesion) indicating that she is currently undergoing radiotherapy treatment (aetiology).

Advanced-level Questions

Which other normal tissues, apart from the skin, are affected by radiation therapy?

Tissues that exhibit early or late damage from radiation therapy include mucosa, spinal cord, bone marrow and lymphoid system. To minimize these effects, radiation is normally delivered in a fractionated manner allowing recovery of normal host tissues (but not of tumour).

What modalities may be used to minimize the side-effects of radiation?

- Fractionation of dose.
- Rendering the tumour more sensitive to radiotherapy by prior chemotherapy and thereby reducing the dose.
- Regional hypothermia (40–42°C) particularly in superficial tumours and relatively bulky non-vascular tumours.

- Radiolabelled antibodies which deliver high levels of radiation locally to the tumour bed.

How is radiotherapy usually delivered?

It is usually delivered either as brachytherapy (where the radiation source is close to the tumour) or as teletherapy (where supervoltage radiotherapy is usually delivered with a linear acclerator).

In which conditions is radiotherapy beneficial?

Malignant conditions:
- Radiotherapy as the sole agent with a curative intent: in Hodgkin's disease, some neoplasms of brain and spinal cord, oral cavity, pharynx, oesophagus, laryngeal tumours permitting cure without loss of voice, tumours of cervix and vagina cavity.
- Radiation with surgery: in cancers of lung, breast, urinary bladder, seminomas, ovary, uterus, sarcomas of soft tissue and testicular seminomas.
- Radiation as adjuvant to chemotherapy: lymphomas, lung cancers and childhood cancers.
- Radiation as palliative therapy for pain and or dysfunction: superior vena caval obstruction, dysphagia of terminal illness, upper airway obstruction, spinal cord compression, pericardial tamponade secondary to malignant pericardial tumours.

Non-malignant conditions:
- Exophthalmos.
- Rheumatoid arthritis (total lymphoid irradiation is an experimental therapeutic procedure).
- Ankylosing spondylitis where local external irradiation of an involved peripheral joint or injected radiation synovectomy can be valuable in ameliorating pain and allowing mobility. Spinal irradiation is no longer used because of the risk of haematological malignancy.

What are the side-effects of radiotherapy?

- Acute toxicity: systemic symptoms including malaise, fatigue, anorexia, nausea and vomiting. Diarrhoea and local skin and mucosal changes. Bone marrow suppression may occur following irradiation to the pelvis and long bones.
- Long-term toxicity: cutaneous hyperpigmentation, impaired function of irradiated viscera, bone necrosis, myelopathy and secondary malignancies.

Reference

Lichter AS & Lawrence TS (1995) Recent advances in radiation oncology. *N Engl J Med* **332** 371–377.

CASE 172 **Tendon Xanthomata**

Instruction

Look at this patient's hands.

Salient features

- Tendon xanthomata seen on the extensor tendons and becoming more prominent when the patient clenches his fist.

Proceed as follows:

- Look at other tendons, particularly the patellar and Achilles tendon.
- Look at the eyes for xanthelasmata and corneal arcus.
- Tell the examiner that you would like to check fasting lipids, in particular for an increase in cholesterol level.

Diagnosis

This patient has tendon xanthomata (lesion) due to hypercholesterolaemia (aetiology).

Questions

In which condition are these seen?

Familial hypercholesterolaemia, an autosomal dominant trait with an excess of low-density lipoprotein (LDL) or β-lipoprotein in the blood. It occurs in 1 in 200–500 of the population.

Advanced-level Questions

What is the basic defect?

Goldstein and Brown, in 1975, showed that this condition was due to a defect or deficiency in LDL cell receptors.

At what age do these patients manifest the condition?

Homozygotes usually have xanthomata at birth or as children. They have a predisposition to ischaemic heart disease which usually results in death before the age of 30 years. About 50% of heterozygotes also present by the same age.

What are xanthomata?

Xanthomata are tumour-like collections of foamy histiocytes within the dermis. There are five types of xanthoma:
- Eruptive xanthoma (seen in types I, IIb, III, IV, V).
- Tuberous xanthoma (types IIa, III, rarely IIb, IV).
- Tendon xanthoma (types IIa, III, rarely IIIb).
- Palmar xanthoma (types III, IIa, associated with primary biliary cirrhosis).
- Xanthelasma (types IIa, III; also without lipid abnormalities).

Michael S Brown (b. 1941) and Joseph L Goldstein (b. 1940), both of the University of Texas Health Science Centre in Dallas, were awarded the 1983 Nobel Prize for their discoveries concerning the regulation of cholesterol metabolism.

CASE 173 Eruptive Xanthomata

Instruction

Examine this patient's skin.
This uncontrolled diabetic has developed a profuse eruption; what are these lesions?

Salient features

- Multiple, itchy, red–yellow vesicles or nodules which are seen over extensor surfaces, i.e. buttocks, back, knees and elbows.

Proceed as follows:

- Tell the examiner that would like to:
  Examine the fundus for lipaemia retinalis.
  Check the urine for sugar.
  Do a lipid profile (remember that eruptive xanthomata signify triglyceridaemia).

Diagnosis

This patient has eruptive xanthomata (lesion) due to hypertriglyceridaemia (aetiology).

Advanced-level Questions

In which conditions are eruptive xanthomata seen?

- Type IV hyperlipidaemia.
    Familial hypertriglyceridaemia.
    Lipoprotein lipase deficiency.
    Apolipoprotein CII deficiency.
- Type I hyperlipidaemia – chylomicronaemia.
- Type V hyperlipidaemia – increased levels of triglycerides and chylomicrons.

Mention some other causes of hypertriglyceridaemia.

- Primary hypertriglyceridaemia (usually greater than 500 mg dl^{-1}): familial hypertriglyceridaemia, familial combined hyperlipidaemia.
- Secondary hypertriglyceridaemia: diet, obesity, excess alcohol intake, diabetes mellitus, hypothyroidism, uraemia, dysproteinaemias, drugs (beta-blockers, oral contraceptives and oestrogens, retinoids).

What is the relationship between hypertriglyceridaemia and coronary artery disease?

The relationship of hypertriglyceridaemia with coronary artery disease is less clear than that with hypercholesterolaemia, but is said to increase risk when levels are greater than 500 mg dl^{-1}, when other risk factors are present or in familial combined hyperlipidaemia.

Of what are patients particularly at risk when serum levels of triglycerides are markedly raised (> 1000 mg dl^{-1})?

They are more susceptible to acute pancreatitis and hyperchylomicronaemia.

How would you manage a patient with raised levels of serum triglycerides?

- Diet: restrict dietary fat, decrease intake of alcohol and simple sugars.
- Weight loss if the patient is overweight.
- Exercise.

- Discontinuation of drugs, e.g. beta-blockers.
- Control secondary causes.

CASE 174 Palmar Xanthomata

Instruction

Examine this patient's hands.

Salient features

- Yellowish-orange discolorations over the palmar and digital creases.

Proceed as follows:

- Look for the following signs:
  Xanthelasmata around the eyes.
  Tuboeruptive xanthomata around the elbows and knees.
- Tell the examiner that this patient probably has a type III hyperlipidaemia.

Note. A more generalized form may be associated with monoclonal gammopathy of myeloma or lymphoma.

Advanced-level Questions

How would you classify hyperlipidaemia?

Fredrickson classification, depending on laboratory findings:
- Type I: raised levels of chylomicrons and triglycerides, normal cholesterol concentration (pancreatitis, eruptive xanthomata and lipaemia retinalis).
- Type IIa: raised LDL and cholesterol levels, normal concentration of triglycerides (premature coronary artery disease, tendon xanthomata and arcus corneae).
- Type IIb: raised levels of LDL, very low density lipoprotein (VLDL), cholesterol and triglycerides (premature coronary artery disease).
- Type III: raised β-VLDL (cholesterol-rich) remnants, cholesterol and triglycerides (premature coronary artery disease, peripheral vascular disease, palmar and tuberous xanthomata).
- Type IV: raised VLDL and triglycerides, normal cholesterol (premature coronary artery disease – in some forms, risk of developing chylomicronaemia syndrome).

- Type V: raised chylomicrons, VLDL, cholesterol and triglycerides (pancreatitis, eruptive xanthoma, lipaemia retinalis).

What are the causes of hypercholesterolaemia?

- Primary hypercholesterolaemia: familial hypercholesterolaemia, familial combined hyperlipidaemia, polygenic hypercholesterolaemia.
- Secondary hypercholesterolaemia: biliary cirrhosis, hypothyroidism, nephrotic syndrome, diet, drugs (thiazides, beta-blockers, oestrogens).

CASE 175 Pseudoxanthoma Elasticum

Instruction

Look at this patient's fundus (*Patient 1*).

Salient features

- Fundus shows angioid streaks, i.e. linear grey or dark red streaks with irregular edges which lie beneath the retinal vessels (roughly 50% of patients with angioid streaks have pseudoxanthoma elasticum, whereas 85% of those with pseudoxanthoma have angioid streaks).

Proceed as follows:

- Look at the neck, antecubital fossae, axillae, groin and periumbilical region for loose 'chicken skin' appearance of skin.

Instruction

Look at this patient (*Patient 2*).

Salient features

- Small yellow papules arranged in a linear or reticular pattern in plaques on the neck, axillae, cubital fossae, periumbilical region and groin.

Proceed as follows:

- Tell the examiner that you would like to examine the fundus.

Diagnosis

This patient has angioid streaks on fundoscopy and 'chicken-skin' appearance in the neck and axillae (lesions) due to pseudoxanthoma elasticum (aetiology).

Advanced-level Questions

In which other conditions are angioid streaks seen?

- Regularly seen in: Paget's disease, sickle cell disease.
- Occasionally seen in: Ehlers–Danlos syndrome, hyperphosphataemia, lead poisoning, trauma, pituitary disorders and intracranial disorders.

What are angioid streaks caused by?

They are caused by abnormal elastic tissue in the Bruch's membrane of the retina.

Which fundal finding is virtually pathognomonic of pseudoxanthoma elasticum?

'Leopard skin spotting' changes which consist of yellowish mottling of the posterior pole temporal to the macula. These may antedate angioid streaks.

What is the triad of pseudoxanthoma elasticum, angioid streaks and vascular abnormalities known as?

Groenblad–Strandberg syndrome.

What are the cardiovascular manifestations of this condition?

- Mitral valve prolapse.
- Restrictive cardiomyopathy
- Renovascular hypertension.
- Premature coronary artery disease resembling accelerated atherosclerosis due to calcification of the internal elastic laminae of arteries. Arterial grafts should not be used for coronary artery bypass surgery in these patients because of possible calcification of the internal elastic laminae of the internal mammary artery.
- Peripheral vascular disease.

What are the gastrointestinal manifestations of this disease?

Gastrointestinal haemorrhage, particularly during the first decade.

Bleeding complications can be prevented by avoiding aspirin in patients with pseudoxanthoma elasticum.

What are the causes of visual loss in pseudoxanthoma elasticum?

Macular involvement by a streak; disciform scarring secondary to choroidal haemorrhage or traumatic macular haemorrhage.

What are cutaneous histological features of pseudoxanthoma elasticum?

The histological diagnosis is made by doing 4-mm punch biopsy of scars or flexural skin of the neck or axillae in patients who have angioid streaks on fundoscopy but no visible skin lesions. The Verhoeff–van Gieson stain (for elastic tissue) reveals characteristic fragmentation and clumping of elastic tissue in middle and deep dermis. The von Kossa stain (for calcium) shows staining of calcified elastic tissue in the middle and deep dermis. Calcified elastic tissue is the hallmark of pseudoxanthoma elasticum.

KWL Bruch (1819–1884), Professor of Anatomy at Giessen, Germany.
EE Groenblad, Swedish ophthalmologist and J Strandberg, Swedish dermatologist.
TL Terry (1899–1946), Head of Ophthalmology at Harvard University, described angioid streaks in Paget's disease.

References

Clarkson JG & Altman RD (1982) Angioid streaks. *Surv Ophthalmol* **26**: 235–246.
Lebwhol M (1993) Pseudoxanthoma elasticum (Images in Clinical Medicine). *N Engl J Med* **333**: 1240. (Candidates are encouraged to refer to this picture for characteristic features of this disease.)
Lebwohl M, Halperin J & Phelps RG (1993) Pseudoxanthoma elasticum in patients with premature cardiovascular disease. *N Engl J Med* **329**: 1237–1239.

CASE
176 **Rosacea**

Instruction

Look at this patient.

Salient features

- Red patch with telangiectasia, acneiform papules, and pustules overlying the flush areas of the face, i.e. cheeks, chin and nose. (The papules and pustules distinguish it from the rash of SLE.)

Proceed as follows:

- Comment on the following:

  Rhinophyma (irregular thickening of the skin of the nose with enlarged follicular orifices).

  Blepharitis, conjunctivitis.

- Tell the examiner that you would like to take a history of unilateral headaches (an increased incidence of migranous headaches accompanying rosacea has been reported).

Diagnosis

This patient has a red patch on the face with papules and pustules (lesion) due to rosacea (aetiology) which is cosmetically disfiguring (functional status).

Advanced-level Questions

How would you distinguish rosacea from acne?

Rosacea is distinguished from acne by age (middle-aged and older people), the presence of a vascular component (i.e. rosy hue, erythema and telangiectasia) and the absence of comedones.

How would you manage such a patient?

- Avoid factors that provoke facial flushing.
- Tetracycline or metronidazole.
- Hydrocortisone cream.
- Retinoids – in resistant disease.
- Yellow light laser for telangiectasia.
- Surgical removal for rhinophyma.

CASE 177 Dermatitis Herpetiformis

Instruction

Look at this patient's skin, who in the past had chronic diarrhoea.

Salient features

- Dry, itchy vesicles and urticarial plaques occurring bilaterally and symmetrically over the extensor surfaces, elbows, knees, posterior neck, back and buttocks.

Proceed as follows:

- Look for similar lesions on the scalp, face, neck, shoulders, buttocks, knees and calves.
- Tell the examiner that you would like to take a history of diarrhoea and gluten intolerance (although these patients rarely have gross malabsorption).

Diagnosis

This patient has itchy vesicles on the elbows (lesion) due to dermatitis herpetiformis (functional status).

Advanced-level Questions

From which other itchy skin disorder should dermatitis herpetiformis be differentiated?

Scabies.

What are the extracutaenous manifestations of dermatitis herpetiformis?

- Gluten-sensitive enteropathy (frequent, asymptomatic).
- Thyroid dysfunction (especially hypothyroidism).
- Lymphoma (especially gastrointestinal).

How would you investigate such a patient?

- Skin biopsy: fibrin and neutrophils accumulate selectively at the *tips of dermal papillae*, forming small microabscesses. Subepidermal vesicle with neutrophilic infiltrate. Immunofluorescence demonstrates granular dermal papillary immunoglobulin (Ig) A deposits.
- Circulating anti-endomysium antibodies are present in all cases.
- Jejunal biopsy: patchy abnormality showing subtotal villous atrophy with increased lymphocyte infiltration in the epithelium.
- Therapeutic test: dapsone dramatically reduces itching in 72 hours, often providing confirmation before the biopsy result is available.
- HLA-B8 and HLA-DRw3 are positive in more than 80% of patients.

How would you treat such a patient?

- Gluten restriction.
- Dapsone or sulphapyridine – neither drug should be given to a patient with glucose-6-phosphate deficiency. Treatment is lifelong; there is usually a rapid relapse if the drug is stopped.

In which foods is gluten found?

Wheat, barley and rye (rice and maize are permitted in these patients).

Is it advisable for these patients to add oats to their gluten-free diets?

Moderate amounts of oats can be ingested without harmful effects in coeliac disease and probably in dermatitis herpetiformis, although there are no studies to support the latter. Oats do not contain gliadin but have avenin. However, avenin comprises only 5–15% of the total seed protein content. Thus, even if avenin in oats were as toxic as gliadin in wheat (a fact that is not universally conceded), the ingestion of large quantities of oats would be required to bring about an equivalent effect, in terms of the amount of protein ingested.

What do you know about gluten?

Gluten is the protein component that persists following the removal of water and starch from defatted flour. Gliadin is a class of protein found in the gluten fraction of flour. There are four gliadin fractions (α, β, γ and ω). α-Gliadin is injurious to the small intestinal mucosa, although there is some disagreement about the toxicity of other peptides. Patients with dermatitis herpetiformis develop IgA and IgG antibodies to gliadin and reticulin (the latter a component of the anchoring fibrils that tether the epidermal basement membrane to the upper dermis).

What are the benefits of a gluten-free diet?

It gradually improves skin lesions, improves any associated manifestations of malabsorptive enteropathy and may reduce the late risk of intestinal lymphoma. It also normalizes histological abnormalities. (**Note**. An elemental diet lacking protein has been reported to benefit patients with dermatitis herpetiformis even in the presence of a gluten challenge.)

Dermatitis herpetiformis was first described in 1884 by LA Duhring (1845–1913), Professor of Diseases of the Skin at the University of Pennsylvania. He studied dermatology in Paris, London and Vienna, and wrote the first American textbook of dermatology. Others believe that dermatitis herpetiformis was first described by F von Hebra, who also wrote a textbook of dermatology.
Samuel J Gee (1839–1911) of St Bartholomew's Hospital, London, provided the first thorough description of coeliac sprue in 1888. Dutch paediatrician, WK Dicke, astutely observed that wheat and rye were harmful in children with this disease.
Parveen Kumar, contemporary Physician, St Bartholomew's Hospital, London, has made major contributions to gastroenterology and, together with Michael Clark,

also a physician at St Bartholomew's Hospital, has made a major contribution to medical education. The book entitled *Clinical Medicine*, which they edited, is the most popular medical textbook in the UK.

References

Dicke WK (1950) *Coeliac disease: investigation of the harmful effects of certain types of cereal on patients with coeliac disease.* Doctoral thesis, University of Utrecht, The Netherlands.

Garioch JJ, Baker BS, Leonard JN & Fry L (1994) 25 years experience of a gluten-free diet in the treatment of dermatitis herpetiformis. *Br J Dermatol* **131**: 541.

Gee S (1888) On the coeliac affection. *St Barth Hosp Rep* **24**: 17–20.

Kadunce DP, McMurray MP, Avots-Avotins A, Chandler JP, Meyer LJ & Zone JJ (1991) The effect of an elemental diet with and without gluten on disease activity in dermatitis herpetiformis. *J Invest Dermatol* **97**: 175–182.

Kumar PJ & Farthing MGJ (1995) Oats and celiac disease. *N Engl J Med* **333**: 1075–1076.

CASE 178 Hairy Leukoplakia

Instruction

Look at this patient's tongue.

Salient features

- Shaggy, hairy, white lesions on the lateral margins of the tongue.

Proceed as follows:

- Tell the examiner that you would like to know whether or not the patient is infected by HIV.

Note. Oral hairy leukoplakia may be difficult to distinguish from oral candidiasis, but in contrast to oral candidiasis it does not rub off, does not respond to antifungal therapy and may change its appearance daily.

Diagnosis

This patient has whitish hairy lesions on the lateral edges of the tongue (lesions) which is oral hairy leukoplakia caused by the Epstein–Barr virus (aetiology).

Questions

What is the cause of this lesion?

Hairy leukoplakia is caused by the Epstein–Barr virus.

Advanced-level Questions

What is the significance of this lesion?

In seropositive subjects, usually it is a harbinger of rapid progression to
AIDS. It is rarely seen in non-HIV immunosuppressed patients.

What are the histological features of this condition?

- Hyperkeratosis.
- Hyperplasia and ballooning of prickle cells.
- Depletion of Langherhans' cells.

How would you treat this condition?

Treatment is seldom indicated, but ganciclovir or acyclovir may be helpful
if treatment is needed.

P Langerhans (1847–1888), German pathologist and dermatologist.

References

Editorial (1989) Oral hairy leukoplakia. *Lancet* **ii**: 1195.
Greenspan D & Greenspan JS (1992) Significance of oral hairy leukoplakia. *Oral
    Surg Oral Med Oral Pathol* **73**: 151.

CASE 179 · Kaposi's Sarcoma

Instruction

Look at this skin lesion.

Salient features

- Plum-coloured violet plaques, either solitary or in crops, on the limbs,
  mouth, tip of the nose and palate.

Proceed as follows:

- Tell the examiner that you would like to check HIV antibody titres.

Diagnosis

This patient has Kaposi's sarcoma (lesion) which has been shown to be due to human herpes virus 8 (aetiology) in patients with AIDS.

Advanced-level Questions

What are the varieties of Kaposi's sarcoma?

- Classic Kaposi's sarcoma: initially described in Jews; indolent; found on the legs of elderly men; confined to the skin and may be present for decades; not fatal.
- AIDS-associated Kaposi's sarcoma: found in approximately one-third of patients with AIDS and more common in homosexuals. The cutaneous lesions respond to α-interferon and cytotoxic chemotherapy. About one-third develop a second malignancy such as lymphoma, myeloma or leukaemia. Patients evenutally die from secondary infection seen in AIDS rather than as a direct consequence of Kaposi's sarcoma.
- African variety: violaceous skin plaques, black under Negroid skin, an aggressive invasive tumour which is ultimately fatal. It occurs in children and younger men. In the former it is often associated with generalized lymphadenopathy.
- Transplantation-associated Kaposi's sarcoma, particularly in patients on high-dose immunosuppressive therapy; these often regress when therapy is stopped.

What is the aetiology of Kaposi's sarcoma?

The aetiology is not known but epidemiological data support a viral infection. Recent reports indicate a herpes-like virus (human herpes virus 8, HHV-8). This new agent has also been found in AIDS-related lymphomas based in body cavities.

What is the histology of Kaposi's sarcoma?

Histologically all varieties are similar.
- The early or 'patch' stage: similar to granulation tissue and characterized by jagged, thin-walled, dilated vascular spaces in the epidermis with interstitial inflammatory cells and extravasated red cells (with haemosiderin deposition).

- Later or 'nodular' lesions: features are more characteristic at this stage and comprise spindle-shaped stromal cells with irregular slit-like spaces filled with red blood cells and lined by recognizable endothelium, intertwined with normal vascular channels.

How would you manage Kaposi's sarcoma in patients with HIV infection?

- Baseline treatment includes a retroviral agent such as zidovudine, which has no direct effect on Kaposi's sarcoma but diminishes the degree of immunosuppression.
- Localized mucocutaneous lesions respond well to radiotherapy, cryotherapy, surgical excision, intralesional vinblastine, bleomycin or interferon α.
- Interferon alpha as systemic treatment is effective in 40–50% of patients with indolent Kaposi's sarcoma and a CD4 count above 0.4 $\times 10^9$ cells per litre who have few systemic symptoms and no opportunistic infections.
- Relatively marrow-sparing chemotherapy (bleomycin, vincristine or low-dose doxorubicin) is used when other treatment fails in patients with aggressive Kaposi's sarcoma. Complete or partial remission may be obtained in over three-quarters of those with Kaposi's sarcoma; shorter survival is associated with low CD4 cell count.

Moritz Kaposi (1837–1902) in 1872 described these as 'idiopathic multiple pigmented sarcoma'. He also described in the rash in SLE as 'butterfly rash' in 1875.

References

Cesarman E, Chang Y, Moore PS, Said JW & Knowles DM (1995) Kaposi's sarcoma-associated herpesvirus-like DNA sequences in AIDS related body cavity-based lymphomas. *N Engl J Med* **332**: 1186-1191.

Kaposi M (1872) Idiopathisches multiples Pigmentsarkom der Haut. *Arch Dermatol Syph* **4**: 265–273.

Moore PS & Chang Y (1995) Detection of herpes-like DNA sequences in Kaposi's sarcoma in patients with and without HIV infection. *N Engl J Med* **332**: 1181-1185.

CASE 180 Peutz–Jeghers Syndrome

Instruction

Look at this patient's face.

Salient features

- Pigmented freckles around the lips.

Proceed as follows:

- Look in the mouth for similar pigmentation and anaemia.
- Tell the examiner that you would like to take a history of the following:
  Pain in the abdomen due to intestinal intussusception.
  Gastrointestinal haemorrhage in the upper gastrointestinal tract, or
    rectal bleeding.
  Family involvement (autosomal dominant).

Diagnosis

This patient has pigmented freckles arounds the lips (lesions) due to
Peutz–Jeghers syndrome (aetiology).

Advanced-level Questions

What are the types of colonic polyps?

- Tubular adenomas: over 60% are in the rectosigmoid colon and may
  cause bleeding or obstruction. The risk of malignancy correlates
  with size. The tubular adenoma is removed endoscopically. Follow-
  up surveillance is by colonoscopy every 2 years.
- Villous adenomas are usually found in the left colon and have a high
  risk of malignancy. Polyps larger than 2 cm have a 50% risk of
  malignancy. They may present with hypokalaemia due to potassium
  loss in the stools. They are removed by colonoscopic resection.
- Hyperplastic polyps are benign and rarely undergo malignant change.
  They are usually detected as an incidental finding at colonoscopy.

What is the histology of polyps in Peutz– Jeghers syndrome?

The polyps, which are large and pedunculated, histologically show an
arborizing network of connective tissue and well-developed smooth
muscle which extends into the polyp and surrounds normal abundant
glands lined by normal intestinal epithelium rich in goblet cells. Polyps are
distributed in the small bowel (100%), stomach (25%) and colon (30%).

What polyposis syndromes do you know?

Familial adenomatous polyposis (FAP) and variants:
- FAP: an autosomal dominant condition with the defect localized to the
  APC gene on chromsome 5q21. There are several thousand polyps in

the colon. The polyps appear between the age of 10 and 35 years. The potential malignant change is 100% by the age of 40 years. Hence all relatives ought to be screened annually from the age of 12 years and all patients ought to have prophylactic colectomy by the age of 30. Recently, a protein assay has been developed that can diagnose the genetic defect in 87% of such families and 150 mg sulindac twice daily has been shown to reduce the number and size of the adenomatous polyps in the rectum.

- Gardner's syndrome: a variant of FAP in which affected members develop extraintestinal soft tissue tumours (osteomas, lipomas, dermoid tumours) and pigmentation of fundi.
- Turcot's syndrome: central nervous system gliomas may also develop. Disruption of any of the three genes – APC, hMLH1 or hPMS2 – can lead to Turcot's syndrome.

Other polyposis syndromes:

- Familial juvenile polyposis: autosomal dominant condition occurring in children and teenagers. It may cause gastrointestinal bleeds, abdominal pain, diarrhoea and intussusception. There is an increased incidence of malignant change in the interspersed adenomatous polyps.
- Peutz-Jeghers syndrome: characterized by mucocutaneous melanosis with gastrointestinal hamartomas. The inheritance is autosomal dominant. The intestinal polyps may give rise to haematemeis, melaena or rectal bleeding, anaemia or intussusception depending on their location. These polyps are usually found in the ileum and jejunum and they rarely undergo malignant change. But these patients tend to have an increased incidence of other malignancy, both of gastrointestinal tract (stomach and duodenum) and other viscera (lung, breasts, pancreas and gonads).
- Cronkhite–Canada syndrome: sporadic, colonic, small bowel or gastric polyps associated with ectodermal changes such as hyperpigmentation, nail atrophy and alopecia.
- Cowden's disease: autosomal dominant; multiple gastrointestinal hamartomas with warty papules on the mucosa, and skin malformations.

What do you know about the genetics of colorectal cancer?

Three separate research groups reported the location of the gene on chromosome 2 in familial colonic cancer, which, it is claimed, may predispose to up to 15% of colorectal cancer. Screening in colorectal cancer should include colonoscopy, and in women pelvic ultrasonography. Those who develop colorectal cancer should be treated by subtotal colectomy.

This condition was originally described by JL Peutz of Holland in 1921 and rediscovered by HJ Jeghers et al of the USA in 1949.
EJ Gardner (b. 1909), US geneticist and Professor of Zoology at Utah University.
J Turcot, Canadian surgeon, J-P Després and F St Pierre first described Turcot's syndrome in 1959. In 1949 HW Crail described a similar syndrome.
LW Cronkhite, physician, Massachusetts General Hospital.
Wilma J Canada, US radiologist.

References

Crail HW (1949) Multiple primary malignancies arising in rectum, brain, and thyroid: report of a case. *US Naval Medical Bull* **49**: 123-128.
Giardiello FM, Hamilton SR, Krush AJ et al (1993) Treatment of colonic and rectal adenomas with sulindac in familial adenomatous polyps. *N Engl J Med* **328**: 1313.
Hamilton SR, Liu B, Parsons RE et al (1995) The molecular basis of Turcot's syndrome. *N Engl J Med* **332**: 839–847.
Morrison PJ & Nevin NC (1993) Peutz–Jeghers syndrome. *N Engl J Med* **329**: 774. (A classical picture of a patient with Peutz–Jeghers syndrome.)
Powell SM, Petersen GM, Krush AJ et al (1993) Molecular diagnosis of familial adenomatous polyposis. *N Engl J Med* **329**: 1982.

CASE 181 Pyoderma Gangrenosum

Instruction

Look at this patient's skin.

Salient features

- Necrotic ulcer with purplish overhanging edges, usually seen on the lower limbs or trunk.

Proceed as follows:

- Tell the examiner that you would like to take a history of the following:
  Diarrhoea (inflammatory bowel disease).
  Joint pains (rheumatoid arthritis).

Diagnosis

These are necrotic ulcers (lesions), which are a feature of pyoderma gangrenosum (aetiology); I would like to investigate for underlying inflammatory bowel disease.

Questions

In which conditions can pyoderma gangrenosum be seen?

- Ulcerative colitis.
- Crohn's disease.
- Chronic active hepatitis.
- Rheumatoid arthritis.
- Acute and chronic myeloid leukaemia.
- Polycythaemia rubra vera.
- Multiple myeloma.
- IgA monoclonal gammopathy.

Advanced-level Questions

How would you manage these lesions?

- High-dose steroids.
- Intralesional steroids.
- Some regress with treatment of the underlying cause.

References

Carr AJ, Percival RC, Rogers K & Harrington CI (1986) Pyoderma gangrenosum after cholecystectomy. *Br Med J* **292**: 729–730.

Mahmood JM & Sneddon IB (1980) Pyoderma gangrenosum complicating non-Hodgkin's lymphoma. *Br J Dermatol* **102**: 223–225.

Powell FC, Schroeter AL, Su WPD & Perry HO (1985) Pyoderma gangrenosum: a review of 86 patients. *Q J Med* **55**: 173–186.

CASE 182
Sturge–Weber Syndrome (Encephalotrigeminal Angiomatosis)

Instruction

Look at this patient's face.

Salient features

- A port-wine stain is present on the face in the distribution of the first and second division of the trigeminal nerve.
- Hypertrophy of the involved area of the face.

Proceed as follows:

- Look for haemangiomas of episclera and iris.
- Tell the examiner that you would like to proceed as follows:
  Examine the fundus for unilateral choroidal haemangiomata.
  Take a history of seizures.
  Do a skull radiograph for intracranial 'tramline' calcification, particularly in the parieto-occipital lobe.
  Check the blood pressure (may be associated with phaeochromocytoma).

Diagnosis

This patient has a port-wine stain on the face in the distribution of the first two divisions of the trigeminal nerve (lesion) which is probably due to Sturge–Weber syndrome (aetiology); these lesions may be cosmetically unacceptable (functional status).

Advanced-level Questions

What is the inheritance in such patients?

This is the only syndrome of the phacomatoses that does not have a hereditary tendency. It occurs sporadically and has no sexual predilection.

What are the neurological manifestations in such patients?

Jacksonian epilepsy, contralateral hemianopia, hemisensory disturbance, hemiparesis and hemianopia, low IQ.

What other ocular manifestations do you know?

Choroidal angioma, glaucoma (in 30% of cases), buphthalmos (large eye), optic atrophy.

What is the histology of port-wine stains?

They are composed of networks of ectatic vessels in the outer dermis, under a normal dermis.

How would you treat such a patient?

- Treatment is aimed at the pharmacological control of seizures.
- The patient should be referred to the ophthalmologist for management of increased intraocular pressure or choroidal angioma.

- Photothermolysis: if port-wine stains are treated in early childhood the psychological burden on the family and child may be alleviated. The 350-μs pulsed dye laser that provides individual 585-nm pulses is the treatment of choice for most port-wine stains particularly in children. Wavelengths of 577–590 nm are optimal as they are minimally attenuated by epidermis and dermis, and strongly absorbed by blood. Pulse durations of 0.5–5 ms produce only transmural injury to the vessel wall, by heat conduction from hot red cells, and hence prevent non-specific dermal injury.

Otto Kalischer, a German pathologist, described post-mortem findings in a case as early as 1901.

William A Sturge (1850–1919), a London physician, described this condition in 1879. He was attached to the The Royal Free Hospital, London, and founded the Society of Prehistoric Archaeology in East Anglia.

Frederick Parkes Weber (1863–1962), a London physician, was the first to describe the radiological appearances in this condition. Two other syndromes to which Weber's name is attached are Weber–Christian disease (relapsing, febrile, nodular, non-suppurative panniculitis) and Osler–Rendu–Weber syndrome (hereditary haemorrhagic telangiectasia).

Reference

Van Gemert MJC, Carruth JAS & Shakespeare PG (1993) Treatment of portwine stains. *Br Med J* **306**: 4–5.

CASE 183 Acne Vulgaris

Instruction

Look at this patient.

Salient features

- Comedones, or blackheads, usually on the chin, face, shoulders and upper chest (due to plugging of hair follicles by keratin) – these are hallmarks of acne.
- Whiteheads (i.e. distended sebaceous glands without a pore).
- Cysts (larger, deeper masses of retained sebum).
- Greasy skin.
- There may be associated scarring.

Proceed as follows:

- Tell the examiner that you would like to take a history of the following:
  Steroid ingestion.
  Isoniazid ingestion.
  Occupational exposure to oils (oil-induced acne).

Remember that acne vulgaris is a multifactorial disease affecting the pilosebaceous follicle and characterized by open and closed comedones, papules, pustules, nodules and scars.

Diagnosis

This patient has blackheads on the face with greasy skin (lesions) which is acne vulgaris caused by *Propionibacterium acnes* (aetiology) and may be cosmetically unacceptable to the patient (functional status).

Advanced-level Questions

What do you know about the pathogenesis of acne?

Follicular keratinization, seborrhoea and colonization of the pilosebaceous unit with *P. acnes* are central to the development of these lesions. Genetic and hormonal factors also play a role, possibly by optimizing the follicular environment suitable for the growth of *P. acnes* or by influencing the inflammatory response and thus the nature of these lesions.

How is the severity of acne graded?

- Mild disease: open and closed comedones and some papules and pustules.
- Moderate: more frequent papules and pustules with mild scarring.
- Severe disease: all of the above plus nodular abscesses; leads to more extensive scarring, which may be keloidal in some instances.

How would you manage acne?

The aims of treatment are to prevent scarring, limit the disease duration and reduce the impact of the psychological stress that may affect over half of sufferers.

- Wash affected parts with soap not more than twice a day.
- Avoid steaming: saunas, Turkish baths.
- Topical therapy: sulphur, benzyl peroxide, retinoic acid, azaleic acid, erythromycin, tetracycline.
- Systemic therapy: tetracycline, erythromycin, isotretinoin.

Have you heard of acne fulminans?

It is a rare but severe variant, seen exclusively in adolescent boys. It is due to an immune complex reaction to *P. acnes*. The lesions eventually become necrotic and form haemorrhagic crusts, causing disfigurement and scarring. There may be associated systemic features such as fever, malaise, arthralgia, arthritis and vasculitis. Osteolytic bone lesions can arise. Inpatient treatment with systemic steroids is necessary.

What do you know about acne conglobata?

It is seen in tall Caucasian males with cystic skin lesions and multiple abscess formation. It rarely regresses.

Reference

Healy E & Simpson N (1994) Acne vulgaris. *Br Med J* **308**: 831–833.

CASE 184 Alopecia Areata

Instruction

Examine this patient's scalp.

Salient features

- Young adult (75% of patients are below the age of 40 years).
- Well-defined patch of hair loss.
- Regrowing hair in the patch appears as a fine, depigmented downy growth.

Proceed as follows:

- Look for patches of hair loss over the eyebrows and beard area.
- Examine the nails for fine pitting, transverse lines, dystrophy, fragmentation (anonychorrhexis) and ridging and 20-nail dystrophy (roughened nail surface and brittle free nail edge).
- Tell the examiner that you would like to:
  Look for and take a history regarding atopy.
  Look for other autoimmune conditions (see below).
  Ask whether there is a family history (25% give a family history).
  Ask the patient whether there are any local symptoms and if the hair loss is cosmetically unacceptable.

Diagnosis

This patient has alopecia areata (lesion) which is suspected to be of autoimmune aetiology and may be cosmetically unacceptable to the patient (functional status).

Advanced-level Questions

What are the signs of disease activity?

At the advancing edge, broken hairs which look like exclamation marks indicate active disease. These are very short hairs, tapering and becoming depigmented as the scalp is approached. Plucking reveals such hair to be in the telogen phase.

Mention some associated disorders.

- Autoimmune conditions (vitiligo, thyrotoxicosis, Addison's disease, pernicious anaemia).
- Down's syndrome.
- Hypogammaglobulinaemia.

What is the difference between alopecia totalis and alopecia universalis?

Both of these conditions can occur in alopecia areata. Alopecia totalis is the loss of all scalp hair and alopecia universalis is the loss of hair from all body sites.

Is alopecia areata associated with scarring?

No.

Mention the causes of hair loss associated with scarring.

Discoid lupus erythematosus, lichen planus.

What is the treatment for alopecia areata?

- Steroids (both topical and systemic).
- PUVA therapy.
- Topical minoxidil.

Cessation of treatment may be associated with recurrent hair loss.

Mention some causes of drug-induced alopecia.

Anticoagulants, retinoids, vitamin A, antithyroid drugs, oral contraceptives, anticancer drugs (invariably reversible).

What do you understand by the term trichotillomania?

It is the self-inflicted pulling out of one's own hair and can be differentiated from alopecia areata as the hair loss is irregular and there is always growing hair, since these cannot be pulled out till they are long enough. These patches are unilateral and are usually on the same side as the patient's dominant hand. The patient may be unaware of this habit.

What do you know about the growth of the hair follicle?

Each follicle has cyclical growth controlled by a constitutional 'time clock'. It has three phases of growth (anagen), a short involutional phase (catagen) and resting (telogen) phase. The anagen phase is 3–5 years and the telogen phase is 2–4 years. Hair found on the pillow and hairbrush is telogen hair and can be recognized by the fact that the club is depigmented as well as expanded, whereas an anagen hair obtained by traction is fully melanized.

How much hair is usually lost by a normal person?

About 70–100 hairs per day. The human scalp contains about 100 000 follicles, 5–10% are in telogen at any time, i.e. 5000–10 000 As telogen lasts for about 100 days, the number of telogen hairs pushed out each day is 70–100.

What is telogen effluvium?

It is a transitory (about 2–4 months) increase in the number of hairs in the resting (telogen) phase of the hair growth cycle. The amount of hair loss exceeds 150 per day. It is associated with high fever, stress, crash dieting, malnutrition, surgery, termination of pregnancy or oral contraceptives. The prognosis is good.

Reference

Healy E & Rogers S (1993) PUVA treatment of alopecia areata. Does it work? A retrospective review of 102 cases. *Br J Dermatol* **129**: 42.

CASE 185 Atopic Dermatitis (Eczema)

Instruction

Look at this patient's skin.

Salient features

- Pruritus.
- Hyperpigmented or hypopigmented lichenified lesions in flexures (including face, neck, upper trunk, wrists, hand, in the antecubital and popliteal folds).

Proceed as follows:

- Tell the examiner that you would like to know whether there is a personal or family history of atopy (asthma, allergic rhinitis, atopic dermatitis) or food allergy.

Diagnosis

This patient has atopic dermatitis (lesion) which is due to atopy as supported by a history of asthma (aetiology), and causes the patient severe itching (functional status).

Questions

How would you treat such patients?

- Foods (typically dairy products and wheat) which cause itching should be avoided.
- Patient should be instructed about skin care including avoiding frequent baths and scratchy fabrics.
- Adequate cutaneous hydration.
- Treatment of infected skin.
- Antihistamines to control itching.
- Corticosteroid lotion, cream or ointment.

CASE 186 Venous Ulcer

Instruction

Look at this patient's leg.

Salient features

- Ulcer located on the medial aspect of leg (around the ankles) with pigmentation.
- Surrounding dermatitis and excoriation due to pruritus (stasis dermatitis).
- White atrophy with scars in the overlying skin.
- The ulcer may be secondarily infected (cellulitis or thrombophlebitis).

Proceed as follows:

- Look for varicose veins.
- Tell the examiner that you would like to take a past history of:
    Deep venous thrombosis.

Diagnosis

This patient has a venous ulcer (lesion) due to varicose veins (aetiology) which has caused severe pigmentation and dermatitis around the ankles (functional status).

Advanced-level Questions

What is the surrounding pigmentation due to?

It occurs as a result of the extravasation of red blood cells and haemosiderin deposition.

What is the white atrophy (atrophie blanche) due to?

It is due to the hyalization of skin vessels, resulting in scars in the overlying skin.

How is the diagnosis confirmed?

When the diagnosis is in doubt, a punch biopsy from the border (not the base) of the lesion is helpful.

How would you manage such an ulcer?

- Reduction of venous hypertension: elevation of the limbs, wearing support bandages, weight reduction in the obese.
- Infection: antibiotics for cellulitis.
- Dermatitis: zinc and salicylic acid paste.
- Ulcers: cleaning with potassium permanganate, debridement, skin grafting.
- Treatment of varicose veins.

CASE 187 Arterial Leg Ulcer

Instruction

Look at this patient's leg.

Salient features

- Tender, punched-out ulcers on leg (usually away from the ankle region).
- Cold atrophic skin.
- Loss of hair.
- Peripheral pulses are not palpable.

Proceed as follows:

- Tell the examiner that you would like to know whether the patient has a history of claudication.

Diagnosis

This patient has an arterial ulcer (lesion) due to vascular insufficiency as evidenced by the absence of popliteal pulses (aetiology).

Questions

How would you investigate such a patient?

- X-rays may show calcification of the arteries of the leg.
- Doppler ultrasonography to define the severity of arterial involvement.
- Aortography shows narrowing and stenosis of the leg arteries.

How would you manage arterial ulcers?

- General: stop smoking, control of diabetes, obesity and hypertension.

- Limbs: should be kept warm (but avoid local heat).
- Feet: chiropodist and foot care.
- Regular exercise to promote development of anastomotic collateral vessels.
- Low-dose aspirin.
- Surgery: balloon dilatation for local iliac or femoral stenoses, aortoiliac bypass, amputation when complicated by gangrene.

Mention other causes of leg ulcers.

- Venous ulcers (see page 490).
- Neuropathic: diabetes mellitus, leprosy.
- Vasculitis: rheumatoid arthritis, SLE, pyoderma gangrenosum.
- Haematological disorders: sickle cell anaemia, spherocytosis.
- Neoplastic: basal cell carcinoma, Kaposi's sarcoma (see page 476)
- Trauma or artefact.
- Infection: postcellulitis, fungal.

CASE 188 Erythema Nodosum

Instruction

Look at this patient's shins.

Salient features

- Poorly defined, exquisitely tender, erythematous nodules (which are better felt than seen).

Proceed as follows:

- Tell the examiner that you would like to elicit a history of:
    Sore throat (β-haemolytic streptococcal infection).
    Drugs (sulphonamides, oral contraceptives).
    Infections (tuberculosis, leprosy, coccidiomycosis, histoplasmosis).
    Sarcoidosis.

Diagnosis

This patient has tender erythema nodosum (lesions) on the shins due to the use of oral contraceptives (aetiology).

Questions

How can a definitive diagnosis be obtained?

By a deep wedge biopsy of the tissue.

Advanced-level Questions

What is the histology?

Erythema nodosum is a panniculitis, which is an inflammatory reaction in the subcutaneous fat.
- In early lesions, there is widening of the connective tissue septa owing to oedema, fibrin exudation and infiltration by neutrophils.
- Later, there is infiltration by lymphocytes, histiocytes, multinucleated giant cells and occasionally eosinophils associated with septal fibrosis.

Note. Vasculitis is absent.

Mention some examples of panniculitis.

Erythema induratum (associated vasculitis), Weber–Christian disease (relapsing febrile nodular panniculitis), factitial panniculitis.

FP Weber (1863–1962), a British physcian who graduated from St Bartholomew's Hospital, London, and was a keen collector of coins and vases. He was an alpinist, like his father Sir HD Weber (1823–1918) who described Weber syndrome.
Henry A Christian (1876–1951), Professor of Medicine and the first Physician-in-Chief of the Peter Bent Brigham Hospital. He also described histiocytosis X (Hand–Schüller–Christian disease).

CASE 189 Fungal Nail Disease

Instruction

Look at this patient's toenails.

Salient features

- Nails are white, green or occasionally black.

Proceed as follows:

- Look at the fingernails.

- Tell the examiner that you would like to look for underlying immunodeficiency states and circulatory disorders (Raynaud's syndrome).

Diagnosis

This patient has fungal nail disease (lesion) which is usually due to *Trichophyton* or *Candida* (aetiology), and is cosmetically unacceptable to the patient (functional status).

Advanced-level Questions

What do you understand by the term onychomycosis?

It refers to a fungal infection of nails.

What are the different causative organisms?

These include:
- Dermatophytes (ringworm, tinea unguium): *Trichophyton rubrum, T. interdigitale.* (Toenails are more commonly affected than fingernails.) *T. rubrum* infection is associated with distal or lateral involvement of the nail plate which spreads proximally, eventually affecting the whole nail, and this may be associated with proximal subungual nail dystrophy associated with separation of the nail from the bed. *T. interdigitale* infection, characteristically seen in patients with AIDS, produces superficial white onychomycosis with crumbly white areas on the nail surface.
- Yeasts: *Candida albicans, C. parapsilosis.* (Fingernails are more commonly affected than toenails.)
- Non-dermatophytes (moulds): *Fusarium, Scopulariopsis brevicaulis.* (Toenails are more commonly affected than fingernails.)

Does the clinical picture vary according to the nature of the infecting organism?

Yes, as follows:
- Dermatophytes: distal or lateral nail involvement spreading proximally, proximal subungual dystrophy, superficial white dystrophy, white or yellow thickened nails, crumbling of nail plate, adjacent web or skin involvement may be present.
- *Candida*: chronic paronychia, shiny red bolstered nail-fold, almost exclusively affects fingernail folds, loss of cuticle, pus exuding from under nail-fold, usually proximal nail involvement, distal nail dystrophy (associated with circulatory disorders), total dystrophic onychomycosis, nails white, green or occasionally black.

- Non-dermatophyte: superficial white onychomycosis, solitary nail involvement, colour of the nail may be influenced by the nature of infecting mould (e.g. *Fusarium* – the nails are white, *S. brevicaulis* – the nails may be white, yellow, brown or green).

What are the patterns of fungal nail involvement?

Distal lateral subungual onychomycosis, superficial white onychomycosis, proximal white subungual onychomycosis, total dystrophic onychomycosis (i.e. all the previous three sites are affected).

Is laboratory diagnosis essential before starting treatment?

Yes, for the following reasons:
- Antifungal treatment is prolonged and the causative organism may be non-fungal.
- To identify contacts of the patient.
- To exclude mixed infection.
- To optimize treatment as certain fungi are less responsive to treatment.

Mention some non-fungal nail infections.

Bacterial nail infection, e.g. *Pseudomonas aeruginosa* (green or blackish discoloration of the nails), *Staphylococcus aureus* (causes acute paronychia or whitlow).

How are specimens obtained for mycological diagnosis?

Scrapings are taken with a blunt scalpel as proximally as possible in the nail:
- In distal and lateral onychomycosis: specimens are taken from the proximal part of the diseased portion of the nail and subungual material.
- In superficial white onychomycosis: the scrapings are taken from the diseased nail surface.
- In proximal white mycosis: the scrapings are taken from the nail surface.

In the laboratory 20–30% potassium hydroxide is added to part of the specimen to macerate nail keratin before direct microscopy and the rest of the specimen is inoculated on different media.

What is the recommended treatment for onychomycosis?

Dermatophyte infections:
- Localized distal nail disease: tioconazole with undecylenic acid paint, amorolfine paint weekly and 40% urea paste for dissolution.
- Proximal or extensive nail disease: terbinafine, itraconazole, griseofulvin and amorolfine nail paint.

Candidal infections:
- Chronic paronychia (localized): imidazole creams or paints, nystatin ointment, terbinafine cream.
- Distal candidal nail infection: tioconazole with undecylenic acid paint, amorolfine nail paint.
- Severe candidal nail infection or severe chronic paronychia: itraconazole.

Non-dermatophyte (mould) onychomycosis:
- Localized nail disease: tioconazole with undecylenic acid paint, amorolfine paint weekly, 40% urea paste for dissolution or even avulsion of the nail.
- Persistent nail disease: itraconazole.

Mention some fungal infections that do not respond to oral treatment.

Scopulariopsis, Scytalidium, Fusarium and *Acremonium*.

Reference

Denning DW, Evans EGV, Kibbler CC et al (1995) Fungal nail disease: a guide to good practice (report of a Working Group of the British Society for Medical Mycology). *BMJ* **311**: 1277–1281.

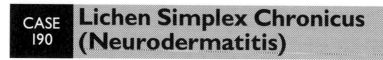

CASE 190 Lichen Simplex Chronicus (Neurodermatitis)

Instruction

Look at this patient's skin.

Salient features

- Several scratch marks (due to pruritus).
- Well circumscribed plaque with lichenified or dry, thickened, leathery skin.

Proceed as follows:

- Look for similar plaques in common areas including the posterior nuchal region, wrists, perineum, dorsum of the feet or ankles.

Diagnosis

This patient has lichen simplex chronicus (lesion) which is due to chronic itching and scratching (aetiology), and is cosmetically disturbing to the patient.

Advanced-level Questions

How would you treat such a patient?

- Break the scratch–itch–scratch cycle by adminstering antipruritic agents.
- High-potency topical steroids (under occlusion or intralesional injection).

What is the prognosis?

The disease tends to remit during treatment; however, it may recur or develop at another site.

CASE 191   Nail Changes

Instruction

Look at these nails.

Salient features

Disorders of the nail bed:
- Terry's nail: brownish-red distal transverse band; occurs normally in the elderly, also seen in cirrhosis and congestive cardiac failure.
- Lindsay's half-and-half nail: distal brown band occupying about 25–50% of the nail bed, and seen in chronic renal failure.
- Muehrcke's nail: pale transverse bands resulting from oedema of the nail bed; seen in hypoalbuminaemia.
- Onycholysis (see page 498).

Disorders of the lunula:
- Blue lunula: in Wilson's disease the normally white lunula becomes blue (see page 325). The lunula has the largest area in the fingers closest to the thumb; in the elderly it becomes smaller or absent.

Disorders of the nail plate:
- Clubbing (see page 519).
- Leukonychia: whitish discoloration which may be diffuse (liver disease, congenital, fungal), punctate or linear (Mees' lines seen in arsenical poisoning).
- Koilonychia (spoon-shaped nails) seen in iron deficiency anaemia, thyrotoxicosis.
- Pitting: seen in psoriasis, alopecia areata.
- Longitudinal brown streaks: junctional naevi seen in black patients.
- Beau's lines: transverse depression due to severe systemic illness. Allows estimation of the date of the illness. Remember the normal nail grows at the rate of 0.1 mm per day and it takes approximately 3–4 months for the nail plate to grow out completely.

Disorders of the nail-fold:
- Nail-fold telangiectasia: seen in dermatomyositis, scleroderma, collagen vascular disease.
- Paronychia: may be acute or chronic, and includes the swelling and inflammation of the proximal or lateral nail-folds.

Disorder of the hyponychium:
- Koenen's subungual angiofibromas seen in tuberous sclerosis (see page 587).
- Warts.

Note. The hyponychium is the most distal region of the nail bed and marks the transition to normal skin.

CASE 192 Onycholysis

Instruction

Examine this patient's hands.

Salient features

- Distal separation of the nail plate from the nail bed.

Proceed as follows:

- Look for nail pitting and silvery white plaques (psoriasis).
- Glance at the neck for goitre and tell the examiner that you would like to exclude thyrotoxicosis, hypothyroidism and diabetes mellitus.
- Tell the examiner that you would like to take a history for excessive

exposure to detergents, alkalis and keratolytic agents, and demeclo-cycline-induced photolysis.
- Tell the examiner that you would like to exclude a fungal infection (see page 493).

Diagnosis

This patient has onycholysis (lesion), probably due to thyrotoxicosis as evidenced by tachycardia, exophthalmos and goitre (aetiology).

Questions

What nail changes are associated with psoriasis?

Yellow, friable nails with pitting and onycholysis (lifting of nail from the bed), distal subungual hyperkeratosis.

How would you manage these nail lesions?

- Manicure and careful debridement.
- Reduction of exposure to irritants (detergents, bleaches, alkalis).
- Intradermal steroids in the area of nail matrix (these are very painful injections).
- Non-surgical removal of dystrophic nails using urea ointments.

What are Plummer's nails?

This term refers to the onycholysis that occurs in hyperthyroidism and typically occurs in the fourth finger.

S Plummer (1874–1936), physician at the Mayo Clinic, Rochester, Minnesota, also described Plummer–Vinson syndrome (iron deficiency anaemia and dysphagia).

Reference

Kechijian P (1985) Onycholysis of finger nails: evaluation and management. *J Am Acad Dermatol* **12**: 552–560.

CASE 193 Malignant Melanoma

Instruction

Look at this skin lesion.

Salient features

- Irregular and asymmetrical, with a fuzzy border where the pigment appears to be leaking into the surrounding skin. (The American Cancer Society mnemonic to suspect malignancy in a mole is ABCD: Asymmetry, Border irregular, Colour variegation and Diameter greater than 6 mm).

Proceed as follows:

- Comment if the mole stands out from the patient's other moles.
- Comment if bleeding and ulceration are present (these are ominous signs).
- Tell the examiner that you would like to:
    Ask the patient whether the mole has changed in colour.
    Ask the patient whether the mole itches and whether it has changed in morphology.
    Examine regional lymph nodes and the liver (for metastatic spread).

Diagnosis

This patient has a malignant melanoma (lesion) as evidenced by its irregular border and, without delay, biopsy and histological examination must be performed to exclude or confirm the diagnosis.

Questions

What are the different types of malignant melanoma?

Depending on the clinical picture and histological findings these include:
- Superficially spreading malignant melanoma (commonest type).
- Nodular malignant melanoma.
- Acral lentiginous melanomas (arising on the palms, soles and nail beds).
- Malignant melanoma on mucous membranes.
- Lentigo maligna melanoma (arising in lentigines in older individuals).
- Amelanotic (non-pigmented) melanoma.
- Miscellaneous: melanoma arising from blue naevi, congenital and giant nevocytic naevi.

Advanced-level Questions

What are the patterns of growth of malignant melanoma?

These include:

- Radial growth: where the growth is horizontal within the epidermis and superficial dermal layers, e.g. lentigo maligna, acral/mucosal lentiginous, superficial spreading types. During this stage of growth the tumour does not have the capacity to metastasize.
- Vertical growth occurs with time, and the melanoma grows downward into the deeper dermal layers as an expansile mass lacking cellular maturation; this correlates with the emergence of a clone of cells with metastatic potential. The nature and extent of this vertical growth phase determines the biological behaviour of malignant melanoma.

What are the predisposing factors?

These include sunlight, the presence of a pre-existing naevus (e.g. dysplastic naevus), hereditary factors.

What is the treatment of such lesions?

- Excision: following histological examination the area is usually re-excised with margins dictated by the thickness of the tumour.
- Elective lymph node dissection is controversial; in general, it is indicated only in melanomas of intermediate thickness with one draining chain of lymph nodes.

What are the prognostic factors in these patients?

- Tumour thickness.
- Level of invasion.
- Sex of the patient.
- Anatomical location: melanomas in the 'TANS' areas (thorax, upper arms, neck and scalp) show a higher relative risk.

Where is the candidate gene in familial atypical mole and melanoma syndrome (FAMM)?

It may be the growth regulator p16 on chromosome 9.

References

Koh HK (1991) Cutaneous melanoma. *N Engl J Med* **325**: 171–182.

Zimmerman GC & Grabski WJ (1994) Malignant melanoma. *N Engl J Med* **331**: 163. (Classical pictures of the different types of melanoma including superficial spreading melanoma lentigo maligna, nodular melanoma, subungual melanoma and amelanotic melanoma.)

CASE 194   Seborrhoeic Dermatitis

Instruction

Comment on this patient's skin.

Salient features

- Greasy scales overlying erythematous plaques or patches affecting the face (eyebrows, eyelids, glabella, nasolabial folds or ears), submammary folds, gluteal clefts. Occasionally it is generalized.
- Severe dandruff on the scalp.

Proceed as follows:

- Tell the examiner that you would like to obtain a history of itching and look for the underlying disorder (Parkinson's disease, HIV and strokes).

Remember that the name is misleading and the condition is unrelated to seborrhoea (excess sebum production).

Diagnosis

This patient has seborrhoeic dermatitis (lesion) with Parkinson's disease, and finds the lesion cosmetically unacceptable (functional status).

Advanced-level Questions

What is the aetiology of this disorder?

It is based on a genetic predisposition mediated by several factors including nutritional status, infection and hormones. Its response to antifungal agents has suggested that it represents an inflammatory reaction to *Pityrosporum ovale* yeasts present in the scalp of humans.

How would you treat these skin lesions?

- Topical glucocorticoids (avoid fluorinated preparations on the face).
- Shampoos containing coal tar and salicylic acid.
- Selenium sulphide shampoos for the scalp.
- Eyelid margins respond to gentle cleaning of lid margins with undiluted Johnson and Johnson baby shampoo using a cotton swab.
- Oral ketoconazole is invaluable in the persistent seborrhoeic dermatitis of AIDS, but should rarely be used otherwise.

What is the prognosis of this condition?

There is a tendency to lifelong recurrences.

CASE 195 Molluscum Contagiosum

Instruction

Look at these skin lesions.

Salient features

- Multiple rounded, dome-shaped, waxy papules that are 2–5 mm in diameter and contain central umbilication with a caseous plug.
- The common sites are face, hands, lower abdomen and genitals.

Proceed as follows:

- Tell the examiner that you would like to investigate for an underlying HIV infection.
- Ask the patient whether there are similar lesions elsewhere (particularly genitals).

Diagnosis

This patient has molluscum contagiosum (lesion) which is of viral aetiology, and you would like to rule out an underlying HIV infection as the lesions are extensive and widely distributed on the face, neck and other parts of the body.

Questions

How do these lesions spread from one part of the body to another?

Probably by autoinoculation.

How is the infection spread from one patient to another?

By direct contact.

What is the histology of these lesions?

Microscopically they show cup-like verrucous epidermal hyperplasia. Large inclusion bodies called 'molluscum bodies' are present in the cells of the stratum corneum and granulosum. These bodies are also seen in the curd-like material which can be expressed from the central umbilication. Numerous virions are present within the molluscum bodies.

What is the aetiology of these lesions?

It is caused by a pox virus which is characteristically brick shaped and has a central dumbbell-shaped DNA core.

How are these lesions treated?

- Curettage or applications of liquid nitrogen to freeze the lesions.
- Light electrosurgery with a needle.

Note. In children these lesions tend to resolve spontaneously.

CASE 196 Urticaria

Instruction

Look at the skin of this patient, who has recurrent lesions.

Salient features

- Wheals that are smooth, oedematous, pin or red, and surrounded by a bright red flare. Clearing of the central area may leave an annular pattern.
- Associated scratch marks, indicating the wheals are itchy.

Proceed as follows:

- Tell the examiner that you would like to:
    Determine physical causes that can precipitate this response (cold urticaria, dermatographism, pressure, sunlight, exercise, hot shower).

Drug history (aspirin and NSAIDs).

Whether any foods precipitate the rash.

Know whether the patient has recurrent angioedema.

Obtain a history of atopy.

Exclude infections (hepatitis, chronic sinusitis) and connective tissue disorders.

Diagnosis

This patient has wheals (lesion) due to chronic urticaria and dermatographism (aetiology), complicated by severe itching (functional status). Tell the examiner that you would like to exclude urticarial vasculitis before making a firm diagnosis.

Note. Systemic lupus erythematosus and Sjögren's sydrome may present with urticarial lesions, which are usually urticarial vasculitis.

Advanced-level Questions

What do you understand by the term dermatographism?

It is the presence of itchy, linear wheals with a surrounding bright red flare at sites of scratching or rubbing.

How would you investigate a patient with chronic urticaria?

- FBC and white count; if eosinophilia is present, examination of the stool for ova and parasites.
- Physical urticaria must be assessed by appropriate challenge testing.
- Serum complement C4 levels when there is a history of repeated cutaneous or mucosal angioedema.
- Thyroid function tests because of diagnostic overlap between chronic urticaria and thyroid disease.

How would you manage patients with chronic urticaria?

- Identify avoidable cause such as food additives. Challenge testing for food additives should be avoided in patients with a history of severe angioedema, asthma or episodes of anaphylaxis.
- Antihistamines: H_1 antihistamines (terfenadine, doxepin) with a low potential for sedation are first-line treatment, 2% ephedrine spray is useful for oropharyngeal oedema.
- Corticosteroids.
- A tepid shower temporarily alleviates itching.
- All patients should be advised to avoid aspirin and other NSAIDs,

angiotensin converting enzyme (ACE) inhibitors, macrolide antibiotics and imidazole antifungal agents.

References

Greaves MH (1995) Chronic urticaria. *N Engl J Med* **332**: 1767.
Hide M, Francis DM, Grattan CEH, Hakimi J, Kochan JP & Greaves MW (1993)
    Autoantibodies against the high-affinity Ig E receptor as a cause of histamine
    release in chronic urticaria. *N Engl J Med* **328**: 1599–1604.

CASE 197 Mycosis Fungoides (Cutaneous T-Cell Lymphoma)

Instruction

Look at this patient's skin.

Salient features

• Itchy, brownish-red plaques on the hips, buttocks and interscapular
  region, usually seen in fifth and sixth decade.

Proceed as follows:

• Tell the examiner that it may also involve the lymph nodes and viscera.

Diagnosis

This patient has itchy brownish-red plaques with lymph node involvement
(lesions), indicating mycosis fungoides (aetiology).

Advanced-level Questions

How would you confirm the diagnosis?

Skin biopsy to detect Pautrier's microabscesses, atypical cells in the nests
in the epidermis, atypical mononuclear cell infiltrates, large hyperchromic
cells with irregular nuclei – the 'mycosis cells'. The hallmark of mycosis
fungoides is the identification of the Sézary–Lautner cells. These are T
helper cells (CD4 antigen positive) that characteristically form band-like
aggregates within the superfical dermis and invade the dermis as single
cells and small clusters (Pautrier's microabscesses).

What is the prognosis?

Very slow progression of skin lesions with eventual tumour formation and systemic dissemination of lymphoma. In most patients this process takes several weeks.

What is the differential diagnosis?

Psoriasis.

How would you treat this patient?

Treatment is palliative with steroids, chemotherapeutic agents and electron-beam therapy.

What are the stages of cutaneous T-cell lymphoma?

- Stage I: eczematoid or psoriasiform erythematous lesions.
- Stage II: infiltrated plaques.
- Stage III: nodules, ulcers, tumours.
- Stage IV: lymph node involvement with or without systemic dissemination.

What is the treatment of mycosis fungoides?

- Various superficial treatments: topical steroids and chemotherapeutic agents (mechlorethamine and carmustine), PUVA and electron-beam radiotherapy improve skin disease, but none has been shown to alter the natural history of the disease.
- Novel approaches being explored include: acyclovir, interferons, retinoids, pentostatin and monoclonal antibodies directed to T-cell antigens.

Have you heard of Sézary's syndrome?

It is a rare leukaemic, erythrodermic variant of mycosis fungoides characterized by lymphadenopathy and large mononuclear cells (Sézary cells) in the skin and blood. It is often resistant to traditional treatment and has a poor prognosis. Extracorporeal photopheresis (which consists of oral administration of methoxsalen, exposure of a lymphocyte-enriched blood fraction to ultraviolet A light and reinfusion of the cells into the patient) has recently shown promise.

Jean Louis M Alibert, a French dermatologist, first described this condition in 1806. A Sézary (1880–1956), a French dermatologist.

CASE 198 Urticaria Pigmentosa

Instruction

Look at this patient's skin.

Salient features

- Itchy reddish-brown macules and papules.
- Telangiectasia.

Proceed as follows:

- Look for hepatosplenomegaly.
- Tell the examiner that you would like to take a history of the following:
  Urticaria with pruritus on trauma, rubbing or heat – Darier's sign.
  Headache.
  Diarrhoea.
  Itching.

Diagnosis

This patient has itchy reddish-brown macules with telangiectasia and Darier's sign (lesions) indicating urticaria pigmentosa (aetiology).

Advanced-level Questions

What do you know about urticaria pigmentosa?

It is the cutaneous manifestation of systemic mastocytosis.

What is the histology of urticaria pigmentosa?

It varies from an increase in the number of spindle-shaped and stellate mast cells about the superficial dermal vessels to large numbers of tightly packed round-to-oval mast cells in the upper and mid dermis. Variable fibrosis, oedema and a small number of eosinophils may also be present.

What do you know about systemic mastocytosis?

It is a condition characterized by mast cell hyperplasia which, in most cases, is neither clonal nor neoplastic. It can occur at any age and is slightly more common in men. Four forms have been recognized:
- Indolent form: does not alter life expectancy and constitutes the majority of cases.

- Associated with frank leukaemia or dysmyelopoiesis: the prognosis is determined by the underlying haematological disorder.
- Aggressive form: the prognosis is determined by the extent of organ involvement.
- Mast cell leukaemia: rare, invariably fatal.

How would you manage such patients?

- H_1 blocker – for flushing and itch (e.g. chlormethiazole).
- H_2 blocker – for gastric and duodenal manifestations (e.g. ranitidine, cimetidine).
- Oral sodium cromoglycate for diarrhoea and abdominal pain.
- NSAID for flushing not responsive to antihistamines.

FJ Darier (1856–1938), a French dermatologist.

MISCELLANEOUS

EXAMINATION OF THE FEET

Inspection

- Comment on deformity: hallux valgus, pes cavus.
- Skin: comment on the colour, ulcers and gangrene, hair loss (remember that hair loss is not a reliable sign of ischaemia).
- Joint: comment on the swelling, e.g. ankle joint, first metatarsophalangeal joint in gout.

Palpation

- Ask the patient whether the foot is sore.
- Feel for temperature difference between the two feet.
- Pulses: dorsalis pedis and posterior tibials (compare with the other side).
- Sensation: check light touch, pain and joint sensation.
- Check the plantar response and the ankle jerk.

CASE 199 Diabetic Foot

Instruction

Examine this patient's legs.
Examine this patient's feet.

Salient features

Neuropathic foot

- Dry, warm and pink with palpable pulses.
- Impaired deep tendon reflexes.
- Reduced pinprick, light touch and vibration sensation.
- Ulcers usually painless and plantar.

Proceed as follows:

- Tell the examiner that you would like to ask:
    Whether there is pain (usually painless neuropathy, but may be painful).
    Whether there is blistering (usually due to an ill-fitting shoe).
    About a previous history of foot ulcers.

Ischaemic foot

- Skin is shiny and atrophic with sparse hair.
- The foot is cold to touch.
- Peripheral pulses are absent.
- Ulcers usually painful and present on the heels and toes.

Proceed as follows:

- Tell the examiner that you would like to:
    Ask whether there is pain (usually painful).
    Check all peripheral pulses.
    Ask about rest pain and claudication.

Neuropathic and ischaemic foot present together

- Ulcer on the foot with callosities at pressure points.
- Loss of the arch of foot.
- Stocking distribution of sensory loss of all modalities.
- Loss of dorsalis pedis and/or posterior tibial pulsations.

Proceed as follows:

- Tell the examiner that you would like to check the urine for sugar.

Note. When asked to examine the feet, remember that the common conditions affecting the feet are diabetes and atherosclerosis. Pay particular attention to the pulses and the skin.

Diagnosis

This patient has features of both an ischaemic and neuropathic foot (lesion) which is due to diabetes mellitus (aetiology); walking is limited by the plantar ulcer (functional status).

Questions

What are the types of diabetic foot?

- Neuropathic foot.
- Ischaemic foot.

Note. Features of both types often occur together.

Advanced-level Questions

What is the pathophysiology of the ischaemic foot?

Occlusive vascular disease involving both microangiopathy and athero-sclerosis of large and medium-sized arteries.

Mention a few conditions in which neuropathic ulcers are seen.

- Progressive sensory neuropathy.
- Tabes dorsalis.
- Leprosy.
- Amyloidosis.
- Porphyria.

How would you manage this patient?

- Patient education: avoid cigarette smoking, inspect the feet daily for blisters, no walking barefoot, avoid tight shoes and cutting toenails straight across.
- Radiograph of the foot.
- Antibiotics.
- Removal of necrotic tissue.
- Removal of weight-bearing and friction from ulcerated areas – appropriate footwear such as moulded insoles or plaster cast, or crutches to avoid weight-bearing.
- Control hyperglycaemia.
- Chiropody.
- Surgical opinion and arteriography if reconstructive vascular surgery or angioplasty is considered. When irreversible arterial insufficiency occurs, it is often quicker and more humane for the patient to undergo early major amputation rather than be subjected to a series of debilitating conservative procedures.

How would you monitor a diabetic at annual review?

- Eyes: visual acuity, fundoscopy.
- Sensory system: touch, pinprick and vibration sense.
- Deep tendon reflexes.
- Cardiovascular system: blood pressure, peripheral pulses.
- Biochemistry: urine and blood sugar, albumin, glycosylated haemoglo-bin, creatinine.

References

Caputo GM, Cavanagh PR, Ulbrecht JS, Gibbons GW & Karchmer AW (1994) Assessment of foot disease in patients with diabetes. *N Engl J Med* **331**:854.

Elkeles RS & Wolfe JHN (1991) ABC of vascular diseases: the diabetic foot. *Br Med J* **303**: 1053.

CASE 200 Swollen Leg I: Deep Vein Thrombosis

Instruction

Look at this patient's leg.

Salient features

- Painful calf.
- Redness.
- Engorged superficial veins.
- Unilateral swollen leg with pitting oedema.
- Pain on the calf on dorsiflexion of the foot – Homans' sign (not a diagnostic sign).

Proceed as follows:

- Check for pitting oedema on both sides (look at the patient's eyes while eliciting this sign, to ensure that you are not hurting the patient).
- Compare the temperature of both the legs (use the dorsum of your fingers to elicit this sign).
- Check the arterial pulses in the leg.
- Tell the examiner that you would like to know whether the swelling is acute or chronic.
- Comment on the heparin pump by the bedside.

Remember to collect your thoughts when asked to examine the legs – do not rush in to grab the patient's legs.

Diagnosis

This patient has a swollen leg resulting from deep vein thrombosis (lesion) which may be due to the oral contraceptives she is taking (aetiology); the leg is oedematous and the patient is at risk of pulmonary embolism (functional status).

Questions

What are the complications of deep vein thrombosis (DVT)?

- Pulmonary embolism.
- Venous gangrene.
- Pain, particularly in iliofemoral thrombosis.

What are the predisposing factors for venous thrombosis?

- Surgery (particularly of leg or pelvis, or after prostatectomy).
- Following cerebrovascular accident (about half of the patients develop DVT).
- Following myocardial infarction (one-third of patients have DVT).
- Obesity.
- Malignancy.
- Varicose veins.
- Oral contraceptives.
- Older age (exponential increase above the age of 50 years).
- Immobilization (paralysed limbs in stroke, paraplegia).
- Previous DVT (risk increases two- to three-fold).
- Pregnancy (risk increased in postpartum period).
- Hypercoagulable states (antithrombin III deficiency, protein C deficiency, protein S deficiency, antiphospolipid syndrome, excessive plasminogen activator inhibitor, polycythemia vera, erythrocytosis).
- Tissue trauma.

How would you investigate a patient with suspected deep vein thrombosis?

As clinical diagnosis is unreliable it is essential to perform the following investigations to assess the extent of thrombosis:
- Duplex ultrasonography scanning and Doppler studies.
- Venography – by injecting contrast into one of the leg veins.

What is the risk of pulmonary embolism in patients with below-knee thrombi?

The risk in such cases is low and many physicians refrain from anticoagulating these patients.

How would you treat these patients?

- Pain relief.
- Control of oedema:

Intermittent elevation of foot and elevation of foot during the night above the level of the heart.

Avoid long periods of standing.

Elastic support stockings from the mid-foot to just below the knee, worn during the day.

- The main aim is to prevent pulmonary emboli and restore venous patency and valvular function in order to prevent postphlebitic syndrome. All patients with thrombi above the knee must be anticoagulated:

  Initial therapy with heparin with the aim of maintaining activated partial thromboplastin time (APTT) 1.5–2.5 times the normal value within the first 24 hours. Failure to achieve this target APTT *within 24 hours* increases the risk of recurrent venous thromboembolism by 15-fold. Heparin therapy is continued for about 5 days

  This is followed by warfarin therapy with the aim of maintaining the international normalized ratio (INR) at 2.0–3.0, recommended for the treatment of venous thromboembolic disease, but substantially less intensive anticoagulation may be effective. Remember that anticoagulants do not affect thrombus that is already present. Oral anticoagulation should be continued for at least 12 weeks to minimize recurrence. Although treatment beyond 3 months is generally not worthwhile, prolonged treatment may be required in prolonged immmbolization or hypercoagulable states.

  When anticoagulation is contraindicated, inferior vena caval filters may be required there is a high risk of pulmonary embolism.

How would you prevent deep venous thrombosis?

- Subcutaneous low-dose heparin should be given to patients:
  who are undergoing surgery to the leg, pelvis or prostatectomy
  with myocardial infarction and
  with cardiac failure.
- Early ambulation within 72 hours after surgery.
- Encourage leg exercise following surgery.
- Elastic supports to patients with a history of thrombosis or obesity.

Advanced-level Questions

What are causes of recurrent venous thrombosis?

- Pregnancy, surgery, trauma, oral contraceptives.

- Abnormalities in antithrombin III, protein C, protein S, fibrinogen or factor V.
- Acquired conditions such as antiphospholipid antibody syndrome, occult cancer, myeloproliferative disorders, some vasculitides.
- Potential abnormalities include thrombomodulin, tissue factor pathway inhibitor, vitronectin associated with heparin and antithrombin III and fibrinolytic receptors.

What do you know of the antiphospholipid antibody syndrome?

The diagnosis of this syndrome requires that a patient have recurrent clinical events (such as thromboses or fetal loss) and an antiphospholipid antibody (such as anticardiolipin antibody or lupus anticoagulant). The 'primary' syndrome has no accompanying autoimmune disease, whereas it is 'secondary' if the patient also has systemic lupus erythematosus or lupus-like disease. Many patients with this syndrome have livedo reticularis, thrombocytopenia and neurological symptoms.

(**Note.** The antiphospholipid antibody can occur in certain drug reactions and infectious diseaes, but only those that occur in patients with autoimmune disease are associated with the clinical syndrome.) The clinical course of the secondary syndrome is independent of the activity and severity of the lupus, but the presence of antiphospholipid antibody worsens the prognosis of the lupus. Warfarin therapy with an international normalized ratio of 3 or more offers the best protection against recurrent thrombosis for patients who have a confirmed major thrombosis.

J Homans (1877–1954) was an American surgeon who worked at Johns Hopkins Hospital with Cushing, initially on experimental hypophysectomy and later on vascular disease.
GRV Hughes, contemporary London physician, Raynes Institute, St Thomas' Hospital, first described the antiphospholipid antibody syndrome.

References

Carson JL, Kelley MA, Duff A et al (1992) The clinical course of pulmonary embolism. *N Engl J Med* **326**: 12140–12145.
Hopkins NF & Wolfe JH (1992) ABC of vascular diseases. Deep venous insufficiency. *Br Med J* **304**: 107.
Hull RD, Raskob GE, Hirsch J et al (1986) Continuous intravenous heparin compared with intermittent subcutaneous heparin in the initial treatment of proximal venous thrombosis. *N Engl J Med* **315**: 1109–1114.
Khamashta MA, Cuadrado MJ, Mujic F, Taub NA, Hunt BJ & Hughes GRV (1995) The management of thrombosis in the antiphospholipid-antibody syndrome. *N Engl J Med* **332**: 993–997.
Nordström M, Lindblad B, Anderson H, Bergqvist D & Kjellström T (1994) Deep

vein thrombosis and occult malignancy: an epidemiological study. *Br Med J* **308**: 891–894.

Weinmann EE & Salzman EW (1994) Deep vein thrombosis. *N Engl J Med* **331**: 1630–1641.

CASE 201 Swollen Leg II: Cellulitis

Instruction

Look at this patient's leg.

Salient features

- Red, inflamed leg with a definite demarcation of erythematous area.
- Oedema.
- Increased temperature.

Proceed as follows:

- Examine the peripheral pulses.
- Ask the patient whether he had fever.
- Look for superficial ulcers.

Diagnosis

This patient has cellulitis of the leg (lesion) which is due to pyogenic bacterial infection (aetiology) and the leg is acutely swollen and painful (functional status).

Questions

How would you manage such a patient?

- Blood cultures.
- Intravenous antibiotics.
- Pain relief and pyretics.
- Surgical referral.

What are the causes of bilateral swollen legs?

- Cardiac failure.
- Renal failure.
- Hypoproteinaemia (due to cirrhosis or nephrotic syndrome).

What are the causes of an acutely swollen leg?

- Deep vein thrombosis.
- Cellulitis.
- Arterial occlusion.
- Trauma.
- Arthritis.

What are the causes of a chronically swollen leg?

- Venous causes: varicose veins, postphlebitic limb.
- Lymphoedema: Milroy's disease, filariasis (in the tropics).
- Congenital.

WF Milroy (1855–1942) described familial lymphoedema of the legs in 1892.

Reference

Reilly DT & Wolfe JHN (1991) ABC of vascular diseases: the swollen leg. *Br Med J* **303**: 1462.

Instruction

Examine this patient's hands.

Salient features

- Increased curvature of the nails, obliteration of the angle of the nail (when in doubt, approximate the dorsal aspects of terminal phalanges of the fingers of both hands which are flexed at the interphalangeal joints. Normally, the angle betwen the nails does not extend more than halfway up the nail bed. In clubbing there is a wide and deep angle – this is known as Schamroth's sign).
- The nails may have a drumstick appearance.

Proceed as follows:

- Look for the following signs:
    Fluctuation at the nail bed.
    Palpate the wrist joints for tenderness seen in hypertrophic pulmonary osteoarthropathy (HPOA). Rapid painful clubbing is nearly always due to bronchogenic carcinoma.

Nicotine (tar) staining of fingers.

Central cyanosis.

Clubbing of the toes.

- Tell the examiner that you would like to examine the following systems:

  Chest (bronchogenic carcinoma; fibrosing alveolitis; mesothelioma; suppurative lung disease such as bronchiectasis, lung abscess and empyema).

  Heart (infective endocarditis, cyanotic heart disease). In infective endocarditis the fingers may be pale and their tips flushed ('pale hands, pink tipped').

  Gastrointestinal tract (cirrhosis, ulcerative colitis, Crohn's disease).

  Thyroid (thyroid acropachy).

- If an underlying cause is not obvious, ask for a family history to confirm the hereditary causes of clubbing.

Diagnosis

This patient has marked clubbing of the fingernails (lesion) and tar staining, indicating that the condition may be due to an underlying bronchial neoplasm (aetiology).

Questions

How is clubbing graded?

There are four grades:

- Grade I: increased glossiness and cyanosis of the skin at the root of the nail associated with increased fluctuation at the base of the nail bed.
- Grade II: the normal angle between the base of the nail and the skin is obliterated (Lovibond's sign) and may even be reversed.
- Grade III: hypertrophy of the soft tissue of the nail pulp and the nail curves excessively longitudinally to give a 'drum-stick' or 'parrot-beak' appearance ('doigts Hippocratique').
- Grade IV: bony changes involving the wrists and ankles, sometimes the elbows and knees (HPOA).

What do you know about pachydermoperiostitis?

This is an unusual variety of idiopathic familial HPOA, in which postpubertal clubbing and bone changes are accompanied by increased sweating of the palms and soles and marked thickening of the skin of the face, forehead and scalp.

Advanced-level Questions

What are the mechanisms for clubbing?

- Increased blood flow in clubbed fingers due to vasodilatation rather than hyperplasia of vessels in the nail bed. The nature of the vasodilator is unclear and many contenders, such as ferritin, bradykinin, prostaglandin and 5-hydroxytryptamine (5-HT), have been implicated. The vasodilator is probably inactivated in the lung in normal persons but when this inactivation is defective, or there is a right-to-left shunt, clubbing occurs.
- Increased growth hormone in disease states causes excessive cellular tissue in the nail bed.
- Clubbing occurs whenever organs supplied by the vagus are affected. It has been shown that, in bronchogenic carcinoma, vagotomy causes reversal of clubbing.
- Tumour necrosis factor has been implicated.
- Megakaryocytes and clumps of platelets may preferentially stream into blood vessels of the digits and release platelet-derived growth factor. The resulting increased capillary permeability, fibroblastic activity and arterial smooth muscle hyperplasia could cause clubbing.

Digital clubbing was first described approximately 2400 years ago by Hippocrates.

References

Adams F (1849) *Hippocrates. The Book of Prognostics. The Genuine Works of Hippocrates*, Vol. 1. London: Sydenham Society.

Burton MD & Wain JC (1993) Clubbing and hypertrophic osteoarthropathy. *N Engl J Med* **329**:1862. (Classical pictures of these conditions.)

Dickinson CJ (1993) The aetiology of clubbing and hypertrophic osteopathy. *Eur J Clin Invest* **23**: 330–338.

Schamroth L (1976) Clubbing of fingers: a method of assessment. *S Afr Med J* **50**: 297.

CASE 203 Dupuytren's Contracture

Instruction

Look at this patient's hands.

Salient features

- Thickening of the palmar fascia, particularly along the medial aspect. (Feel for thickening before you comment on it.)

- In almost all cases, the fourth finger is affected with associated involvement of fifth, third and second fingers in decreasing order of frequency.

Proceed as follows:

- Tell the examiner that you would like to:
  Check the feet for contracture of the plantar fascia.
  Take a family history (as there is a genetic predisposition).
  Look for signs of alcoholism and cirrhosis.

Diagnosis

This patient has Dupuytren's contracture (lesion) associated with chronic alcoholic liver disease (aetiology) and has developed disabling contractures (functional status).

Advanced-level Questions

What do you know about Dupuytren's contracture?

It is due to the thickening and shortening of palmar fascia; the plantar fascia may also be affected. Fibrous nodules are often the earliest abnormality resulting from a contracture of the proliferating fibroblasts in the superficial compartment of the palm. The nodules consist of mature-appearing fibroblasts surrounded by dense collagen. Ultrastructurally many of these cells are myofibroblasts and thus may be contractile.

What other structures are involved?

There does not appear to be any direct involvement of the muscles, joints, tendons (and their sheaths), and nervous or vascular tissue. However, the dermis is frequently invaded by fibroblastic cells, resulting in fixation to deeper structures.

What is the natural history of this condition?

It is unpredictable, with little change or disability over a period of many years in some individuals. In others, the contraction of the fascia occurs rapidly, resulting in severe deformity and loss of hand function.

What do you know about the epidemiology of Dupuytren's contracture?

There may be a hereditary predisposition (usually autosomal dominant) and the disorder is about five times more frequent in men, more common in whites and in Europe. There is a gradual increase in the incidence with age.

With which other conditions is Dupuytren's contracture associated?

- Alcoholism.
- Chronic antiepileptic therapy.
- Systemic conditions such as cirrhosis, diabetes, epilepsy, tuberculosis.
- Thickening of the corpora cavernosa of the penis (Peyronie's disease).
- Garrod's knuckle pads.
- Retroperitoneal fibrosis.

Why is the deformity caused by this condition usually well tolerated?

Because it exaggerates the normal position of function of the hand.

How would you manage such patients?

Treatment depends on the severity of findings and includes:
- Periodic examination of patients in early stages. If the palmar thickening is growing rapidly, local injections of triamcinolone into the growing nodule may be of benefit.
- Surgery is indicated when there are disabling flexion contractures, although recurrences are common.

Baron Guillaume Dupuytren (1777–1835), Surgeon-in-Chief, Hôtel-Dieu, Paris, is reported to have been the first to achieve successful removal of the lower jaw.
Sir AE Garrod (1857–1936), physician at St Bartholomew's Hospital, London, succeeded Osler as Regius Professor at Oxford.
F de la Peyronie (1678–1747), a French surgeon who influenced Louis XVI in his decision to issue an ordinance banning barbers from practising surgery.

Reference

Pojer J, Radiwojevic M & Williams TF (1977) Dupuytren's disease: its association with abnormal liver function in alcoholism and epilepsy. *Arch Intern Med* **129**: 561–566.

CASE 204 Cataracts

Instruction

Examine this patient's eyes.

Salient features

- Bilateral cataracts (shine light obliquely across the lens).

Proceed as follows:

- Tell the examiner that you would like to:
  Check the urine for sugar.
  Take a drug history (steroids, chloroquine, phenothiazines, chlorambucil, busulphan).
  Take a history of gradual deterioration of vision.
  Inquire about smoking and alcohol consumption (cigarette smoking and heavy alcohol consumption increases the risk of cataract formation).

Diagnosis

This patient has premature bilateral cataracts (lesion) due to diabetes mellitus (aetiology) and has had a gradual deterioration of vision (functional status).

Questions

Mention a few causes of cataracts.

Common causes:
- Old age (look for arcus senilis). The Framingham study reported that 13% of people aged 65–74 years and about 40% of those over the age of 75 years had cataracts.
- Diabetes mellitus (non-enzymatic glycosylation of lens protein is twice as high in diabetics as in age-matched controls and may contribute to the premature occurrence of cataracts).
Uncommon causes:
- Trauma.
- Metabolic: Cushing's syndrome, Wilson's disease (stellate cataracts), galactosaemia.
- Chromosomal disorders: dystrophia myotonica, Turner's syndrome.
- Congenital infections (rubella or cytomegalovirus).
- Drugs (see above).

- Dermatological disorders: atopic dermatitis, ichthyosis.
- Radiation: infra-red (glass-blower's cataract), X-ray radiation, micro-wave radiation.

Advanced-level Questions

How are cataracts treated?

Cataract extraction is performed by removing the lens nucleus and cortex from within the lens capsule. In most adults, a plastic lens is implanted within the capsule. Multifocal intraocular lens implants in some instances have reduced the need for both reading and distance spectacles. Lens extraction improves vision in 95% of instances. In the remaining, prior retinal disease or postoperative complications such as haemorrhage, glaucoma, infection or retinal detachment may be the cause.

How is early cataract detected using direct ophthalmoscopy?

Examination of the red reflex with + 4 dioptres at approximately 20 cm from the patient will reveal a black opacity in the lens against the reddish hue of the reflex. If this opacity appears to move down on upward gaze, it is located in the posterior half of the lens, but if it appears to move up then it is located in the anterior half of the lens.

References

Christen WG, Manson JE, Seddon, JM et al (1992) A prospective study of cigarette smoking and risk of cataract in men. *JAMA* **268**: 989–994.
Ritter LL, Klein BE, Klein R et al (1993) Alcohol use and lens opacities in Beaver Dam Eye Study. *Arch Ophthalmol* **111**: 113.

CASE 205 **Anaemia**

Instruction

Would you like to ask this anaemic patient (*Patient 1*) a few questions?

Salient features

Proceed as follows:

- Ask about the following:
  Blood loss such as bleeding per rectum, melaena, haematemesis.

Menstrual blood loss (duration of periods, the occurrence of clots, and the number of sanitary towels or tampons used).

Drug history – NSAIDs, phenytoin, chloramphenicol.

Associated symptoms such as weight loss, shortness of breath, chronic diarrhoea.

Diet – in vegans, alcoholics, elderly patients.

Past history of gastrectomy.

Diagnosis

This patient's anaemia is due to severe melaena which indicates bleeding in the upper gastrointestinal tract and is probably due to peptic ulcer or bleeding varices (aetiology).The patient is currently receiving a blood transfusion, indicating that the anaemia was severe (functional status).

Instruction

Would you like to examine this anaemic patient (*Patient 2*)?

Salient features

Proceed as follows:

- Examine the following:
    Nails for koilonychia or iron deficiency anaemia, and (rarely) for clubbing of infective endocarditis.

    Comment on the pallor of the face and conjunctiva, looking for the lemon-yellow hue of pernicious anaemia.

    Tongue for glossitis of vitamin B_{12} deficiency.

    Mouth for angular stomatitis of severe malnutrition, and ulcers of neutropenia.

    Lymph nodes in the neck, axillae and groin (secondaries, lymphoproliferative disorders).

    Skin for bruising associated with bone marrow depression seen in leukaemia and aplastic anaemia.

    Abdomen for hepatomegaly, splenomegaly and other masses.

    Legs for ulcers seen in haemoglobinopathies.
- Comment on the ethnic origin (thalassaemia).
- Tell the examiner that you would like to:
    Do a rectal examination and inspect the stool for occult blood.

    Do an FBC including a peripheral smear and ESR.

Diagnosis

This patient has koilonychia and anaemia indicating an iron deficiency anaemia. I would like to exclude a gastrointestinal cause for the blood loss (aetiology).

Questions

Mention a few causes of anaemia.

- With a low mean corpuscular volume (MCV):
    Iron deficiency anaemia.
    Thalassaemia.
    Sideroblastic anaemia.
- With a high MCV:
    Vitamin B_{12} deficiency (pernicious anaemia, vegans, alcoholics, coeliac disease).
    Folate deficiency (pregnancy, phenytoin, sprue, coeliac disease, malignancy, haemolysis).
    Other: myxoedema, liver disease, alcoholics.
- With a normal MCV:
    Uraemia.
    Malignancy.
    Rheumatoid arthritis.
    Aplastic anaemia (myelofibrosis, chloramphenicol, phenylbutazone, gold, anticancer drugs).

What do you know about the Paterson – Kelly syndrome?

It comprises iron deficiency anaemia and dysphagia due to oesophageal webs in middle-aged women. The clinical significance of this syndrome is uncertain. It is also known as Plummer–Vinson syndrome.

What are the common causes of iron deficiency anaemia?

Occult gastrointestinal bleeding from the following:
- Peptic ulcer.
- Carcinoma located anywhere in the gastrointestinal tract.
- Excessive anticoagulation.
- Hereditary haemorrhagic telangiectasia.
- Angiodysplasia of the colon.

How would you investigate microcytic anaemia?

- FBC.
- Serum ferritin.
- Faecal occult blood.

- Upper gastrointestinal endoscopy.
- Barium enema, colonoscopy.
- International normalized ratio (INR), prothrombin time and platelet count.
- Haemoglobin electrophoresis in susceptible ethnic groups (Asians, Afro-Caribbeans).

How would you investigate macrocytic anaemia?

- Peripheral smear.
- Vitamin B_{12} and red-cell folate and serum folate concentrations.
- Serum ferritin, plasma iron and total iron-binding capacity (for associated iron deficiency).
- Schilling test.
- Gastric parietal cell and intrinsic factor antibodies.
- Upper gastrointestinal endoscopy.
- Reticulocyte count (a high MCV could be present when the reticulocyte count is over 50%).
- Bone marrow examination.

RF Schilling (b. 1919), Chairman of the Department of Medicine and haematologist at the University of Wisconsin.

CASE 206 Lymphadenopathy

Instruction

Perform a general examination.
Examine this patient's neck.

Salient features

As soon as you feel a group of lymph nodes, examine drainage areas for obvious pathology. For example:
- Inguinal lymph nodes: examine the lower limbs and external genitalia.
- Axillary lymph nodes: examine the chest, breasts and upper limbs.
- Upper cervical lymph nodes: examine the chest, breast and upper limbs. Also, perform an ear, nose and throat (ENT) examination for nasopharyngeal carcinoma.
- Lower cervical and supraclavicular lymph nodes: examine the thyroid, chest, abdomen for gastric carcinoma (Virchow's nodes) and testis.
- Examine other lymph node areas in a systemic manner: submental,

submandibular, deep cervical (upper and lower), occipital, posterior triangle, supraclavicular, axillary, epitrochlear and inguinal.
- Examine the mouth for the following signs:
  Tonsillar lymph nodes.
  Palatal petechiae and pharyngitis (glandular fever).
  Neoplastic tumours or ulcers.
- Tell the examiner that you would like to proceed as follows:
  Examine the abdomen for liver and spleen.
  Examine the chest and do a CXR (for bronchogenic carcinoma, TB).

Diagnosis

This patient has generalized lymphadenopathy, probably a lymphoma – either Hodgkin's or non-Hodgkin's (aetiology) – and has severe disease as evidenced by alopecia, presumably due to chemotherapy (functional status). I would like to discuss other causes of generalized lymphadenopathy.

Questions

What are the causes of generalized lymphadenopathy?

Lymphomas, chronic lymphatic leukaemia, acute lymphoblastic leukaemia.
Glandular fever, cytomegalovirus.
AIDS, toxoplasmosis.
SLE, rheumatoid arthritis, sarcoid.
Chronic infections such as TB, secondary syphilis, brucellosis.
Drugs – phenytoin.

What do you understand by the term Hodgkin's disease?

Hodgkin's disease is a group of neoplasms characterised by Reed–Sternberg cells in an appropriate reactive cellular background. It is divided into several subtypes histologically: lymphocyte predominance, nodular sclerosis, mixed cellularity and lymphocyte depletion. The Reed–Sternberg cell is a giant cell with two or more nuclear lobes and huge eosinophilic inclusion like nucleoli. The classic Reed–Sternberg cell has a symmetrical, mirror image nucleus that creates an 'owl-eye' appearance.

Advanced-level Questions

What is the mode of presentation of Hodgkin's disease?

- Usually as a painless lymphadenopathy.
- Other presenting symptoms include systemic symptoms such as fever,

weight loss, drenching night sweats, generalized pruritus or pain in the affected lymph node following the ingestion of alcohol.

How is Hodgkin's disease staged?

Stage I: one lymph node region involved.
Stage II: more than two lymph node regions involved on one side of the diaphragm.
Stage III: lymph nodes involved on both sides of the diaphragm.
Stage IV: disseminated disease with bone marrow or liver involvement.

In addition they are designated as Stage A when systemic symptoms are absent or as Stage B when there is significant weight loss, fever or night sweats.

How is a patient with Hodgkin's disease treated?

- Localized disease (i.e. Stages IA, IIA) is treated with radiotherapy. Five-year cure rates are in excess of 80% and relapses are treated with chemotherapy.
- Disseminated disease (Stages IIIB, IV) is treated with combination chemotherapy with an ABVD (Adriamycin, bleomycin, vincristine, dacarbazine) regimen alternating with a MOPP regimen (mechlorethamine, oncovin, procarbazine and prednisolone). Five-year survival rates are about 50%. Patients who relapse after initial chemotherapy may be cured with autologous bone marrow transplantation.
- In Stages IIB and IIIA, optimal management is controversial but current evidence suggests an advantage to combination chemotherapy.

What do you understand by the term non-Hodgkin's lymphomas?

These are a heterogeneous group of cancers of lymphocytes. They are variable in their presentation and natural history, varying from a slow indolent course to a rapidly progressive illness.

How are non-Hodkin's lymphomas classified?

A working classification is as follows:
- Low grade or favourable: slow, indolent course with good response to minimal therapy and long survival. These include small lymphocytic, plasmocytoid, follicular small cleaved cell and follicular mixed cell. Patients are usually treated with alkylating agents such as chlorambucil or a CVP regimen (cyclophosphamide, vincristine and prednisolone).

- High grade or unfavourable: including immunoblastic, small non-cleaved (Burkitt's and non-Burkitt's), lymphoblastic and true histiocytic. The mainstay of therapy is combination chemotherapy; traditionally the CHOP regimen (cyclophosphamide, doxorubicin, vincristine and prednisolone) is used. In highly aggressive lymphomas autologous bone marrow transplantation may increase the chances of cure.
- Intermediate grade: follicular large cell, diffuse small cleaved cell, diffuse mixed cell, diffuse large cell.
- Other: cutaneous T cell (mycosis fungoides, adult T cell leukaemia/lymphoma).

RLK Virchow (1821–1902), successively Professor of Pathology at Würzberg and Berlin. He also described Virchow cell (lepra cell), Virchow space (perivascular space of Virchow–Robin) and Virchow triad of the pathogenesis of thrombosis.

Thomas Hodgkin (1798–1866), an English physician at St Thomas's Hospital, London. He was the Curator of the Pathology Museum at Guy's Hospital before this.

Dorothy Reed (1874–1964) graduated from Johns Hopkins Hospital, Baltimore, and worked successively in New York and Wisconsin.

K Sternberg (1872–1935), an Austrian pathologist who described the cells in 1898.

Burkitt's lymphoma was described by Dennis Burkitt in children in West Africa who presented with a lesion in the jaw, extranodal abdominal involvement and ovarian tumours. Most patients have Epstein–Barr antibodies in the serum.

References

Armitage JO (1993) Treatment of non-Hodgkin's lymphoma. *N Engl J Med* **328**: 1023.

DeVita VT, Jr and Hubbard SM (1993) Hodgkin's disease. *N Engl J Med* **328**: 560.

Mack TM, Cozen W, Shibata DK et al (1995) Concordance for Hodgkin's disease in identical twins suggesting genetic susceptibility to the young-adult form of the disease. *N Engl J Med* **332**: 413–418.

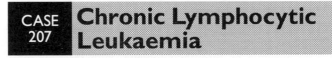

CASE 207 Chronic Lymphocytic Leukaemia

Instruction

Perform a general examination of this patient

Salient features

- Usually men over the age of 40 years (male:female ratio is 2:1).

- Symmetrical, painless, rubbery lymph nodes.
- Liver or spleen may be palpable.

Proceed as follows:

- Tell the examiner that you would like to do a full blood count and examine the peripheral smear (lymphocytosis $>15\,000\,\mu l^{-1}$, with mature appearance of small lymphocytes).

Remember that chronic lymphocytic leukaemia (CLL) manifests clinically with organ infiltration with lymphocytes, immunosuppression (hypogammaglobulinaemia) and bone marrow failure.

Diagnosis

This elderly male patient with painless enlargement of lymph nodes probably has chronic lymphocytic leukaemia (lesion). He has severe pallor, indicating he is in Binet Stage C (functional status).

Questions

What are the causes of anaemia in CLL?

Bone marrow infiltration, autoimmune (Coombs' positive) haemolysis.

How may this patient present?

About 25% of cases are asymptomatic; some complain of generalized malaise, wieght loss and loss of appetite; and others complain of bleeding.

Advanced-level Questions

How is chronic lymphocytic leukaemia staged?

Binet staging (evaluates the enlargement of spleen, liver and lymph nodes in the head and neck, axillae and groin):
> Stage A – no anaemia or thrombocytopenia and less than three areas of lymphoid enlargement.
> Stage B – no anaemia or thrombocytopenia, with three or more involved areas.
> Stage C – anaemia and/or thrombocytopenia, regardless of the number of areas of lymphoid enlargement.

Rai staging:
> Stage 0 – lymhocytosis only (in blood and bone marrow).
> Stage I – lymphocytosis plus lymphadenopathy.

Stage II – lymphocytosis with hepatic and/or splenic enlargement.
Stage III – lymphocytosis with anaemia.
Stage IV – lymphoctyosis with thrombocytopenia.

Note. Although clinical staging is useful for prognosis, it does not provide information on the likelihood of progression in a given patient.

How are patients with CLL treated?

- Specific treatment may not be indicated until Stage B or C. Patients with Stage A disease should be reassured that, despite the frightening diagnosis of leukaemia, they will be able to live a normal life for many years with a median survival of 8 years.
- Patients with Stage B and C will require specific and supportive therapy, i.e. correction of anaemia and folic acid deficiency, and correction of bone marrow infiltration initially with prednisolone and oxymetholone and subsequently with chemotherapeutic agents such as chlorambucil. Purine analogues such as fludarabine, 2-chlorodeoxyadenosine and pentostatin are currently being investigated. Combination chemotherapy (CHOP regimen) and radiotherapy have also been used. Intravenous immunoglobulin reduces the incidence of infection.

What is Richter's syndrome?

This is when an isolated lymph node in CLL is transformed into an aggressive large cell lymphoma. There is a median survival of less than 1 year after its appearance.

Which lymphomas can convert to leukaemias?

Small cell lymphoma (chronic lympocytic leukaemia).
Burkitt's lymphoma (B-cell acute lymphoblastic leukaemia).
Lymphoblastic lymphoma (T-cell acute lymphoblastic leukaemia).

Reference

Rozman C & Montserrat E (1995) Chronic lymphocytic leukemia. *N Engl J Med* **333**: 1052–1057.

CASE 208 Crohn's Disease

Instruction

These patients have chronic diarrhoea.
Examine this patient's face (*Patient 3*).
Examine this patient's abdomen (*Patients 1 and 2*).
Comment on this patient's perianal area (*Patient 4*).

Salient features

- Mass in the right iliac fossa (*Patient 1*).
- Multiple fistulous openings in the right iliac fossa (*Patient 2*).
- Swollen lips (*Patient 3*).
- Multiple perianal fistulous tracts (*Patient 4*).

Proceed as follows:

- In all four patients, examine for the following:
    In the mouth for aphthous ulcers.
    Uveitis.
    Anaemia.
    Arthropathy.
    Skin lesions (erythema nodosum, pyoderma gangrenosum).
    Liver disease.

Remember that Crohn's disease may affect any part of the gastrointestinal tract from the mouth to the anus, but has a tendency to involve the terminal ileum. The inflammation is transmural (extending through all layers of bowel) with relatively normal bowel in between (skip lesions).

Diagnosis

This patient has multiple anal fistulas (lesions) due to Crohn's disease (aetiology), indicating that the disease is active (functional status).

Questions

What investigations would you do?

- Sigmoidoscopy and biopsy.
- Small bowel study.
- Barium enema.
- Colonoscopy.

Mention some complications.

- Iritis.
- Arthritis.
- Erythema nodosum.
- Pyoderma gangrenosum.

Mention some associated diseases.

- Ankylosing spondylitis (HLA-B27 positive).
- Sacroiliitis.
- Cholangitis, hepatitis, cirrhosis.

Advanced-level Questions

Mention some ocular features of Crohn's disease.

Eye lesions are seen in about 5% of cases.
- Common: conjunctivitis, anterior uveitis.
- Rare: scleritis, keratitis, keratoconjunctivitis sicca, choroiditis, retinal vasculitis, optic neuritis and orbital pseudotumour.

How would you treat Crohn's disease?

- Sulphasalazine or rectal steroids for colonic disease.
- Oral steroids for small bowel disease.
- Metronidazole for perianal disease and fistulas.
- 6-Mercaptopurine may be useful in severe cases.
- Surgery is reserved for intestinal fistulas and intestinal obstruction that does not respond to medical management. Proctocolectomy and ileostomy is the standard operation. (**Note.** Ileorectal anastomosis or ileoanal anastomosis should be avoided in Crohn's disease.)

Burrill Bernard Crohn (b. 1884) was a physician in Mount Sinai Hospital, New York; he described the condition in 1932 and pointed out the non-tuberculous aetiology.

Anne Ferguson, contemporary Professor of Gastroenterology at the Western General Hospital in Edinburgh, whose chief interest is inflammatory bowel disease.

References

Carethers JM & McDonnell WM (1994) Extraintestinal manifestations of Crohn's disease. *N Engl J Med* **330**: 1870. (Classical pictures of aphthous ulcers and perianal fistulas.)

Crohn BB, Ginzburg L & Oppenheimer GD (1972) Regional ileitis: a pathologic and clinical entity. *JAMA* **99**:1323–1329.

Greenberg GR, Feagan BG, Martin F et al and the Canadian Inflammatory Bowel Disease Study Group (1994) Oral budesonide for active Crohn's disease. *N Engl J Med* **331**: 836–41.

Rutgeerts P, Löfberg R, Malchow H et al (1994) A comparison of budesonide with prednisolone for active Crohn's disease. *N Engl J Med* **331**: 842–845.

CASE 209   Dysphagia

Instruction

Patient 1 has difficulty in swallowing; would you like to ask her a few questions?

Proceed as follows:

- Ask about the following:
  The duration of symptoms.
  Whether the difficulty is in swallowing liquids or solids, or both.
  Nasal regurgitation.
  Whether or not the patient coughs on swallowing.
  The level at which the food sticks (suprasternal notch or mid-sternal)
  Associated heart burn.
  Weight loss.

Instruction

Patient 2 has difficulty in swallowing; would you like to examine him?

Proceed as follows:

- Examine:
  Mouth for ulcers, thrush and pallor; check the gag reflex.
  Neck for lymph glands and goitres.
  For scleroderma.
- Tell the examiner that you would like to look for an underlying neurological deficit (evidence of stroke, motor neuron disease, myasthenia gravis).

Diagnosis

This patient with dysphagia is recovering from a stroke (aetiology) and his functional status is best determined by videofluoroscopy and assessment by a speech therapist.

Questions

Mention a few causes of dysphagia.

- Benign oesophageal stricture.
- Carcinoma of the oesophagus.
- Peptic ulcer of the oesophagus.
- Achalasia cardia.
- Pharyngeal pouch.
- Retrosternal goitre, bulbar palsy, myasthenia gravis, Plummer–Vinson syndrome (Paterson–Kelly syndrome).

Remember that oesophgeal dysphagia is due either to mechanical narrowing or to a motor disorder affecting normal peristalsis.

How would you investigate such a patient?

- FBC, ESR.
- Barium swallow.
- Gastroscopy.

What do you understand by the term presbyoesophagus?

It is a condition that occurs in the elderly, characterized by impaired motor function of the oesophagus.

HS Plummer and PP Vinson, both physicians at the Mayo Clinic, Rochester, Minnesota.
DR Paterson and A Brown Kelly, both British ENT surgeons.

CASE 210 Diarrhoea

Instruction

Patient 1 has diarrhoea; would you like to ask him a few questions?

Salient features

Proceed as follows:

- Ask about the following:
    Onset.
    Duration of diarrhoea.

Frequency.

Whether or not it is nocturnal.

Blood (seen in ulcerative colitis, shigellosis, diverticulitis, carcinoma of the colon) and mucus in the stools; blood on the toilet paper.

Nature of the stools (pale and bulky and difficult to flush away in steatorrhoea).

Associated pain in the abdomen.

Appetite (increased in thyrotoxicosis).

Weight loss (marked in chronic diarrhoea).

Associated nausea and vomiting.

Drug ingestion (including antibiotics and laxatives).

Foreign travel.

Instruction

Patient 2 has diarrhoea, would you like to examine her?

Salient features

Proceed as follows:

- Look for the following signs:
  Anaemia.
  Clubbing.
  Aphthous ulcers.
  Abdominal tenderness, abdominal masses.
- Tell the examiner that you would like to do a rectal examination and check for faecal occult blood.

Diagnosis

This patient has chronic diarrhoea with aphthous ulcers and abdominal tenderness indicating that she has inflammatory bowel disease (aetiology).

Questions

What do you understand by the term 'diarrhoea'?

It implies passing of increased amounts of loose stool (more than 300 g per day).

How would you investigate a patient with diarrhoea?

- FBC, ESR.
- Serum albumin.

- Sigmoidoscopy.
- Stool chart, stool cultures, faecal cultures.
- Barium enema, small bowel barium studies.

Advanced-level Questions

What are the mechanisms of diarrhoea?

- Osmotic diarrhoea: the mucosa of the gut acts as a semipermeable membrane; the diarrhoea stops when the patient fasts, e.g. diarrhoea due to magnesium sulphate, lactulose, malabsorptive states.
- Secretory diarrhoea: there is active secretion of intestinal fluid, e.g. *Escherichia coli* diarrhoea.
- Inflammatory diarrhoea: there is mucosal damage, e.g. shigellosis, ulcerative colitis.
- Increased gut motility, e.g. irritable bowel syndrome.

What are the poor prognostic factors in ulcerative colitis?

Anaemia (Hb < 10 g dl^{-1}), raised ESR (30 mm in the first hour), fever (37.5°C), increased frequency of stools (more than six per day), tachycardia (> 90 beats min^{-1}) and hypoalbuminaemia (< 30 g l^{-1}).

CASE 211 Marfan's Syndrome

Instruction

Look at this patient.
Examine this patient's heart.

Salient features

- Disproportionately long limbs compared with the trunk – the arm span will exceed the height.

Proceed as follows:

- Examine the following:
  Hands, for hypermobile joints and spidery fingers or arachnodactyly (confirm by: (1) *thumb sign* – asking the patient to clench his thumb in his fist; the thumb should not exceed beyond the ulnar side of the hand in normal subjects but because of hypermobility and laxity of the joint in Marfan's disease it

protrudes beyond his clenched fingers; and (2) *wrist sign* – put the patient's fingers around the other wrist: normal subjects cannot overlap the thumb and little finger around the wrist but in Marfan's syndrome the little finger will overlap by at least 1 cm in 80% of patients).

Eyes, for iridodonesis or ectopia lentis (subluxation upwards) – the patient may be wearing thick spectacles; blue sclera.

Head, for long-headedness (dolichocephalic with bossing of frontal eminences and prominent supraorbital ridges).

Palate, for high arched palate.

Skin, for small papules in the neck (Miescher's elastoma).

Chest, for pectus excavatum, cystic lung disease.

Heart, for mitral valve prolapse, aortic aneurysm and aortic regurgitation.

Spine, for scoliosis and kyphosis.

- Tell the examiner that you would like to take a family history (autosomal dominant).

Remember that each patient should be referred for ophthalmic examination, annual echocardiography and genetic counselling to maximize the preventive potential in this disease.

Diagnosis

This patient has Marfan's syndrome and aortic regurgitation (lesion) and is limited by cardiac failure (functional status).

Questions

What are the criteria for Marfan's syndrome?

- People with no family history require, apart from skeletal features, involvement of at least two other systems and one of the major criteria (these include ectopia lentis, dilatation of the aortic root or aortic dissection).
- Patients with a family history need features in at least two systems.

What is your differential diagnosis?

Homocystinuria (recessively inherited inborn error of amino acid metabolism due to a deficiency of cystathionine β-synthetase) in which the skeletal features are similar.

How would you differentiate the two?

In homocystinuria the lens is dislocated downwards and there is homocystine in the urine.

Advanced-level Questions

Why do these patients need annual echocardiography?

To monitor aortic diameter and mitral valve function. Prophylactic replacement of the aortic root with a composite graft when the diameter reaches 50–55 mm (normal < 40 mm) prolongs life. Untreated patients commonly die in the fourth or fifth decade from dissection of the aorta or from cardiac failure due to aortic regurgitation. Chronic beta-blockade to produce a negative inotropic effect retards the rate of aortic dilatation. Also, patients should be advised regarding infective endocarditis prophylaxis.

What is the common cause of mortality in Marfan's syndrome?

Cardiovascular complications cause 95% of deaths in such patients and reduce mean life expectancy by 40%.

What are the ocular features of Marfan's syndrome?

- Subluxation of lens.
- Small and spherical lens.
- Glaucoma.
- Hypoplasia of dilator pupillae, making pupillary dilatation difficult.
- Flat cornea.
- Myopia.
- Retinal detachment.

What are the complications of pregnancy in women with Marfan's syndrome?

- Early premature abortion.
- Risk of maternal death from aortic dissection. Pregnancy is not dangerous when the aortic diameter is less than 40 mm.

Is there a gene implicated in Marfan's syndrome?

The Marfan syndrome appears to be caused by mutations in a single fibrillin gene on chromosome 15. Fibrillin is a glycoprotein produced by fibroblasts; it aggregates in conjunction with other proteins or alone in the extracellular matrix. The microfibrillary fibres form the framework on which elastin is deposited. These microfibrillary fibres are particularly abundant in the ciliary zonules that support the lens, in ligaments and in the aorta. Dilatation of the aorta occurs due to cystic medionecrosis.

B-JA Marfan (1858–1942), a French paediatrician, wrote his paper in 1896. He was appointed Foundation Professor of Hygiene at the Clinic of Infantile Diseases in Paris in 1914.

Victor McKusick, contemporary Professor of Medicine at Johns Hopkins Hospital, Baltimore, whose chief interest is genetics.

American President Abraham Lincoln is suspected to have had Marfan's syndrome.

References

Dietz HC, McIntosh I, Sakai LY et al (1993) Four novel FBNI mutations: significance for mutant transcript level and ECF-like domain calcium binding in pathogenesis of Marfan syndrome. *Genomics* **17**: 468–475.

Shores J et al (1994) Progression of aortic dilatation and the benefit of long-term beta-adrenergic blockade in Marfan's syndrome. *N Engl J Med* **330**: 1335.

Tsipuras P, Del-Mastro R, Safarazi M et al (1992) Genetic linkage of the Marfan syndrome, ectopia lentis, and congenital contractural arachnodactyly to fibrillin genes on chromosomes 15 and 5. *N Engl J Med* **326**: 905.

Walker BA & Murdoch JL (1970) The wrist sign. *Arch Intern Med* **126**: 276.

Wood JR, Bellamy D, Child AH & Citron KM (1984) Pulmonary disease in patients with Marfan's syndrome. *Thorax* **39**: 780–784.

CASE 212 **Nephrotic Syndrome**

Instruction

Look at this patient.

Salient features

* Generalized oedema – puffiness of face, pitting oedema of legs and hands.
* Look at the nails for ridges of hypoproteinaemia.
* Comment on the pallor.

Proceed as follows:

* Tell the examiner that you would like to examine:
    The abdomen for ascites.
    The urine for protein and sugar. (Urine microscopy may show oval fat bodies which consist of degenerating tubular epithelial cells having cholesteryl esters. These appear as 'grape clusters' with light microscopy and have a 'Maltese-cross' appearance under polarized light.)

Diagnosis

This patient has nephrotic syndrome (lesion) due to diabetes mellitus (aetiology), and has developed gross anasarca indicating hypoalbuminaemia and marked urinary protein loss (functional status).

Questions

What do you understand by the term 'nephrotic syndrome'?

It consists of albuminuria (more than 3.5 g per day) and hypoalbuminaemia accompanied by generalized oedema, hyperlipidaemia (due to increased hepatic production) and lipiduria.

What causes this syndrome?

- Glomerular disease: minimal-change glomerulonephritis, membranous glomerulonephritis, proliferative glomerulonephritis.
- Systemic disease: diabetes mellitus, SLE, amyloidosis, drugs (captopril, gold, penicillamine, street heroin), Hodgkin's disease, syphilis, malaria, HIV, cancer, hepatitis B.

How would you investigate these patients?

- 24-hour urinary protein, creatinine clearance, urine electrophoresis.
- FBC, ESR.
- Urea and electrolytes, serum creatinine, albumin, cholesterol.
- DNA antibody, antinuclear factor, complement levels.
- Renal biopsy.

What complications may such a patient suffer?

- Thromboembolic events, including renal vein thrombosis and deep vein thrombosis (due to loss of antithrombin III and other proteins involved in the coagulation and fibrinolytic cascade).
- Protein malnutrition.
- Acclerated atherosclerosis.
- Infection.

Advanced-level Questions

What is orthostatic proteinuria?

It is usually seen in adolescents and occurs when standing and resolves on lying down. The long-term prognosis is good.

What do you know about Tamm – Horsfall protein in the urine?

Normal individuals excrete less than 150 mg protein per day. Of this, about 5–15 mg is albumin and the remainder consists of different plasma proteins and glycoproteins derived from renal cells. Tamm–Horsfall mucoprotein is the most abundant protein that is not derived from plasma but from the cells of the ascending limb of the loop of Henle, and is excreted at the rate of 50–75 mg per day. Pathological proteinuria occurs when daily excretion exceeds 150 mg protein.

I Tamm, scientist, Rockefeller University, New York.
FL Horsfall, Professor of Microbiology, Sloan Kettering Institute and Cornell University, New York.
Nephrotic syndrome was clearly described by R Bright (1789–1858), an English physician in the 19th century. He qualified from Edinburgh and worked at Guy's Hospital, London. Chronic nephritis is known as Bright's disease. Three of his renal specimens are still preserved at Guy's Hospital.

Reference

Ritz E (1994) Pathogenesis of idiopathic nephrotic syndrome. *N Engl J Med* **330**: 61–62.

CASE 213 Uraemia

Instruction

Patient 1: Would you like to ask this uraemic patient some questions?

Salient features

Proceed as follows:

- Anorexia, nausea, vomiting and hiccups.
- Fatigue.
- Polyuria, nocturia, dysuria, haematuria, difficulty in passing urine.
- Swelling of the face and feet.
- Shortness of breath (due to secondary left ventricular failure).
- Itching.
- Drug history, in particular NSAIDs, tetracycline.
- History of diabetes, hypertension, recurrent urinary tract infections.
- Family history of renal disease, in particular polycystic kidneys.
- Tell the examiner that you would like to take a history for impotence.

Instruction

Patient 2: Would you like to examine this uraemic patient?

Salient features

- Examine the nails (for Lindsay's 'half-and-half' nails where the proximal portion is whitish while the distal portion is brownish red; the lunula is usually obscured).
- Comment on the lemon tinge of the skin, the pallor and scratch marks. Rarely, there may be 'uraemic frost'.
- Examine the arms for asterixis (flapping tremor), haemodialysis fistula.
- Comment on the vascular shunts, if any.
- Comment on hyperventilation of Kussmaul's respiration secondary to metabolic acidosis.
- Examine the abdomen for palpable kidneys (hydronephrosis, polycystic kidneys) and palpable bladder.
- Check for pitting leg oedema.
- Tell the examiner that you would like to proceed as follows:
   Check the blood pressure (hypertension, hypotension).
   Look for pericardial friction rub.
   Look for evidence of peripheral neuropathy.
   Do a rectal examination.
   Examine the urine for sugar, albumin, specific gravity, microscopy.

Diagnosis

This patient has chronic renal failure (aetiology) due to diabetes mellitus (aetiology), and is currently requiring dialysis as evidenced by the arteriovenous fistula in the arm (functional status).

Questions

How would you investigate a patient with renal failure?

- Urine: glucose, microscopy, specific gravity, creatinine clearance, 24-hour urinary protein.
- Blood: FBC, ESR.
- Serum: urea, electrolytes, creatinine, protein, calcium phosphate, uric acid.
- Ultrasonography of the abdomen for kidneys, bladder.
- Special investigations: pyelography, protein electrophoresis, kidney biopsy.

What do you understand by the term 'azotaemia'?

Azotaemia indicates a raised level of urea and creatinine without symptoms (glomerular filtration rate (GFR) about 20–35% of normal).

What do you understand by the term 'uraemia'?

Uraemia implies a deterioration of renal function associated with symptoms (GFR below 20% of normal).

What are the common causes of chronic renal failure?

- Glomerulonephritis.
- Diabetes mellitus.
- Hypertensive nephropathy.
- Pyelonephritis.
- Polycystic kidney disease.
- Analgesic nephropathy.

Advanced-level Questions

Mention a few drugs that you would avoid in renal failure.

Aminoglycosides, frusemide with cephalosporins, potassium salts, tetracycline.

What are the consequences of renal failure?

- Metabolic: sodium imbalance, hyperkalaemia, metabolic acidosis, hyperuricaemia, hypocalcaemia, hypermagnesaemia, hyperphosphataemia.
- Cardiovascular: cardiac failure, hypertension, accelerated atherosclerosis, pericarditis.
- Haematological: anaemia, clotting disorders, leukocyte abnormalities.
- Skin: itching, hyperpigmentation, bruising.
- CNS: encephalopathy, peripheral neuropathy.
- Gastrointestinal: anorexia, nausea, vomiting, peptic ulcer, diarrhoea.
- Endocrine: vitamin D disorders, secondary hyperparathyroidism, impotence, amenorrhoea, glucose intolerance.

When would you consider dialysis?

- Hyperkalaemia (potassium concentration > 7 mmol l^{-1}).
- Bicarbonate concentration less than 12 mmol l^{-1}.
- Urea level greater than 20 mmol l^{-1}.
- Creatinine concentration greater than 500 μmol l^{-1}.

What are the bone changes in chronic renal failure?

● Osteomalacia (renal rickets).
● Osteitis fibrosa cystica (secondary hyperparathyroidism): subperiosteal erosions especially of the phalanges, long bones and distal end of clavicles.
● Osteosclerosis where there is enhanced density of the bone in the upper and lower margins of vertebrae (rugger-jersey spine).

Is there any benefit in restricting dietary protein in chronic renal disease?

A large randomized controlled trial suggests no benefit from protein restriction.

What is Bricker's trade-off hypothesis?

Early in the course of renal failure, the kidney fails to excrete phosphorous causing a rise in the level of phosphorous in the body. To normalize this rise in serum levels of phosphorous and calcium, the serum parathyroid hormone level rises, but the 'trade-off' is bone disease (osteitis fibrosa cystica). This is the basis for secondary hyperparathyroidism in renal failure.

PG Lindsay, an American physician.
Neil S Bricker, a US nephrologist.
NP Mallick, contemporary Professor of Renal Medicine at the Manchester Royal Infirmary.

References

Klahr S, Andrew S, Levey MD et al (1994) The effects of dietary protein restriction and blood pressure control on the progression of chronic renal disease *N Engl J Med* **330**: 877–884.
Mallick NP (1994) Dietary protein and progression of chronic renal disease. *Br Med J* **309**: 1101–1102.

CASE 214 Paget's Disease

Instruction

Examine this patient's face.
Examine this patient's legs.

Salient features

Face:

- Comment on the hearing aid, if any. Test hearing and determine whether the deafness is a conduction defect (due to involvement of the ossicle) or neural (due to compression of the eighth nerve).
- Typical appearance of the skull and increased skull diameter (more than 55 cm is abnormal).

Proceed as follows:

- Tell the examiner that you would like to examine the fundus for optic atrophy or angioid streaks.

Neck:

- Look for platybasia.
- Raised JVP (cardiac failure in Paget's disease is due to hyperdynamic circulation).

Spine:

- Deformity of the spine – kyphosis; auscultate over the vertebral bodies for bruits. In up to one-third of patients the third and fourth lumbar vertebrae are involved, and in 20% the lower thoracic vertebrae are involved.

Legs:

- Comment on the anterior bowing of the tibia and the lateral bowing of the femur.
- Feel the bone for warmth.

- Tell the examiner that you would like to examine the joints for osteoarthritis (limitation of hip movement, in particular abduction, and fixed flexion deformity of the knees).
- Tell the examiner that you would like to:
  Do a urine analysis (high incidence of renal stones).
  Measure the patient's height (for serial follow-up).
  Compare the patient's appearance with a previous photograph.
  Ask the patient whether there is an increase in hat size.

Remember that Paget's disease is a remodelling disease of isolated areas of the skeleton.

Diagnosis

This patient has Paget's disease (lesion) with hyperdynamic cardiac failure and sensorineural deafness (functional status).

Questions

What are complications of Paget's disease?

- Diminished mobility.
- Fractures.
- Cord compression due to basilar invagination.
- Root lesions due to vertebral damage.
- Hypercalcaemia.
- High-output cardiac failure.
- Sarcomatous changes are seen in less than 2% of patients.

Advanced-level Questions

Mention the neurological complications of Paget's disease.

- Headache.
- Fits.
- Platybasia.
- Hydrocephalus.
- Cerebellar signs.
- Cranial nerve palsies.
- Cord compression.

What are the mechanisms of hearing loss in such patients?

- It is usually due to the disease process involving the ossicles.
- Less commonly it is due to the progressive closure of the skull foramina compressing the eighth cranial nerve.

What is the basic defect in bone metabolism?

Increased osteoclastic activity resulting in bone resorption and increased osteoblastic activity.

What are the radiological manifestations of this disease?

- Skull: 'honeycomb' appearance with underlying osteoporosis circumscripta, 'cottonwool' appearance.
- Pelvis: thickening of the iliopectineal line 'brim-sign', enlargement of ischial and pubic bones.
- Long bones: increased trabeculation.
- Vertebra: sclerotic margins giving a 'picture frame' appearance.
- Remember that a bone scan is more sensitive than an X-ray in determining the extent of disease.

What is the prevalence of Paget's disease?

The exact prevalence is not known but several reports indicate a 3% prevalence in patients over the age of 40 years and increases with age to reach a maximum of 10% by the ninth decade. Males predominate by a ratio of about 2:1.

What factors have been implicated in the aetiology of Paget's disease?

- Slow viral infection – measles syncytial virus, paramyxovirus (canine distemper).
- Genetic factors have been described in Italy.

What are the biochemical features of this disease?

- Serum calcium concentration is normal (except in prolonged immobilization or malignancy).
- Increased bone serum alkaline phosphatase level (indicates increased osteoblastic activity).
- Increased urinary hydroxyproline secretion (indicates increased bone resorption).

Which drug is commonly used in the treatment of this disease?

- Diphosphonates (they inhibit osteoclast-mediated bone resorption).
- Calcitonins (act by reducing osteoclastic activity).

To which patients would you offer therapy?

Treatment is offered to patients with any of the following symptoms:
Agonizing bone pain.
Severe deformity.
Hypercalcaemia.
Cardiac failure.

Sir James Paget (1814–1899), Surgeon, St Bartholomew's Hospital, London. He also described Paget's disease of the nipple (carcinoma involving the areola and the nipple), Paget's disease of the skin (skin cancer involving the apocrine glands) and Paget–Schroetter syndrome (venous thrombosis of the axillary veins, of unknown cause).

Reference

Paget J (1877) On a form of chronic inflammation of bones (osteitis deformans). *Med Chir Trans* **60**: 37.

CASE 215 — Parotid Enlargement

Instruction

Look at this patient's face.

Salient features

- Bilateral parotid enlargement.

Proceed as follows:

- Ask the patient whether the parotids are painful.
- Look for the following conditions:
  Dry mouth.
  Lupus pernio.
  Rheumatoid arthritis.
- Tell the examiner that you would like to know whether the patient has gritty eyes or dry mouth.

Remember that unilateral parotid enlargement with associated facial nerve palsy is more likely to be malignant tumour of the parotids; it is very rare for facial weakness to occur with benign tumours.

Diagnosis

This patient has parotid enlargement, which is painless, and has a dry mouth (lesion) probably due to Sjögren's syndrome (aetiology). The dry mouth is making swallowing difficult (functional status).

Questions

What are the causes of painless bilateral parotid enlargement?

- Sarcoidosis.
- Sjögren's syndrome or keratoconjunctivitis sicca.
- Lymphoma and leukaemia.

How would you test objectively for dry eyes?

Schirmer's test: filter paper is hooked over the lower eyelid; in normal people at least 15 mm is wet in 5 minutes whereas a value of less than 5 mm is seen in sicca syndrome.

What do you know about keratoconjunctivitis sicca?

It is a condition characterized by decreased production of tears by lacrimal glands.

Advanced-level Questions

Mention a few causes of keratoconjunctivitis sicca.

- Primary keratoconjunctivitis sicca is common and characterized by involvement of the lacrimal gland alone.
- Primary Sjögren's syndrome is an autoimmune disorder which is usually positive for rheumatoid factor, antinuclear antibodies and hypergammaglobulinaemia. Less frequently, autoantibodies to DNA, salivary gland, smooth muscle and gastric parietal cells are present. There may be associated dry mouth and bronchial epithelium, and the vagina may also be affected. Histopathogically the glands show intralobar ductal epithelial hyperplasia and lymphocytic infiltration of the gland.
- Secondary Sjögren's syndrome is the presence of keratoconjunctivitis sicca in association with a systemic disorder such as the following:
  Rheumatoid arthritis.
  Psoriatic arthritis.
  Connective tissue disorder.
  Sarcoidosis.
  Crohn's disease.

How would you manage such patients?

- Artificial tears (e.g. hypromellose) are instilled frequently for dry eyes.
- Artificial saliva for dry mouth.

Which are the other salivary glands?

These include submandibular, sublingual and minor salivary glands in the oral cavity, pharynx and larynx.

What do you know about superficial anatomy of the salivary gland?

The gland lies on the lateral surface of the ramus of the mandible and folds itself along the posterior mandibular border. It is usually not palpable as a discrete structure. Clenching the teeth tenses the masseter and makes the anterior border of the gland more prominent (as the gland lies just behind the masseter muscle).

How are parotid secretions carried into the oral cavity?

By Stensen's duct, which opens just opposite the upper second molar tooth.

What is Mikulicz's disease?

It is the enlargement of salivary and lacrimal glands (due to sarcoidosis, lymphoma or tuberculosis) associated with dry mouth and dry eyes but not arthritis.

Which neoplasm may be associated with Sjögren's syndrome?

Usually B cell-derived non-Hodgkin's lymphoma.

OWA Schirmer (1864–1917) a German ophthalmologist.
J von Mikulicz-Radecki (1850–1905) was successively Professor of Surgery at Könisberg and Breslau.
HSC Sjögren (1899–), Swedish Professor of Ophthalmology in Gothenburg.
N Stensen (1638–1686), Danish anatomist and Professor of Anatomy at Copenhagen. He was then appointed the Catholic Bishop of Titiopolis in 1677 and was an international authority on geology. He described the tetralogy of Fallot before Fallot, in 1672.

CASE 216 Superior Vena Caval Obstruction

Instruction

Look at this patient.

Salient features

- Tortuous, visible and dilated veins on the chest wall and neck.
- The neck veins are non-pulsatile.
- The face may be plethoric and suffused. The patient may be short of breath.

Proceed as follows:

- Look for signs of Horner's syndrome and for radiation marks.
- Tell the examiner that you would like to examine for signs of bronchogenic carcinoma, i.e. clubbing, tar staining, lymph nodes and chest signs.

Diagnosis

This patient has superior vena caval obstruction (lesion) which is usually due to bronchogenic carcinoma (aetiology), and is tachypnoeic at rest (functional status).

Questions

What symptoms might the patient have?

- Shortness of breath.
- Dysphagia.
- Blackouts.
- Facial oedema.

What are the causes of superior vena caval obstruction?

- Bronchogenic carcinoma is the commonest cause.
- Lymphoma – in young adults.
- Other causes:
    Aortic aneurysm.
    Mediastinal goitre.
    Mediastinal fibrosis.
    Constrictive pericarditis.

How would you manage this patient?

This condition is a medical emergency and an urgent CT scan of the chest should be requested. Emergency treatment consists of the following:
- Intravenous frusemide to relieve the oedematous component of vena caval compression.
- Intravenous anticancer chemotherapy, e.g. cyclophosphamide.
- Mediastinal irradiation within 24 hours.
- More recently, expandable metal stents have been used to relieve the obstruction.
- Mechanical thrombectomy with an Amplatz thrombectomy device.

Obstruction of the superior vena cava was first described in 1757 by William Hunter in the case of syphilitic aortic aneurysm.

References

Abner A (1993) Approach to a patient who presents with superior vena cava obstruction. *Chest* **103** (suppl 4): 394S.
Kovacs RG & Aguayo SM (1993) Superior vena caval syndrome. *N Engl J Med* **329**: 1007. (Classical picture of this condition.)

Robinson L, Jackson J, Bloom SR, Pride N & Hughes J (1994) New approaches to superior vena caval obstruction: mechanical clearance of thrombus may help *Br Med J* **308**:1697–1699.

Sculier JP & Field R (1985) Superior vena caval obstruction syndrome. Recommendations for management. *Cancer Treat Rev* **12**: 209.

CASE 217 | **Glass Eye**

Instruction

Look at this patient's fundus.
Examine this patient's eyes.
Check this patient's vision or visual fields.

Salient features

- Glass eye which is obvious.
- The patient is blind on the affected side.
- The light reflex is absent.

Proceed as follows:

- Tell the examiner that you would like to take a history for trauma.

Note. Suspect malignant melanoma if asked to examine the abdomen and the liver is palpable (due to metastases).

Diagnosis

This patient has a glass eye (lesion) which is secondary to trauma in childhood (aetiology).

Advanced-level Questions

What is sympathetic ophthalmitis?

It is inflammation that attacks the sound eye after injury (usually perforating wound) of the other. It is almost always a plastic iridocyclitis; rarely it manifests as neuroretinitis or choroiditis. It never occurs after exicison of an injured eye unless it has already commenced at the time of operation. Steroids have improved the prognosis if such treatment is commenced early.

Mention any fungus that can invade the globe.

Rhizopus mucormycosis, originating in the paranasal sinuses and nose, occurs predominantly in patients with poorly controlled diabetes mellitus, malignancy, organ transplantation and those who are receiving long-term desferrioxamine therapy. This fungus can invade the globe or ophthalmic artery to cause blindness.

From which tissues do ocular melanomas arise?

They arise from a variety of ocular tissues including the conjuctiva, uveal tract (iris, ciliary body and choroid), eyelid, orbit and nasolacrimal ducts. Iris melanomas rarely metastasize, whereas ciliary body and choroidal melanomas readily disseminate.

What is the histology of ocular melanomas?

Unlike cutaneous melanomas, the ocular type consists of two distinct cell types – spindle and epithelioid. Lesions composed of completely or predominantly spindle cells have low aggressiveness, do not tend to metastasize and are associated with a 75% survival rate at 15 years. Thus ophthalmologists tend to avoid enucleation. The epithelioid type is associated with only a 35% survival rate despite enucleation, because of late metastases.

CASE 218 Turner's Syndrome

Instruction

Look at this patient.

Salient features

- Webbing of the neck in a female patient.
- Abnormal angulation of both elbows – increased carrying angle (cubitus valgus).
- Dwarfism.
- Receding chin.
- Low hairline over the back of the neck.
- Shield-shaped chest – nipples are widely separated.
- Short fourth metacarpal.
- Lymphoedema of the hands and feet.

Proceed as follows:

- Tell the examiner that you would like to:
    Check for radiofemoral delay (coarctation of the aorta).
    Examine genitalia for infantilism.
    Measure serum FSH and LH levels (these will be high, confirming
        primary hypogonadism).

Diagnosis

This patient has Turner's syndrome (lesion) which is due to the absence of
one of the X chromosomes (aetiology). She has amenorrhoea and skeletal
abnormalities (functional status).

Questions

What constitutes a web?

Either a fan-like fold of skin extending from the shoulder to the neck, or an
abnormal splaying out of the trapezius.

Advanced-level Questions

Which other cardiovascular lesions are associated with webbing of the neck?

Noonan's syndrome or Ullrich's syndrome with pulmonary stenosis.

What is the chromosomal defect in Turner's syndrome?

It is due to the absence of one of the X chromosomes (blood karyotype
showing 46,XO). Other variants of the syndrome include 46,X (with
abnormal X), 45,XO/46,XX mosaics and 45,XO/46,XY mosaics.

What are the facial features of Turner's syndrome?

Ptosis, micrognathia, low-set ears, epicanthal folds.

What are the renal abnormalities associated with Turner's syndrome?

Horseshoe kidney, hydronephrosis.

How would you manage such patients?

The treatment is supportive and includes replacement hormone therapy on
attaining puberty, primarily to prevent osteoporosis and induce sexual
maturation and menses.

What do you know about Lyon's hypothesis?

In 1961, geneticist Mary Lyon outlined that only one of the X
chromosomes is genetically active, whereas the other is inactive. The
inactivation of either the maternal or paternal X chromosome occurs at
random among all the cells of the blastocyst around the 16th day of
embryonic life, and inactivation of the same X chromosome persists in all
cells derived from each precursor cell.

More recent studies, however, have shown that many genes escape X
chromosome inactivation and that both X chromosomes are important for
normal growth, as evidenced by severe abnormalities in Turner's syndrome
with a monosomy of X chromosome. It is now believed that a gene which
maps Xq13 serves as a master switch that is critical for 'switching-off'
most of the genes on the active chromosome 13. This gene is known as X-
inactive-specific transcript gene (XIST).

Henry H Turner (b.1892), an American endocrinologist, described this condition in
1938.
Mary Lyon (b. 1925), contemporary geneticist working for the Medical Research
Council in Oxford.

CASE 219 Yellow Nail Syndrome

Instruction

Look at this patient's hands.

Salient features

• Yellow discoloration of all the nails. The nails are often smooth,
  thickened and overcurved. There is no involvement of the skin.

Proceed as follows:

• Tell the examiner that you would like to:
    Examine the chest (for pleural effusion, bronchiectasis).
    Examine the legs for lymphoedema.
    Ask about past history of sinusitis.

Diagnosis

This patient has yellow nail syndrome (lesion) complicated by severe
bronchiectasis (functional status).

Advanced-level Questions

What is the pathogenesis?

The pathogenic mechanism underlying the yellow nail syndrome has not been defined. Abnormality of lymphatic vessels was suggested as the cause by Samman and White in their original description of the syndrome. This theory is supported by lymphangiographic findings which in most patients showed few, hypoplastic or dilated, deficient lymphatics. Electron microscopy in two cases noted dilated but otherwise normal lymphatics.

Mention some associations with this syndrome.

- Malignancy (melanoma, carcinoma of larynx, lung and breast, Hodgkin's disease).
- Thyroid disease (Hashimato's thyroiditis, hypothyroidism, thyrotoxicosis).
- Hypogammaglobulinaemia.
- Rheumatoid arthritis.

This syndrome was first described in 1964 by PD Samman and WF White.

References

Nordkild P, Kromann-Andersen H & Struve-Christensen E (1986) Yellow nails syndrome – the triad of yellow nails, lymphoedema and pleural effusions. *Acta Med Scand* **219**: 221–227.

Pavlidakev GP, Hashimato K & Blum D (1984) Yellow nails syndrome. *J Am Acad Dermatol* **11**: 509–512.

Runyon BA, Forker EL & Sopko JA (1979) Pleural fluid kinetics in a patient with primary lymphoedema, pleural effusion and yellow nails. *Am Rev Respir Dis* **119**: 821.

Samman PD & White WF (1964) The yellow nails syndrome. *Br J Dermatol* **76**: 153–157.

Solal-Celigny P, Cormier Y & Purnier M (1983) The yellow nail syndrome. Light and electron microscopy aspects of the pleura. *Arch Pathol Lab Med* **107**: 183–185.

Venecie PY & Dicken CH (1984) Yellow nails syndrome: report of five cases. *J Am Acad Dermatol* **10**: 187–192.

CASE 220 Osteogenesis Imperfecta

Instruction

Look at this patient's eyes.

Salient features

- Blue sclera.

Proceed as follows:

- Look for the following signs:
    Hearing loss due to otosclerosis.
    Signs of old fractures.
    Defective dentine formation in the teeth.
    Kyphosis and scoliosis.
    Joint hypermobility.
    Hernias.
    Aortic regurgitation.
- Tell the examiner that you would like to ask some questions:
    About previous fractures.
    Whether or not the condition runs in the family.

Diagnosis

This patient has blue sclera with abnormalities of skeleton and teeth (lesion) due to osteogenesis imperfecta tarda (aetiology), and is disabled by the condition (functional status).

Questions

Why is the sclera blue?

Because the choroid pigment is visible.

Mention other conditions in which the sclera is blue.

- Marfan's syndrome.
- Ehlers–Danlos syndrome.

Advanced-level Questions

What is the inheritance?

Usually autosomal dominant, although some cases may be autosomal recessive.

What are the clinical types?

- Osteogenesis imperfecta congenita (fetal type), in which the fractures occur *in utero* and skeletal abnormalities are present at birth.
- Osteogenesis imperfecta tarda, in which the fractures and deformities occur after birth.

Reference

Editorial (1986) Molecular genetics and osteogenesis imperfecta. *Lancet* **ii**: 496.

 CASE 221 Down's Syndrome

Instruction

Look at this patient.

Salient features

- Collapse of the bridge of the nose.
- Low-set ears.
- Epicanthic folds.

Proceed as follows:

- Look at the iris for Brushfield's spots, i.e. yellow speckles seen in young children.
- Tell the examiner that you would like to:
  Examine the hands for simian palmar crease.
  Examine for short inward curving of the little finger (Siegert's sign).
  Examine the heart for murmur of mitral regurgitation (endocardial cushion defects), and atrial septal defect (ASD) (ostium primum type).
  Check mental status quotient (MSQ) and formal IQ testing (80% have an IQ between 25 and 50).
  Ask the mother at what age she delivered the child (it occurs once in 1550 live births in women under the age of 20 years, in contrast to 1 in 25 live births for mothers over the age of 45 years).

Diagnosis

This patient has features of Down's syndrome (lesion) which is usually due to trisomy 21 (aetiology) and is associated with a reduced life expectancy (functional status).

Questions

What complications can be seen in such patients?

- Increased incidence of acute leukaemia.
- Presenile dementia of Alzheimer type (occurs in the fourth and fifth decades and reduces life expectancy).
- Atlantoaxial subluxation.
- Duodenal atresia in children.

Advanced-level Questions

Mention two chromosomal abnormalities seen in this condition.

- Trisomy 21.
- Mosaicism (46,XY/47,XY, +21). Approximately 1% are mosaics due to mitotic non-dysjunction.

What are the underlying genetic mechanisms?

- Non-dysjunction (occurs during meiosis, particularly in the ovum, and correlates with maternal age).
- *De novo* translocation.
- Familial translocation usually robertsonian translocation of the long arm of chromosome 21 to another acrocentric chromosome, e.g. 22 or 14.

Which maternal serum markers are used for prenatal screening of Down's syndrome?

Serum α-fetoprotein, chorionic gonadotrophin and oestriol.

J Langdon Down (1828–1896) wrote an article in *Clinical Lectures and Reports of the London Infirmary* (now the Royal London Hospital) in 1866 entitled 'The ethnic classification of idiots'.
T Brushfield (1858–1937), a British physician.
Ferdinand Siegert (1865–1946), a German paediatrician.
Hyman Isaac Goldstein (1887–1954), an American physician, described Goldstein's sign which is a wide space between the great toe and the adjoining toe seen in Down's syndrome.

Reference

Antonrakis SE (1991) Parental origin of the extra chromosome 21 as indicated by analysis of DNA polymorphisms. *N Engl J Med* **324**: 872.

CASE 222 Late Congenital Syphilis

Instruction

Look at this patient.

Salient features

- Collapsed bridge of the nose (saddle nose or Zaufal's sign).
- Corneal opacity (interstitial keratitis).
- Rhagades (linear scars at the angles of the mouth).
- Peg-shaped incisors (Hutchinson's teeth).
- Perforation of the palate.
- Frontal bossing.

Proceed as follows:

Check for deafness (nerve deafness).
Look at the shins for sabre tibia.
Look for Clutton's joints (bilateral knee effusions).
Look at the fundus for optic atrophy.

Diagnosis

This patient has a saddle nose and peg-shaped incisors (lesions) due to congenital syphilis caused by maternal *Treponema pallidum* infection (aetiology).

Advanced-level Questions

What is Hutchinson's triad?

- Interstitial keratitis.
- Deafness.
- Typical dental change, i.e. peg-shaped incisors (Hutchinson's teeth).

What are the ocular features of congenital syphilis?

- Interstitial keratitis.

- Retinopathy – fine pigmentation, 'salt and pepper fundus'.

Sir Johnathan Hutchinson (1828–1913) was simultaneously a surgeon at The London Hospital (now the Royal London Hospital), an ophthalmologist at Moorfields Hospital and a dermatologist at Blackfriars Hospital (now closed).
H Clutton (1850–1901), an English surgeon who worked at St Thomas's Hospital, London.
Emanuel Zaufal (1833–1910), a Czechoslovakian rhinologist.

CASE 223 Arteriovenous Fistula

Instruction

Look at this patient's arms.

Salient features

- Hypertrophy of the affected arm.
- Prominent, dilated, tortuous veins.
- Continuous thrill over the fistula; listen for continuous bruit.
- Collapsing pulse; increased pulse pressure indicating hyperdynamic circulation.

Proceed as follows:

- Look for signs of cardiac failure.
- Elicit Branham's sign, i.e. slowing of the pulse on occluding the feeding vessel of the fistula.
- If the fistula is in the upper limb, then perform Allen's test: the radial and ulnar arteries are occluded at the wrist and the hand is exercised; the arteries are then released one at a time to establish which is the dominant feeding vessel.
- Look for signs of chronic renal failure.

Diagnosis

This patient has an arteriovenous fistula (lesion) which has been surgically created (aetiology) for haemodialysis and is functioning well.

Advanced-level Questions

How are arteriovenous malformations classified?

Angiographically, as follows:
- Group 1 – predominantly arterial or arteriovenous lesions: present with pain, hypertrophy of the digit or limb, deformity, distal ischaemia, venous hypertension; large lesions can cause symptoms and signs of cardiac failure.
- Group 2 – lesions affecting tiny vessels including capillaries: for example, port-wine stain, epistaxis in hereditary haemorrhagic telangiectasia, gastrointestinal haemorrhage with colonic dysplasia.
- Group 3 – predominantly venous lesions: local oedema, pain and venous ulceration; there may be a history of trauma.

How would you manage a patient with an arteriovenous malformation?

- Referral to a vascular surgeon.
- Doppler ultrasonography.
- Angiography.

When and how is an arteriovenous malformation treated?

Arteriovenous malformations are treated when they cause discomfort, disfigurement and danger to the patient. The patient should be jointly assessed by a vascular surgeon and an interventional radiologist for embolization. The temptation to ligate the feeder vessel should be resisted as subsequent embolization may be difficult. Complete exicision of the fistula is accepted treatment in resistant cases.

EV Allen (1900–1961), Professor of Medicine at the Mayo Clinic, Rochester, Minnesota, introduced coumarin anticoagulants into clinical practice and edited one of the first comprehensive textbooks on peripheral vascular disease.
HH Branham, an American surgeon in the nineteenth century.

Reference

Allison DJ & Kennedy A (1991) ABC of vascular diseases: peripheral arteriovenous malformations. *Br Med J* **303**:1191–1194.

CASE 224 Carotid Artery Aneurysm

Instruction

Examine this patient's neck.

Salient features

- Pulsatile swelling along the course of the carotids, usually unilateral (the swelling may be firm) and at the base of the neck.

Proceed as follows:

- Auscultate over the mass for a bruit.
- Look for Horner's syndrome.
- Tell the examiner that you would like to proceed as follows:
  Examine all peripheral pulses.
  Examine the heart and blood pressure.

Diagnosis

This patient has a carotid artery aneurysm (lesion) due to atherosclerosis (aetiology), and may require surgery before the lesion ruptures (functional status).

Advanced-level Questions

How would you manage this patient?

- All patients must be referred to a vascular surgeon.
- Check urine for sugar.
- Serum lipids.
- Intravenous carotid digital subtraction angiography.

CASE 225 Retro-orbital Tumour

Instruction

Examine this patient's eyes.

Salient features

- Unilateral exophthalmos.

- Impaired extraocular movement (due to either muscle or nerve involvement).
- Chemosis, conjunctival oedema.
- Radiation marks may be present.

Proceed as follows:

- Examine the visual acuity and visual fields.
- Look for pulsations over the globe.
- Palpate the orbital margin for erosion of the underlying bone.
- Auscultate over the globe for bruit.

Diagnosis

This patient has a retro-orbital tumour with a bruit over the globe (lesion) indicating a pulsatile structure such as an arteriovenous fistula in the orbit (aetiology). The tumour is causing considerable distress to the patient (functional status).

Advanced-level Questions

What is your differential diagnosis?

- The commonest cause of unilateral exophthalmos is Graves' disease.
- Other causes are as follows:
    Retro-orbital tumour (primary or metastatic).
    Arteriovenous fistula (carotico-cavernous fistula).
    Cavernous sinus thrombosis.
    Orbital cellulitis.

What investigations would you do?

- T_4, TSH, free T_3.
- Orbital ultrasonography.
- Cranial CT, in particular the orbits.

How would you manage such a patient?

- Ophthalmology opinion.
- Therapy – radiation to the orbit and steroids, and surgical decompression, depending on the underlying aetiology.

What are the causes of a unilateral pulsating proptosis?

- Arteriovenous fistula between the carotid artery and cavernous sinus – stops with pressure on the artery in the neck.

- Aneurysm of the ophthalmic artery.
- Cirsoid aneurysm of the orbit.
- Vascular neoplasms in the orbit growing rapidly.

CASE 226 Achondroplasia

Instruction

Look at this patient.

Salient features

- Dwarfism.
- Bulging forehead.
- Depression of the root of the nose.
- Shortened proximal extremities.
- Trunk of normal size.

Proceed as follows:

- Tell the examiner that you would like to take a family history (autosomal dominant inheritance; however, 80% are new mutations).

Diagnosis

This patient with short stature and normal trunk size has achondroplasia (lesion), which is due to mutation of the fibroblast growth factor receptor gene (aetiology).

Questions

Is the life span reduced in these subjects?

No, they have a normal life span.

How is the IQ affected in these patients?

The IQ in these patients is normal.

Is the reproductive status affected?

No, they have a normal reproductive status.

What do you know about the genetics of achondroplasia?

It is inherited as an autosomal dominant trait with complete penetrance. Mutations of the fibroblast growth factor receptor 3 (FGFR-3) gene with the transition from guanine to adenine or a guanine to cytosine transversion at nucleotide 1138 is the defect in these patients.

CASE 227 Breast Lump

Instruction

Examine this patient's breasts.

Salient features

- Breast lump which is non-tender and poorly delineated margins. Asymmetry of the breasts and retraction or dimpling of the skin can often be accentuated by having the patient raise her arms overhead or press her hands on her hips to contract the pectoralis muscle.

Proceed as follows:

- Examine axillary and supraclavicular lymph nodes.
- Look for oedema of the ipsilateral arm (due to metastatic infiltration of regional lymphatics).
- Examine the chest (metastases, lymphangitis carcinomatosa).
- Examine for hepatomegaly (metastases).
- Tell the examiner that you would like to take a history of:
    Breast pain, nipple discharge, erosion, enlargement or itching of the nipple.
    Back or bone pain, jaundice or weight loss (indicate systemic metastases).

Diagnosis

This patient has a breast lump which is infiltrating the skin and axillary lymph nodes (lesion) indicating malignant breast carcinoma (aetiology).

Questions

How would you investigate such a patient?

- FBC and ESR (ESR is consistently raised).
- Urea and electrolytes, liver function tests (hypercalcaemia, raised alkaline phosphatase level indicates bone or liver metastases).
- Biopsy: large needle-core biopsy, fine-needle aspiration or open biopsy under local anaesthesia.
- Carcinoembyronic antigen (CEA) could be a marker for recurrence.
- Imaging for metastases:
  Chest X-ray for lung secondaries.
  CT scan of liver or brain when metastasis is suspected in these areas.
  Bone scanning (if patient has bone pain or raised alkaline phosphatase level).

Advanced-level Questions

How would you investigate a patient with a suspicious mammogram but no clinical evidence of mass?

Although a mass cannot be palpated, the patient should undergo a mammographic localization biopsy.

What are the histological types of breast cancer?

They are of two main types which may be invasive or *in situ*:
- Ductal: arising from the epithelial lining of large or intermediate-sized ducts. Most arise from intermediate ducts and are invasive (e.g. invasive ductal, infiltrating ductal). When ductal carcinoma has not invaded extraductal tissue, it is intraductal or *in situ* ductal.
- Lobular: arising from the epithelium of the terminal ducts of the lobules.

How are patients with breast cancer managed?

- Surgery:
  Breast-conserving surgery (lumpectomy, axillary dissection and radiation therapy) is usually offered to patients with single tumours less than 4 cm in diameter, because the cosmetic outcome of excising larger tumours is poor. However, in 80% of patients with large tumours and in 25% of those with locally advanced breast cancers, breast conservation is possible if the size of the tumour is reduced by a course of primary systemic treatment (such as combination chemotherapy and hormonal therapy).
  Modified radical mastectomy (total mastetcomy, removal of the overlying skin, nipple as well as the underlying pectoralis

fascia with axillary lymph node dissection). The major
advantage is that radiation is not necessary, but many patients
suffer from the psychological trauma of breast loss.

- Adjuvant therapy:
  CMF regimen (cyclophosphamide, methotrexate and fluorouracil).
  MMM regimen (mitozantrone, methotrexate and mitomycin C).
  Doxorubicin and cyclophosphamide.
  Tamoxifen.
- Palliative therapy:
  Radiotherapy (may be complicated by brachial plexus neuropathy),
  hormonal treatment (tamoxifen, diethylstilboestrol, megestrol
  acetate, aminoglutethimide).

Which breast cancers are suitable for treatment by conservative breast surgery?

- Single clinical and mammographic lesion.
- Tumours less than 4 cm in diameter (or those greater than 4 cm in a
  large breast).
- No sign of local advancement.

Which patients are best treated by mastectomy?

- Those who prefer mastectomy.
- Those in whom breast conservation would produce an unacceptable
  cosmetic result.
- Those with either clinical or mammographic evidence of more than one
  focus of cancer in the breast.

What factors are associated with increased rates of local recurrence after mastectomy?

Axillary lymph node involvement, lymphatic or vascular invasion by
cancer, grade III carcinoma or tumours greater than 4 cm in diameter.

Which patients are more likely to respond to hormone therapy?

Women with high levels of oestrogen receptors in the tumour, when there
is a long interval from initial surgery to time of relapse, and those with
metastatic disease in bone and soft tissue (unlike those with liver or
lymphangitis carcinomatosa).

Are women with fibroadenomas at increased long-term risk of breast cancer?

Not all patients with fibroadenomas are at increased risk, but those with a family history of breast cancer, complex fibroadenomas or proliferative disease have an increased long-term risk of breast cancer.

What is the role of implants for breast augmentation?

In breast cancer, silicone gel implants were used for augmentation, but with new evidence that these may cause autoimmune reactions or connective tissue disorders, doctors have stopped using these implants. Saline implants do not work well for reconstruction after surgery for breast cancer or for very thin women. If silicone gel implants are removed from the market, these patients will have no alternative.

Which genes have been implicated in familial breast cancer?

There may be more than five genes causing familial breast cancer; the most important of these is *BRCA1* located on the long arm of chromosome 17. The gene *p53* on the short arm of chromosome 17 has been implicated in the rare breast cancer family syndrome (the Li Fraumeni syndrome, in which breast cancer occurs at a younger age associated with soft tissue sarcoma, osteosarcoma, adrenal tumours, gliomas and other childhood tumours).

In 1894 William Halsted published his seminal report on radical mastectomy for the cure of cancer of the breast.
RAGE (Radiotherapy Action Group Exposure) is a pressure group formed by patients who suffered the side-effects of radiotherapy including brachial plexus neuropathy, often resulting in severe pain and the loss of use of the arm.

References

Dixon JM (1995) Surgery and radiotherapy for early breast cancer. *Br Med J* **311**: 1515–1516.
Dupont WD, Page DL, Parl FF et al (1994) Long-term risk of breast cancer in women with fibroadenoma. *N Engl J Med* **331**: 10–15.
Henderson IC (1995) Paradigmatic shifts in the management of breast cancer. *N Engl J Med* **332**: 951–952.
Sainsbury JRC, Anderson TJ, Morgan DAL & Dixon JM (1994) Breast cancer. *Br Med J* **309**: 1149–1154.
Spittle MF (1995) Brachial plexus neuropathy after radiotherapy for breast cancer. *Br Med J* **311**: 1516–1517.

CASE 228 Gingival Hypertrophy

Instruction

Look at this patient's mouth.

Salient features

- Hypertrophy of the gums.

Proceed as follows:

- Look for other features of chronic phenytoin therapy (coarsening of facial features, hypertrichosis, hirsutism, generalized lymphadenopathy, rash, cerebellar syndrome, peripheral lymphadenopathy).
- Tell the examiner that you would like to take a history of:
  Drugs (phenytoin, cyclosporin, nifedipine).
  Leukaemia (myelomonocytic leukaemia).

Diagnosis

This patient has poor oral hygiene and gingival hypertrophy (lesion) due to chronic ingestion of phenytoin (aetiology).

Questions

What are the other long-term side-effects of phenytoin?

Coarsening of facial features, rashes, systemic lupus erythematosus, blood dyscrasias, generalized lymphadenopathy, induction of hepatic microsomal enyzmes, folic acid deficiency, peripheral neuropathy, cerebellar syndrome (ataxia, nystagmus and dysarthria), hypertrichosis, osteomalacia and encephalopathy. When taken during pregnancy may result in cleft lip and palate in the child.

In which types of seizure is phenytoin generally used?

Generalized clonic–tonic seizures.

Reference

van Uum SH & Keuning J-J (1994) Gingival hypertrophy in myelomonocytic leukaemia. *N Engl J Med* **330**: 826. (A classical picture of gingival hypertrophy.)

CASE 229 Haemophilia A

Instruction

Examine this patient's knee (or elbow) joint; he has a bleeding disorder.

Salient features

- Male patient.
- Fixed deformity of the joint (haemarthrosis causes bone and joint destruction).

Proceed as follows:

- Tell the examiner that you would like to know whether there is a family history of bleeding (X-linked recessive disorder).

Diagnosis

This patient has a fixed deformity of the elbow (lesion) due to bleeding into the joint as a complication of haemophilia A (aetiology). The joint is now undergoing osteoarthritic changes (functional status).

Questions

What is the inheritance of haemophilia?

One-third are sporadic and the rest are X-linked (defects include deletions, point mutations and insertions on the X chromosome).

What is deficient in haemophilia?

It is Factor VIII:C – the clinical manifestations depend on its level. Levels less than 1% are associated with spontaneous bleeding, whereas patients with levels lower than 5% have severe bleeding after trauma and occasionally spontaneous bleeding. When levels are above 5%, bleeding occurs after trauma.

Advanced-level Questions

How are bleeding episodes treated?

- Factor VIII concentrates: for minor bleeding, factor VIII concentrates should be raised to 20–30% of normal, and for severe bleeding to at least 50%. For major surgery, levels should be raised to 100% and maintained at over 50% until healing has occurred. Patients can stock Factor VIII in domestic refrigerators for self-adminstration to start treatment immediately on bleeding. It is given twice daily and intravenously.

- DDAVP, administered intravenously, can increase factor VIII levels depending on the initial level.

What is the commonest cause of mortality?

Currently, it is HIV infection, transmitted by contaminated Factor VIII concentrate administered in the past. HIV-associated immune thrombocytopenia may worsen the bleeding tendency.

Queen Victoria's descendants are said to have suffered from haemophilia.

In 1803 John Conrad Otto emphasized its inheritance as an X-linked disorder in his description of a New Hampshire family.

In 1964 Pool and co-workers discovered that Factor VIII is concentrated in cryoprecipitate.

In 1984 the Factor VIII gene was cloned and expressed in tissue culture.

Robert Gwyn Macfarlane, Professor at Oxford, did pioneering work on the care of haemophiliacs and was the first to propose the cascade hypothesis of blood coagulation.

Reference

Hoyer LW (1994) Haemophilia A. *N Engl J Med* **330**: 38.

CASE 230 Klinefelter's Syndrome

Instruction

Examine this patient and give us your diagnosis

Salient features

- Male patient with eunuchoid body habitus with abnormally long legs.
- Elongated body with an increase in length between the soles and pubic bone.
- Lack of a beard, and the voice is not masculine.

Proceed as follows:

- Tell the examiner that you would like to:
    Examine the external genitalia (small atrophic testes, lack of male distribution of pubic hair).

Test the IQ (usually lower than normal, although mental disability is
uncommon).
Elicit a history of infertility.
Check for hypo-osmia (Kallman's syndrome).

Diagnosis

This patient has Klinefelter's syndrome (lesion) due to an excess of X and
Y chromosomes (aetiology), and has infertility (functional status).

Questions

How would you investigate such a patient?

- Plasma gonadotrophins (FSH levels are consistently raised).
- Plasma testosterone concentration (variably reduced).
- Plasma oestradiol level (raised).
- Chromosomal analysis (two or more X chromosomes and one or more
  Y chromosomes).

What is the commonest karyotype?

Eighty-two per cent of patients have 47,XXY which results from non-
dysjunction during meiosis in one of the parents.

Advanced-level Questions

What is Kallman's syndrome?

It is idiopathic hypogonadotrophic hypogonadism with involvement of the
hypothalamus. Patients have hypo-osmia and other defects of the
rhinencephalon (cleft lip/palate, congenital deafness and blindness).
Replacement therapy with both gonadotrophins and gonadotrophin
releasing hormone (GnRH) ensures fertility in many of the affected
individuals.

HF Klinefelter (b. 1912), an American physician who worked at Johns Hopkins
Hospital in Baltimore. He described this syndrome with Fuller Albright (1900–
1969) while he was a visiting fellow at Massachusetts General Hospital and
Harvard Medical School. Albright described Albright's syndrome and was stricken
with Parkinson's disease at the age of 36 years, and was rendered invalid in 1953
following surgical attempts to improve his Parkinson's disease.

CASE 231 Macroglossia

Instruction

Examine this patient's mouth.

Salient features

- Protrusion of the resting tongue beyond the teeth or alveolar ridge. The impressions of the teeth may be obvious along the edges of the tongue on either side.

Proceed as follows:

- Tell the examiner that you would like to:
  Ask whether there is any difficulty in breathing or swallowing.
  Look for an underlying cause such as hypothyroidism.

Diagnosis

This patient has macroglossia (lesion) of which the cause is not obvious by clinical examination (aetiology), and which is complicated by heavy breathing (functional status).

Questions

What do you understand by the term macroglossia?

It is a resting tongue that protrudes beyond the teeth or alveolar ridge. It is usually used to indicate long-term painless enlargement rather than the rapid growth of acute parenchymatous glossitis.

What are the types of macroglossia?

- True macroglossia – definitive histopathological findings:
  Primary – characterized by hypertrophy or hyperplasia of tongue muscles.
  Secondary – the result of infiltration of normal tissue with anomalous elements.
- Pseudomacroglossia – relative enlargement secondary to a small mandible with no histological abnormalities.

Advanced-level Questions

What are the causes of true macroglossia?

- In children:
    Hypothyroidism.
    Lymphangioma.
    Haemangioma.
    Idiopathic hyperplasia.
    Metabolic disorders.
    Beckwith–Wiedmann syndrome.
- Secondary macroglossia
    Amyloidosis.
    Acromegaly.
    Angioedema.
    Lymphoma.
    Chronic infections: TB, syphilis.
    Space-occupying lesions: cystic hygroma, cysts in lingual thyo-glossal ducts, rhabdomyosarcoma.

What are the causes of pseudomacroglossia?

Down's syndrome, Pierre Robin syndrome, cerebral palsy.

What are the complications of macroglossia?

- Prolonged exposure can cause ulceration and necrosis of the mouth and tip of the tongue.
- Noisy breathing, drooling and unsightly appearance, particularly in children.
- Maxillofacial defects such as anterior open bite, prognathism.
- Difficulty in swallowing and, as a consequence, poor weight gain.
- Difficulty in the articulation of consonants requiring the tip of the tongue to be in contact with the alveolar ridge or roof of the mouth.
- Airway obstruction which can be life threatening.

How would you manage macroglossia?

- Medical:
    Treatment of the underlying systemic cause, e.g. thyroxine in hypothyroidism, bromocriptine in acromegaly.
    Steroids – in life-threatening airway obstruction or postoperative oedema.

- Surgical:
    Reduction glossectomy for symptomatic macroglossia.
    Excision for neoplastic lesions.
- Rehabilitation of physical and psychological problems:
    Secondary orthodontic care and speech therapy.
    Psychological and psychiatric support.

Reference

Murthy P & Laing MR (1994) Macroglossia. *Br Med J* **309**: 1386.

CASE 232 **Osteoporosis of the Spine (Dowager's Hump)**

Instruction

Examine this patient's spine.

Salient features

- Elderly patient (usually a woman).
- Marked kyphosis.
- Loss of height.
- Protuberant abdomen.

Proceed as follows:

- Look for spinal tenderness, demonstrate straight-leg rising sign.
- Tell the examiner that you would like to know whether the patient:
    Has a history of back pain (usually the onset is sudden with severe pain in the dorsal spine).
    Has been on long-term corticosteroid therapy.
    Is postmenopausal or has had an oopherectomy.
    Is a smoker and consumes alcohol.
    Has a family history.

Diagnosis

This elderly patient with marked kyphosis (lesion) has postmenopausal osteoporosis (aetiology) complicated by frequent fractures and loss of height (functional status).

Questions

What do you understand by the term osteoporosis?

It is a disorder resulting from the combination of low bone mass (osteopenia) and low trauma fractures.

Advanced-level Questions

What are the types of osteoporosis?

- Type I: results from accelerated bone loss, particularly trabecular bone, and is probably due to oestrogen deficiency. It typically results in fractures of vertebral bodies and the distal forearm in women in their 60s and 70s.
- Type II: results from age-related bone loss and is much slower. It occurs in both sexes and typically results in fracture of the proximal femur in the elderly.
- Secondary osteoporosis: accounts for about 20% of cases in women and 40% of cases in men.

What are the typical sites of fracture in osteoporosis?

Vertebrae, neck of femur, distal radius (Colles' fracture).

What are the clinical consequences of osteoporosis?

Increased mortality rate (increases by 20% in the first year after hip fracture), pain, deformities (kyphosis, loss of height and abdominal protrusion) and loss of independence.

What are the risk factors for osteoporosis?

Smoking, high alcohol consumption, thin body type in women, heredity, premature menopause, prolonged secondary amenorrhoea, primary hypogonadism, corticosteroid therapy, anorexia nervosa, malabsorption, primary hyperparathyroidism, organ transplantation, chronic renal failure, hyperthyroidism, prolonged immobilization.

How would you investigate such a patient?

- X-rays and bone scans looking for fractures and to exclude metastases.
- Serum calcium and phosphates, alkaline phosphatase and creatinine (remember osteoporosis is not a disorder of calcium metabolism).

- 24-hour urinary calcium and creatinine excretion.
- Urinary Bence Jones protein concentration and serum protein electrophoresis.
- Thyroid-stimulating hormone concentrations.
- Serum testosterone level in men.
- Dual-energy X-ray absorptiometry (DEXA) scanning, which determines bone density.

How would you prevent osteoporosis?

- Life-style advice: exercise, stop smoking and reduce alcohol consumption.
- Replacement oestrogen therapy in postmenopausal women.
- Dietary calcium intake increased to 1.5 g per day.
- Alendronate, which is a new bisphosphonate. It is 1000 times more potent than etidronate in inhibiting bone resorption and hence is able to provide effective inhibition at a dosage that does not affect bisphosphonates. Long-term safety profile is awaited. Other new bisphosphonates currently being evaluated include tiludronate and residronate.

What is the pathology of osteoporosis?

It is characterized by a decrease in the amount of bone present, so that the structural integrity of the skeleton is compromised. The rate of bone formation is normal but the rate of bone resorption is increased. This results in greater loss of trabecular bone than compact bone, accounting for the clinical features of the disease.

A Colles (1773–1843), Professor of Anatomy and Surgery at the College of Surgeons (Ireland).

References

Liberman UA, Weiss SR, Bröll J et al (1995) Effect of oral alendronate on mineral density and the incidence of fractures in post-menopausal osteoporosis. *N Engl J Med* **333**:1437–1443.

Peel N & Eastell R (1995) Osteoporosis. *Br Med J* **310**: 989–992.

Reid IR, Ames RW, Evans MC, Gamble GD & Sharpe SJ (1993) Effect of calcium supplementation of bone loss in postmenopausal women. *N Engl J Med* **328**: 460–464. (This study showed that calcium supplementation significantly slows axial and appendicular bone loss in normal postmenopausal women.)

Sambrook P, Birmingham J, Kelly P et al (1993) Prevention of corticosteroid osteoporosis. *N Engl J Med* **328**:1747–1752. (This study showed that calcitriol and calcium used prophylactically, with or without calcitonin, prevent corticosteroid-induced bone loss in the lumbar spine.)

CASE 233   Pressure Sores (Bedsores)

Instruction

Look at this leg.

Salient features

- Pressure sore over the sacrum.
.

Proceed as follows:

- Look for pressure sores elsewhere, particularly the skin overlying the occiput, ears, elbows, hips and ankles.
- Comment on any obvious paralysis or incontinence (the latter contributes to ulcers in the sacral areas).
- Comment on skin traction or any orthopaedic splints (as 70% are orthopaedic patients).
- Tell the examiner that you would like to culture and biopsy the ulcer if it has not been healing properly or looks suspicious.

Questions

What are the causes of pressure sores?

- Loss of sensation and when circulation or nutrition to the skin and underlying tissue are compromised: diabetes mellitus, malnutrition, peripheral vascular disease, oedema, arthritis, anaemia, general debility.
- Others: sedation, urinary or faecal incontinence, sedation and anaesthesia.

How are pressure sores best prevented?

- Good nursing care, nutrition and maintenance of skin hygiene.
- Moribund, paralysed patients should be turned frequently (at least every hour) and pressure points should be inspected for areas of redness and tenderness.
- Water-beds, alternating pressure mattresses and sheep skins are useful.

Advanced-level Questions

How are pressure sores graded?

- Grade I: erythema, skin intact.
- Grade II: skin loss, epidermis or dermis (abrasion, blister, shallow crater).
- Grade III: full thickness loss and damage to subcutaneous tissues.
- Grade IV: extensive destruction, tissue necrosis or damage to the underlying muscle or bone.

CASE 234 Sickle Cell Disease

Instruction

Examine this patient's hands who has recurrent episodes of abdominal pain, precipitated by infection.

Salient features

- Afro-Caribbean patient.
- Anaemia.
- Digits of varying lengths (may be painful).

Proceed as follows:

- Tell the examiner that you would like to ask about:
    Bone pain.
    Past history of strokes, fits.
    Priapism.
    Family history of similar problem.
    Precipitating factors (infection, dehydration, cold, acidosis or hypoxia).
- Tell the examiner that you would like to examine the:
    Urine for haematuria (renal papillary necrosis).
    Leg for arterial ulcers.
    Abdomen for hepatomegaly.
    Heart for cardiomegaly and hyperdynamic circulation.
    Retina (for neovascularization which may cause blindness).

Diagnosis

This African black patient has evidence of old dactylitis (lesions) due to sickle cell anaemia (aetiology) which has caused severe deformity of the hand. She has difficulty buttoning her clothes (functional status).

Questions

What is the abnormality in this patient?

This patient has a structural abnormality of the haemoglobin chain where there is a single base mutation from adenine to thymine which produces a substitution of valine for glutamine at the sixth codon of the β-globin chain. This results in the characteristic sickle appearance of haemoglobin. Sickling can produce a shortened red cell survival and impaired passage of cells through the microcirculation leading to obstruction of small vessels and tissue infarction.

What do you know about the genetics of this syndrome?

In the homozygous state, i.e. sickle cell anaemia, both genes are abnormal (Hb SS), whereas in the heterozygous state, i.e. sickle cell trait, only one chromosome carries the gene (Hb AS). The disease does not manifest until the Hb F decreases to adult levels at about 6 months of age.

Does the haemoglobin level fall during a sickle cell crisis?

The patient has 'steady state' anaemia and the haemoglobin level does not fall unless there is parvovirus-induced bone marrow aplasia, drug-induced haemolysis or sequestration of sickle cells in the liver and spleen.

Is the spleen enlarged in these patients?

The spleen may be enlarged, in childhood, due to haemolysis but in adult life patients often undergo autosplenectomy (due to infarcts) which increases their susceptibility to infection by *Streptococcus pneumoniae* (pneumonia, meningitis) and salmonella osteomyelitis.

What are the other complications of this disease?

Chronic leg ulcers (due to ischaemia), pigmentary gallstones (due to persistent haemolysis), aseptic necrosis of femoral heads and chronic renal disease.

How would you investigate these patients?

- FBC: haemoglobin 6–8 g dl^{-1}, with raised reticulocyte count.
- Blood smear shows signs of hyposplenism (Howell–Jolly bodies, target cells).
- Sickling of red cells can be introduced by sodium metabisulphite.

- Haemoglobin electrophoresis: there is no haemoglobin A, 80–95% Hb SS and 2–20% Hb F. High Hb F levels are associated with a more benign progress. The parents of the patient will show features of sickle cell trait (remember that sickle cell trait protects against *Plasmodium falciparum* malaria).
- Hydroxyurea and erythropoietin are given to increase synthesis of Hb F.

How would you manage an acute sickle cell crisis?

Supportive therapy with intravenous fluids, oxygen, antibiotics and analgesia. Folic acid is given for those with severe haemolysis.

What is the role of blood transfusion in these patients?

Steady-state anaemia requires no treatment and regular blood transfusions are given only when the anaemia is severe or if the patient has frequent episodes of crisis, particularly during pregnancy (to suppress endogenous production of Hb S).

What is the prognosis of this condition?

It is variable with some having a normal life span while others succumb in the first few years of life to infection or episodes of sequestration. Median age of death is 42 years for homozygotes.

WH Howell (1860–1945), Professor of Physiology at Johns Hopkins Hospital, Baltimore, who also discovered and isolated heparin.
JMJ Jolly (1870–1953), French Professor of Histology.

Reference

Griffin TC, McIntire D & Buchanan GR (1994) High-dose intravenous methylprednisolone therapy for pain in children and adolescents with sickle cell disease. *N Engl J Med* **330**: 733–737.

CASE 235 Thrush

Instruction

Look at this patient's tongue.

Salient features

- Superficial white patches or large fluggy membranes that are easily detachable, e.g. by a tongue depressor, leaving underlying erythema.

Proceed as follows:

- Look for other sites of candidal infection (eczematoid lesions in moist areas of the skin, such as inframammary folds, inguinal creases, between the fingers and toes).
- Look for id reactions (which are hypersensitivity cutaneous reactions remote from the site of infection).
- Ask the patient about dysphagia (oesophagitis).
- Tell the examiner that you would like to investigate for underlying:
  Diabetes mellitus.
  Neutropenia (secondary to chronic granulomatous disease, leukaemia, anticancer therapy or immunosuppressive drugs).
  Drugs (steroids, broad-spectrum antibiotics and oral contraceptives).
  HIV infection.
  Polyendocrine deficiencies (including hypoparathyroidism, hypoadrenalism and hypothyroidism).

Diagnosis

This patient has oral thrush or candidal infection (lesion), which is a complication of the use of the broad-spectrum antibiotic tetracycline (aetiology), and has dysphagia (functional status).

Questions

What is the most common species that causes human infection?

Candida albicans.

How would you confirm your diagnosis?

- Wet preparation of a smear with potassium hydroxide will confirm spores and may show non-septate mycelia.
- Biopsy will show intraepithelial pseudomycelia.

With which type of antibiotics is candidal infection common?

Broad-spectrum antibiotics, e.g. tetracycline, chloramphenicol.

Which candidal species usually colonizes skin?

C. parapsilosis.

How would you treat candidal infection?

Effective antifungal therapy may be achieved with fluconazole, ketoconazole, clotrimazole or nystatin.

What are the features of disseminated candidiasis?

Disseminated candidiasis manifests with systemic features including fever, toxicity, pulmonary involvement, endocarditis and retinal abscesses. Very rarely, it may cause focal manifestations including pustular skin abscesses, osteomyelitis, myositis, brain abscess or meningitis. It often causes sepsis associated with intravenous catheterization. Patients with blood cultures with *Candida* should receive intravenous amphotericin B.

References

Laine L (1994) The natural history of oesophageal candidiasis after successful treatment in patients with AIDS. *Gastroenterology* **107**: 744.

Roth JS & Grossman E (1994) Cutaneous lesions of disseminated candidiasis. *N Engl J Med* **330**: 1650.

Walsh TJ, Hathorn JW, Sobel JD et al (1991) Detection of circulating candida enolase by immunoassay in patients with cancer and invasive candidiasis. *N Engl J Med* **324**: 1026–1031.

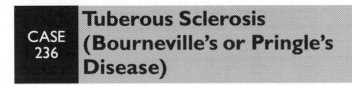

CASE 236

Tuberous Sclerosis (Bourneville's or Pringle's Disease)

Instruction

Look at this patient who has a history of seizures and mental retardation.

Salient features

- Angiofibromas (adenoma sebaceum) distributed in a butterfly pattern over the cheeks, chin and forehead.

- Shagreen patches (leathery thickenings in localized patches over the lumbosacral region).
- Ash-leaf patches (hypopigmented areas).
- Subungual fibromas.

Proceed as follows:

- Tell the examiner that you would like to:
  Examine the fundus (retinal glial hamartomas).
  Take a family history (autosomal dominant inheritance with variable penetrance).

Diagnosis

This patient has adenoma sebaceum (lesions) due to tuberous sclerosis. I would like to know his IQ and elicit a history of seizures to determine his functional status.

Advanced-level Questions

What other lesions may be present?

- Hamartomas within the CNS occurring as cortical tubers and subependymal hamartomas.
- Renal angiomyolipomas.
- Cardiac rhabdomyomas and pulmonary myomas.
- Cysts in the liver, kidney and pancreas.

How would you manage such patients?

Symptomatically, with anticonvulsant therapy for seizures and genetic counselling. When severe epilepsy and mental retardation is present the prognosis for life beyond the third decade is poor. Death is usually due to seizures, associated neoplasms or intercurrent illness.

Do you know on which chromosome the gene is localized?

Linkage studies have localized the gene to chromosomes 9 and 16.

DM Bourneville (1840–1909), a French neurologist.
JJ Pringle (1855–1922), an English dermatologist who was also the editor of the *British Journal of Dermatology.*

FUNDUS

EXAMINATION OF THE FUNDUS

1. Tell the patient, 'Look straight ahead with your right or left (R/L) eye while I look into your L/R eye'. (The candidate need not remove his or her spectacles while the fundus is being examined.) The candidate should use his or her own R/L eye to examine the patient's R/L eye.

2. Look at the eye from a distance of at least 50 cm and check for the red reflex. (The presence of a red reflex indicates that the media in front of the retina is transparent and that the retina is firmly in apposition with the underlying choroid. Red reflex may be absent when there is a lens opacity, vitreous haemorrhage or retinal detachment.)

3. Look systematically at the following:
   - The optic discs (comment on the colour, contour, cup and lamina cribrosa).
   - The macula (one or two disc diameters away from and a little below the temporal margin of the optic disc). It appears darker than the surrounding retina, and in young individuals has a central yellow point called the fovea centralis.
   - The nasal and temporal halves of the fundus.
   - The retinal vessels (remember that the retinal artery has four main branches and the normal ratio of the artery to the vein is 2:3). The candidate should assess the transparency of the vessels (the arteries usually have a shiny central reflex stripe), the presence of pressure effects such as AV nicking, the presence of focal narrowing of arteries as well as tortuosity of the venules.

Note.
- Lesions in the fundus are measured using the disc diameter as the reference size.
- Elevation of any lesion is measured by noting the difference between lens powers that focus clearly on the top of the lesion and an adjacent normal area of the fundus. Elevation of 3-dioptres lens changes is approximately equal to 1 mm in actual elevation.

CASE 237 Diabetic Retinopathy

Instruction

Examine the fundus in these patients.

Salient features

You will be expected to comment on whether it is background or proliferative retinopathy. You may have a clue about the underlying diabetes, either from a diabetic chart or from the presence of diabetic fruit juices at the bedside.

Patient 1 has background retinopathy, caused by microvascular leakage into the retina.
- Microaneurysms, usually seen in the posterior pole temporal to the fovea.
- Dot and blot haemorrhages.
- Hard exudates.
- Cottonwool spots.

Diagnosis

This patient has dot and blot haemorrhages, and cottonwool spots (lesions), probably due to diabetic retinopathy (aetiology), and good visual acuity (functional status).

Questions

What symptoms will this patient have?

The patient will be asymptomatic as the macula is spared.

How would you manage such a patient?

- Treat diabetes and associated hypertension.
- Annual fundal examination.

The Early Treatment of Diabetic Retinopathy Study (ETDRS) has established that early peripheral (panretinal) argon laser photocoagulation is not indicated for mild to moderate non-proliferative retinopathy. Early treatment in the form of argon laser photocoagulation applied directly to leaking microaneurysms, as well as grid photocoagulation applied to diffuse areas of leakage and thickening, is highly beneficial.

Salient features

Patient 2 has diabetic maculopathy, caused by oedema and/or hard exudates.

- Signs of background retinopathy with hard exudates or oedema of the macula.

Questions

What symptoms may this patient have?

There will be a gradual impairment of central vision, such as difficulty in reading small print or seeing road signs.

Advanced-level Questions

What are the signs of macular oedema?

Macular oedema includes any of the following signs:
- Retinal thickening at or within 500 μm of the centre of the macula.
- Retinal thickening of one disc area or larger, in any part of the retina which is within the one-disc diameter from the centre of the macula.
- Hard exudates at or within 500 μm of the centre of the macula.

How will you manage this patient?

Non-urgent referral to an ophthalmologist for photocoagulation which will stabilize (seldom improve) visual acuity in 50% of patients. The ability to alter the course of visual loss in diabetic macular oedema favourably is a major advance but patients must be cautioned that the most likely result of treatment is stabilization, not improvement, of visual acuity.

What is the principal mechanism of visual loss in non-proliferative retinopathy?

The principal mechanism of visual loss in non-proliferative retinopathy is through macular oedema, which results from focal vascular leakage from microaneurysms in the macular capillaries, as well as diffuse vascular leakage. With time, areas of leakage progress to macular thickening associated with hard exudates or cystoid changes.

What are the different types of clinical presentation?

Patients may present with no visual symptoms, paracentral scotomata or various degrees of central visual loss. Consequently, the diagnosis and management of macular oedema depend crucially on the determination of macular thickening by fundus examination. Ophthalmoscopy detects intraretinal haemorrhages and hard exudates but does not deter substantial retinal thickening. A critical evaluation of retinal thickening requires stereoscopic examination of the retina by slit-lamp biomicroscopy with lens for retinal visualization or stereoscopic fundus photography.

Salient features

Patient 3 has preproliferative retinopathy which is uncommon and is caused by retinal hypoxia.

- Cottonwool spots.
- Venous dilatation, beading, looping or sausage-like segmentation.
- Arteriolar narrowing.
- Haemorrhages – large dark blots.
- Intraretinal microvascular abnormalities.

Questions

What symptoms may this patient have?

Asymptomatic if the macula is spared.

How would you manage this patient?

Semiurgent referral to the ophthalmologist for close follow-up to enable early detection and treatment of proliferative retinopathy.

Salient features

Patient 4 has proliferative retinopathy caused by retinal hypoxia, usually seen in insulin-dependent diabetic retinopathy.

- Neovascularization around the disc (NVD) or away from the disc – in early stages the vessels are bare and flat and easily missed. In later stages they are elevated and may be associated with a white fibrous component.
- Presence of laser burns (in treated cases).

Questions

What symptoms may this patient have?

Asymptomatic in the absence of complications.

How would you manage this patient?

Urgent referral to an ophthalmologist for laser treatment.

What are the complications of proliferative retinopathy?

- Vitreous haemorrhage.
- Traction retinal detachment.
- Rubeosis irides.
- Rubeotic glaucoma – some of these patients can have partial restoration of vision by microsurgery called pars plana vitrectomy.

Advanced-level Questions

What is the prevalence of retinopathy in diabetes?

The overall prevalence is about 25%. It is 40% in insulin-dependent diabetes mellitus (IDDM) and 20% in non-insulin-dependent diabetes mellitus (NIDDM).

What is the relationship between the duration of diabetes and retinopathy?

There is a close relationship: in patients diagnosed to have diabetes before the age of 30 years, the incidence of retinopathy is about 50% after 10 years and 90% after 30 years. It is unusual for retinopathy to develop within 5 years of onset of diabetes; however, 5% of patients with NIDDM have background retinopathy at presentation.

What associated systemic conditions worsen diabetic retinopathy?

- Pregnancy.
- Hypertension.
- Anaemia.
- Renal failure.

What is the relationship between diabetic control and retinopathy?

The Diabetes Control and Complications Trial compared intensive treatment for blood glucose control with conventional treatment in patients with and without retinopathy at baseline who were followed for a mean of 6.5 years. Intensive treatment has profound benefits in both subgroups and was associated with a reduction in the incidence of both the development of new retinopathy and the risk of progression of existing retinopathy.

How often would you screen diabetic patients for retinopathy?

- Non-insulin-dependent diabetics: annually.
- Insulin-dependent diabetics:
    Newly diagnosed: no screening for the first 5 years.
    Five to ten years from initial diagnosis: annually.
    Over 10 years after initial diagnosis: every 6 months.

What is the earliest sign of retinal change in diabetes?

An increase in capillary permeability, evidenced by the leakage of dye into the vitreous humour after fluorescein injection, is the earliest sign of retinal change in diabetes mellitus.

What do you know about the pathogenesis of retinal new vessel formation?

It is not completely understood and current theories emphasize the production of angiogenic factors by areas of ischaemic and hypoxic retina. More recently vascular endothelial growth factor (VEGF) has been isolated from ocular fluid and is an endothelial cell-specific angiogenic factor whose production is increased by hypoxia; it has been implicated in the neovascularization seen in diabetic retinopathy and retinal vein occlusion.

What do you know about photocoagulation?

Photocoagulation is a technique whereby several thousand lesions are produced over a 2-week therapy period with lasers. Panretinal photocoagulation reduces the risk of severe visual loss. The laser is used to ablate a portion of the retina and does not directly cauterize the neovascularization. It is believed that the regression of neovascularization due to laser is a result of the destruction of ischaemic and hypoxic retina with reduction in angiogenic factors. Photocoagulation decreases the incidence of haemorrhage or scarring in proliferative retinopathy.

Photocoagulation is also useful in the treatment of microaneurysms, haemorrhages and oedema. Some loss of peripheral vision may be inevitable with this technique.

What surgical technique may be used for a non-resolving vitreous haemorrhage and retinal detachment?

Pars plana vitrectomy may be used but is often complicated by retinal tears, retinal detachment, glaucoma, infection, cataracts and loss of the eye.

Reference

Aiello LP, Avery RL, Arrigg PG et al (1994) Vascular endothelial growth factor in ocular fluid of patients with diabetic retinopathy and other retinal disorders. *N Engl J Med* **331**: 1480–1487.

CASE 238 **Hypertensive Retinopathy**

Instruction

Examine this patient's eyes.
Examine this patient's fundus.

Salient features

- Arteriovenous nipping.
- Arteriolar narrowing.
- Macular star.
- Flame-shaped and blot haemorrhages.
- Cottonwool exudates.
- Papilloedema may or may not be present.

Proceed as follows:

- Tell the examiner that you would like to:
    Check the blood pressure.
    Examine the urine for proteinuria.
    Examine the heart for left ventricular hypertrophy.

Diagnosis

This patient has flame-shaped haemorrhages with a macular star (lesions) due to hypertension (aetiology).

Advanced-level Questions

How would you grade hypertensive retinopathy?

Keith–Wagener–Barker classification:
- Stage I – arteriolar narrowing.
- Stage II – irregular calibre of arterioles.
- Stage III – cottonwool exudates; flame and blot haemorrhages, retinal oedema.
- Stage IV – papilloedema.

Note. Subsequent studies have shown that the clinical features and prognosis of patients with stage III and stage IV disease were similar whether or not papilloedema was present; consequently the terms 'malignant' and 'accelerated' can be used interchangeably. Instead 'hypertensive crisis' is used to refer to the syndrome of raised blood pressure complicated by end-organ damage (e.g. stroke, renal failure, myocardial ischaemia or infarction, stage III or IV hypertensive retinopathy).

Mention some causes of cottonwool spots.

- HIV infection *per se.*
- Anaemias.
- Infective endocarditis.
- Leukaemias.
- Diabetic retinopathy (see page 590).

Mention a few causes of hypertension.

- In 90% of cases it is essential hypertension with no underlying cause and this may represent the 'normal' spread.
- In 10% of cases there is an underlying cause:
  Renal causes: renal artery stenosis, polycystic kidneys, chronic glomerulonephritis, polyarteritis nodosa, chronic pyelonephritis.
  Endocrine causes: Cushing's syndrome, Conn's syndrome, phaeo-chromocytoma, acromegaly, diabetes mellitus.
  Eclampsia and pre-eclamptic toxaemia of pregnancy.
  Coarctation of the aorta.

How would you investigate a patient with hypertension?

- Urine for protein, glucose, casts.
- Mid-stream urine for microscopy and culture.
- Urea and electrolytes, fasting lipids.
- CXR.
- ECG.
- Urine catecholamines.
- Intravenous pyelography.
- Renal artery digital subtraction angiography (DSA).

How would you treat hypertension?

- Salt restriction.
- Drug therapy.
- First line:
  In women and smokers – bendrofluazide.
  In non-smoking men – beta-blockers.
- Advise the patient to stop smoking.

Sir CT Dollery, was Dean, Royal Postgraduate Medical School, Hammersmith Hospital, London; his interests include clinical pharmacology, hypertension and medical education.
John Swales, contemporary Professor of Medicine, Leicester; his chief interest is hypertension.
James C Petrie, contemporary Professor and Head of Medicine and Therapeutics, Aberdeen; his interests include hypertension and cardiovascular prevention.

References

Ahmed ME, Walker JM, Beevers DG & Beevers M (1986) Lack of difference between malignant and accelerated hypertension. *Br Med J* **292**: 235–237.

Dollery CT, Ramalho PS, Patterson JW et al (1965) Retinal microemboli: experimental production of 'cottonwool' spots. *Lancet* **i**: 303.

Keith NM, Wagner HP & Barker NW (1939) Some different types of essential hypertension: their course and prognosis. *Am J Med Sci* **197**: 332–343.

Swales JD (1990) First line treatment in hypertension. *Br Med J* **301**: 1172.

Webster J, Petrie JC, Jeffers TA & Lovell HG (1993) Accelerated hypertension – patterns of mortality and clinical factors affecting outcome in treated patients. *Q J Med* **86**: 485–493.

CASE 239 Papilloedema

Instruction

Examine this patient's fundus.

Salient features

- There is swelling of the optic disc (look for haemorrhages and soft exudates).

Note. Remember that the common causes are:
Intracranial space-occupying lesion.
Hypertensive retinopathy.
Benign intracranial hypertension.

Diagnosis

This patient has bilateral papilloedema (lesion) and I would like to investigate for an intracranial space-occupying lesion (aetiology).

Questions

What do you understand by the term 'papilloedema'?

Papilloedema is the swelling of the nerve head as seen on ophthalmoscopy. The colour of the disc becomes redder, approximating to that of the rest of the retina; its contour becomes blurred and the cup and cribrosa are filled in.

What is the first manifestation of papilloedema?

The earliest manifestation of papilloedema is the engorgement of the veins.

What is the nature of the field defect in papilloedema?

Papilloedema is always associated with enlargement of the blind spot, with a consequent diminution of visual fields and gradual loss of visual acuity, bu a fair acuity may remain until papilloedema is marked.

Advanced-level Questions

Mention a few causes of papilloedema.

- Raised intracranial pressure resulting from one of the following conditions:
  Impaired circulation of the CSF due to aqueduct stenosis.
  Meningitis.
  Subarachnoid haemorrhage.
- Cerebral oedema:
  Following head injury.
  Following cerebral anoxia.
- Metabolic causes:
  Carbon dioxide retention.
  Steroid withdrawal.
  Thyroid eye disease.
  Vitamin A intoxication.
  Lead poisoning.
- Increased protein in the CSF due to one of the following:
  Guillain–Barré syndrome.

Spinal cord tumours.
Any spinal block.
- Haematological and circulatory disorders:
  Central retinal vein thrombosis.
  Superior vena caval obstruction.
  Polycythaemia vera.
  Multiple myeloma.
  Macroglobulinaemia.

Mention a few conditions simulating papilloedema.

- Deep optic cup:
  Nasal edge appears heaped up.
  Vessels plunge into the optic cup.
  Temporal edge is quite normal.
- Medullated nerve fibres, seen on the disc or even on the retina. The appearance is typically flared and on focusing will reveal fibres traversing the area. Field defects are due to the retinal vessels being obscured. Since these are present from birth, the patient is unaware of the defect.
- Bergmeister's papilla, in which there is a whitish elevation of the centre of the disc with venous and arterial sheathing. It is common and seen at all ages. There is an equal sex and racial incidence.
- Pseudopapilloedema, i.e. congenitally elevated discs secondary to hyaloid tissue (drüsen) or hyperopia.

Note. Elevation or swelling on the optic disc occurs in the following conditions:
  Papilloedema.
  Papillitis.
  Drüsen.
  Infiltration of the nerve head by malignant cells.

What do you know about Foster Kennedy syndrome?

Unilateral papilloedema with or without 'secondary' optic atrophy on the other side suggests a tumour of the opposite side on the olfactory lobe or orbital surface of the frontal lobe or of the pituitary body.

What do you understand by the term 'papillitis'?

- Demyelination of the optic nerve (multiple sclerosis).
- Inflammation.
- Degeneration (Leber's optic atrophy).

- Vascular disorders of the nerve head.
- Malignant infiltration.

How do you differentiate papillitis from papilloedema?

Papillitis	Papilloedema
Usually unilateral	Usually bilateral
Visual acuity is considerably reduced in relation to the degree of swelling of the disc	Visual acuity only slightly reduced until late stages
Visual field defect is usually central, particularly for red and green	Peripheral constriction or enlargement of the blind spot
Marcus Gunn pupil may be present	Marcus Gunn pupil is absent
Eye movements may be painful	Eye movements are never painful

Note. A Marcus Gunn pupil is one that shows better constriction to an indirect response than to direct light.

What are the stages of papilloedema?

- Stage I – increase in venous calibre and tortuosity.
- Stage II – optic cup becomes pinker and less distinct, the vessels seeming to disappear suddenly on the surface of the disc.
- Stage III – blurring of the discs on the nasal side. (**Note.** In many normal discs the nasal edge is less distinct and one of the most frequent false-positive signs is questionable blurring of the nasal disc margins.)
- Stage IV – the whole disc becomes suffused and slightly elevated. The margins may disappear and the vessels seem to emerge from a mushy swelling. The optic cup is filled and there are haemorrhages around the disc.

Foster Kennedy (1884–1952) was born in Belfast. He was Professor of Neurology at Cornell University. He described his syndrome in 1923.

Reference

Sanders MD & Senneham RH (1980) Differential diagnosis of the optic disc oedema. *Trans Ophthalmol Soc UK* **100**: 123–131.

CASE 240 Optic Atrophy

Instruction

Examine this patient's eyes.
Examine this patient's fundus.

Salient features

- Pale disc with sharp margins.
- Intact consensual light reflex but impaired direct light reflex – Marcus Gunn pupillary response (seen in asymmetrical involvement of the two eyes).
- Central scotoma on testing of visual fields.

Proceed as follows:

- Tell the examiner that you would like to look for cerebellar signs (remember that multiple sclerosis is the commonest cause of optic atrophy).

Diagnosis

This patient has primary optic atrophy (lesion) due to multiple sclerosis (aetiology). I would like to check the visual fields for central scotoma (functional status).

Questions

What is your diagnosis?

The differential diagnosis is as follows:
- Demyelinating disorders (multiple sclerosis).
- Optic nerve compression by tumour or aneurysm.
- Glaucoma.
- Toxins: methanol, tobacco, lead, arsenical poisoning.
- Ischaemia, including central retinal artery occlusion due to thrombo-embolism, temporal arteritis, idiopathic acute ischaemic optic neuropathy, syphilis.
- Hereditary disorders: Friedreich's ataxia, Leber's optic atrophy (sex linked, seen in young males).
- Paget's disease.
- Vitamin B_{12} deficiency.
- Secondary to retinitis pigmentosa.

Advanced-level Questions

What is the difference between primary and secondary optic atrophy?

Primary	Secondary
White and flat with clear-cut edges	Greyish-white, edges indistinct
Visible lamina cribrosa	Cup filled and lamina cribrosa not visible
Arteries and veins normal	Arteries thinner than normal
	Veins may be dilated
Capillaries decreased in number (fewer than seven) – Kestenbaum's sign	Capillaries decreased in number

What is consecutive optic atrophy?

Consecutive optic atrophy is a controversial term and is best avoided. Some use it as an equivalent or alternative for what has been described above as secondary optic atrophy, but others use the term to indicate an atrophy complicating or, rarely, a retinitis such as Tay–Sachs disease or retinitis pigmentosa.

What is glaucomatous optic atrophy?

Glaucomatous optic atrophy denotes loss of disc substance, referred to as increased cupping.

How would you investigate a patient with optic neuropathy?

- FBC, ESR.
- Blood glucose.
- Serology for syphilis.
- Vitamin B_{12} and B_1 levels.
- Skull X-ray of pituitary fossa, optic foramina and sinuses, or CT scan of the brain and orbit.
- ECG.
- Pattern-stimulated visual evoked responses.
- Electroretinography.

R Marcus Gunn (1850–1909), a Scottish ophthalmologist who worked at Moorfields Eye Hospital, London.
T von Leber (1840–1917), Professor of Ophthalmology at the University of Heidelberg, Germany.
W Tay (1843–1927), a British ophthalmologist, Moorfields Eye Hospital, London.
BP Sachs (1858–1944), a German neuropsychiatrist who worked in New York. He described this condition independent of Tay.

CASE 241 Retinal Vein Thrombosis

Instruction

Examine this patient's eyes.
Examine this patient's fundus.

Salient features

Patient 1 has central retinal vein occlusion (i.e. occlusion is behind the cribriform plate):

- Multiple retinal and preretinal haemorrhages surround the optic nerve head. There is marked dilatation and tortuosity of the veins, hyperaemia or oedema of the nerve head and soft exudates – 'blood and thunder' appearance.
- Visual acuity is only slightly reduced.

Patient 2 has branch vein occlusion (the occlusion is in front of the cribriform plate):

- These occur just distal to the arteriovenous crossing. The superior temporal vein is most commonly involved. Haemorrhages are seen surrounding the occluded vein.
- May cause a quadrantic field defect.
- Visual prognosis is good if the haemorrhages do not extend to the macula with accompanying macular oedema.

Proceed as follows:

- Tell the examiner that you would like to check for the following conditions:
  Diabetes (urine sugar).
  Hypertension.
  Chronic simple glaucoma.
  Hyperviscosity syndromes (Waldenström's macroglobulinaemia, multiple myeloma).

Diagnosis

This patient has multiple retinal haemorrhages (lesions) due to central retinal vein occlusion with underlying diabetes mellitus (aetiology).

Advanced-level Questions

What are the usual sites of occlusion in branch retinal vein occlusion?

- At arteriovenous crossings, causing classical quadrantic or small macular occlusions.
- Along the main veins, as in diabetes mellitus.
- At the edges of the optic disc, resulting in occlusion of the hemisphere.
- Peripherally, as in sickle cell disease.

What are the vascular responses to retinal vein occlusion?

These include dilatation of retinal capillaries, abnormal vascular permeability and retinal capillary closure.

What is the prognosis in branch retinal vein occlusion?

It varies from complete resolution with no residual visual deficits to a progressive deterioration resulting in permanent loss of vision.

What is the clinical course in central retinal vein occlusion?

- In mild cases, there is minimal dilatation of veins and haemorrhages with little or no oedema of the macula and no visual deficit.
- In severe instances, the vision may deteriorate to hand motions, with extensively deep and supericial haemorrhages with stagnation of blood in the markedly dilated veins and several cottonwool spots.

What are the complications of central retinal vein occlusion?

These include neovascularization of the retina, rubeosis iridis (usually visible by 1 month) and rubeotic glaucoma (usually by 3 months).

How would you manage such eyes?

- Treat the underlying condition.
- Fluorescein angiography to determine areas of retinal ischaemia.
- Regular follow-up by the ophthalmologist as secondary neovascularization is a common sequela and may need laser therapy. Panretinal photocoagulation prevents the dreaded complications of neovascular glaucoma.

JG Waldenström (b. 1906), Professor of Medicine, Uppsala University, Sweden.

CASE 242 Subhyaloid Haemorrhage

Instruction

Examine this patient's fundus.

Salient features

- A large, solitary subhyaloid haemorrhage (there may be no fluid level if the patient is lying flat).
- There may be associated retinal haemorrhage.
- 20% have mild papilloedema.

Proceed as follows:

- Comment on any obvious hemiplegia.

Note. When the subhyaloid (preretinal) haemorrhage extends into the vitreous humour it is called Terson's syndrome.

Diagnosis

This hemiplegic patient has a subhyaloid haemorrhage (lesion) due to subarachnoid haemorrhage (aetiology).

Advanced-level Questions

What is the commonest cause of subhyaloid haemorrhage?

Subarachnoid haemorrhage.

What are the other causes of haemorrhage into the vitreous?

- Local injury.
- Blood diseases.
- Hypertension.
- Diabetes.
- Idiopathic.

Mention some causes of neck stiffness.

- Subarachnoid haemorrhage.
- Meningitis.
- Posterior fossa tumours.
- Local neck pathology such as cervical spondylosis.

What are causes of deterioration in a patient with subarachnoid haemorrhage?

- Rebleeds.
- Cerebral infarction due to reflex vasospasm of cerebral vessels (hence the rationale to use nimodipine).
- Secondary hydrocephalus.

How would you investigate such a patient?

CT head scan, and if this rules out intracranial hypertension then a lumbar puncture to diagnose minor leaks.

Reference

Ostergaard JR (1990) Warning leak in subarachnoid haemorrhage. *Br Med J* **301**: 190.

CASE 243 **Retinitis Pigmentosa**

Instruction

Examine this patient's fundus.
Examine this patient's eyes.

Salient features

- Peripheral retina shows perivascular 'bone spicule pigmentation' and arteriolar narrowing. The retinal veins (never the arteries) often have a sheath of pigmentation for part of their course. The pigment spots which lie near the retinal veins are seen to be anterior to them, so that they hide the course of the vessel. (In this respect they differ from the pigment around the spots of choroidal atrophy in which the retinal vessels can be traced over the spots.)
- Optic disc is pale.
- Maculopathy which is atrophic or cystoid.

Proceed as follows:

- Look for polydactyly in the hands and feet (Laurence–Moon–Biedl syndrome).
- Comment on the white walking aid (if any) used by the registered blind.
- Tell the examiner that you would like to check visual fields and take a family history (can be autosomal recessive, which is more severe, or autosomal dominant, which is more benign).

Diagnosis

This patient is obese, has polydactyly and retinitis pigmentosa (lesion) due to Laurence–Moon–Biedl syndrome (aetiology) and is registered blind (functional status).

Questions

What is the prognosis in retinitis pigmentosa?

Most patients are registered blind by the age of 40 years, with central field less than 20 degrees in diameter. Almost all patients lose central vision by the seventh decade.

What do you know about retinitis pigmentosa?

Retinitis pigmentosa is a slow degenerative disease of the retina. It occurs in both eyes, begins in early childhood, and often results in the loss of sight by middle or advanced age. The degeneration primarily affects the rods and cones, in particular the rods.

How may it present?

It may present with defective vision at dusk (night blindness), which may occur several years before the pigment is visible in the retina.

Advanced-level Questions

Mention a few systemic disorders associated with retinitis pigmentosa.

- Laurence–Moon–Biedl–Bardet syndrome, which is a recessively inherited disorder characterized by mental disability, polydactyly, syndactyly, hypogonadism and obesity.
- Bassen–Konzweig syndrome (abetalipoproteinaemia), characterized by fat malabsorption, abetalipoproteinaemia, acanthocytosis and spinocerebellar ataxia.
- Refsum's disease (phytanic acid storage disease), an autosomal recessive disorder characterized by hypertrophic peripheral neuropathy, deafness, ichthyosis, cerebellar ataxia, raised CSF protein levels in the absence of pleocytosis.
- Kearns–Sayre syndrome, a triad of retinitis pigmentosa, progressive external ophthalmoplegia and heart block.
- Usher's disease, a recessively inherited disorder characterized by congenital, non-progressive, sensorineural deafness.
- Friedreich's ataxia (see page 192).

Which ocular conditions are associated with retinitis pigmentosa?

- Open-angle glaucoma.
- Posterior subcapsular cataracts.
- Myopia.
- Keratoconus.

What is secondary retinitis pigmentosa?

Secondary retinitis pigmentosa is a sequela to inflammatory retinitis. It is often ophthalmoscopically indistinguishable from the primary condition, the electroretinographic and electro-oculographic responses are slightly subnormal unless the condition is far advanced. (In the primary type the response is markedly subnormal to the electroretinogram and electro-oculogram.)

What is retinitis pigmentosa sine pigmento?

A variety of retinitis pigmentosa but without visible pigmentation of the retina.

What is inverse retinitis pigmentosa?

Bone corpuscles are visible in the perifoveal area, whereas the retinal periphery is normal.

JZ Laurence (1830–1874), an English ophthalmologist.
RC Moon (1844–1914), a US ophthalmologist.
A Biedl (1869–1933), a Czech physician.
G Bardet (b. 1885), a French physician.
FA Bassen (b. 1903), physician, and AL Kornzweig (b. 1900), ophthalmologist, Mount Sinai Hospital, New York.
S Refsum, a Norwegian physician.

References

Cogan DG, Rodrigues M, Chu FC et al (1984) Ocular abnormalities in abeta-lipoproteinaemia. *Ophthalmology* **91**: 991.
Dryja TP, McGhee TL, Hahn LB et al (1990) Mutations within the rhodopsin gene in patients with autosomal dominant retinitis pigmentosa. *N Engl J Med* **323**: 1502.
Fishman GA, Kumar A & Joseph Me (1983) Usher's syndrome. *Arch Ophthalmol* **101**: 1367.
McKechnie NM, King M & Lee WR (1985) Retinal pathology in Kearns Sayre syndrome. *Br J Ophthalmol* **69**: 63.

CASE 244 Old Choroiditis

Instruction

Examine this patient's fundus.

Salient features

- Old or inactive retinochoroiditis appears as white, well-defined areas of chorioretinal atrophy with pigmented edges (due to proliferation of retinal pigment epithelium).
- The retinal blood vessels pass over the lesions undisturbed.

Diagnosis

This patient has areas of retinal atrophy with pigmented edges (lesion) due to old choroiditis complicating cytomegalovirus infection (aetiology).

Questions

What may be the aetiology?

- Reactivation of congenital toxoplasmosis.
- Cytomegalovirus infection.
- AIDS.
- Sarcoidosis.
- TB.
- Syphilis.
- Behçet's disease.

What is the prognosis?

Prognosis varies according to the underlying aetiology. It is poor if the fovea is involved.

What does the presence of pigment on fundoscopy indicate?

A chronic lesion of the retina or choroid.

In which other conditions is the retinal pigment seen?

- Normally – racial (tigroid fundus).
- Retinitis pigmentosa.
- Malignant melanoma.

H Behçet (1889–1940), Professor of Dermatology in Turkey, described this syndrome in 1937 based on three patients he observed between 1924 and 1936.

CASE 245 Cholesterol Embolus in the Fundus

Instruction

Examine this patient's fundus.

Salient features

- Presence of a cholesterol embolus (Hollenhorst plaques) in one of the branches of the retinal artery.

Proceed as follows:

- Look for a cherry-red spot at the fovea (the ischaemic retina at the posterior pole becomes milky white and swollen, and the choroid is seen through the fovea as a cherry-red spot).
- Tell the examiner that you would like to check for visual field defects.

Remember that retinal artery occlusion results in infarction of the inner two-thirds of the retina, reflex vasoconstriction of the retinal arterial tree and stasis in the retinal capillaries.

Diagnosis

This patient has a cholesterol embolus in one of the branches of the retinal artery (lesion) due to underlying atherosclerotic disease (aetiology).

Questions

What are the complications of such an embolus?

Retinal artery occlusion causing field defects or loss of vision.

Where is the likely origin of this embolus?

The most likely origin is an atherosclerotic plaque in the carotid circulation.

What are the causes of retinal arterial occlusion?

Commonest cause:

- Emboli arising from the major arteries supplying the head or from the left side of the heart. Embolic particles consist of platelet clumps, cholesterol crystals or Hollenhorst plaques and others (mixed thrombus, calcific or septic material from cardiac valves, fat, myxoma, talc in intravenous drug abusers or silicone in those who receive injections for cosmetic purposes).

Other causes:

- Temporal arteritis.
- Collagen vascular diseases.
- Increased orbital pressure, e.g. retrobulbar haemorrhage, Graves' exophthalmos.
- Sickle cell disease.
- Syphilis.

What do you understand by the term 'amaurosis'?

Amaurosis means blindness from any cause.

What do you understand by the term 'amblyopia'?

Amblyopia means that impaired vision is not due to refractive error or ocular disease.

What do you understand by the term 'amaurosis fugax'?

Amaurosis fugax is a retinal artery transient ischaemic attack (TIA) which manifests with a painless, unilateral loss of vision that usually lasts a few minutes.

How would you manage this patient?

- Aspirin.
- Ophthalmology opinion.
- Ultrasonography of the carotid arteries.
- Advise the patient to stop smoking.
- Control of hypertension.
- Carotid angiography with a view to performing carotid endarterectomy.

What is the effect of cholesterol crystals?

Cholesterol crystals rarely cause significant obstruction to the retinal arterioles.

What manoeuvre would you use to make the cholesterol crystals more apparent?

Mild lateral pressure on the globe may make the presence of unobtrusive crystals clearly visible when the retinal arteries pulsate.

How would you manage an acute occlusion of the retinal artery?

- Lie the patient in a supine position to ensure adequate circulation.
- Intermittent ocular massage is applied for 15 minutes to dislodge the emboli, lower intraocular pressure and improve circulation.
- Intravenous acetazolamide to lower intraocular pressure.
- Inhalation of a mixture of 5% carbon dioxide and 95% oxygen.
- Anterior chamber paracentesis.

If the investigation of a patient with amaurosis fugax comes up with no evidence of carotid artery disease, embolism or other recognized causes of the disorder, then the diagnosis by exclusion should be vasospasm. In such cases a calcium channel blocker should be tried.

What do you know about the 'purple-toe syndrome'?

This was first described with warfarin therapy by Feder and Auerbach in 1961 and was shown to be due to showers of atheroemboli. Now, with the increasing use of coronary angioplasty and thrombolytic therapy in the elderly, cholesterol emboli are increasingly reported. They result in 'purple-toes', amaurosis fugax, and atheroembolic disease of kidneys, skin and gastrointestinal tract.

References

Feder W & Auerbach R (1961) Purple toes: an uncommon sequela of oral coumarin therapy. *Ann Intern Med* **55**: 911–917.
Gautier J (1993) Amaurosis fugax. *N Engl J Med* **329**: 427.

CASE 246 Vitreous Opacities

Instruction

Examine this patient's fundus.

Salient features

- Small white opacities which are present in front of the retinal vessels.
- The patient may complain of diplopia (monocular diplopia).

Proceed as follows:

- Tell the examiner that you would like to:
  Test for monocular diplopia.
  Check urine for sugar.
  Check the blood pressure.

Diagnosis

This patient has vitreous opacities (lesions) with monocular diplopia (functional status), and has underlying diabetes mellitus (aetiology).

Questions

What are the causes of vitreous opacities?

- Blood: diabetes, retinal vein occlusion, trauma, subarachnoid haemorrhage, sickle cell retinopathy.
- Cholesterolosis bulbi: where free floating, highly refractile, crystals are seen in liquified vitreous and in patients with severe intraocular disease.
- Asteroid hyalitis (Benson's disease): where whitish yellow solid bodies, containing calcium palmitate and stearate, are suspended in normal vitreous.
- Other: e.g. retinoblastoma, primary amyloidosis.

What are the other causes of monocular diplopia?

- Opacities in the lens.
- Corneal opacities.
- Retinal detachment.

CASE 247 Myelinated Nerve Fibres

Instruction

Examine this patient's fundus.

Salient features

- White, streaky patches which extend from the disc and terminate peripherally in a feather-like pattern. It may cover the retinal vessels.

Diagnosis

This patient has white streaky patches in a feather-like pattern (lesion); these are medullated nerve fibres (aetiology) and are benign (functional status).

Questions

What is the pathology?

Occasionally, the myelination of the optic nerve does not stop at the lamina cribrosa but extends on to nerve fibres surrounding the optic disc. This condition is a benign congenital abnormality known as medullated or myelinated nerve fibres. It terminates peripherally in a feather-like margin with fine striations from the course of the nerve fibre layer.

CASE 248 Retinal Changes in AIDS

Instruction

At a distance from the patient, the examiner will say that this patient has HIV, examine his fundus.

Patient 1
- Cottonwool spots.

Proceed as follows:

- Tell the examiner that you would like to exclude diabetes and retinal vascular disease.

Questions

How would you treat these lesions?

In a patient with known HIV infection, such infarcts require no specific therapy.

Patient 2: Cytomegalovirus (CMV) retinitis.
- An area of retinitis with nerve fibre layer infarcts, haemorrhages, retinal opacification and perivascular sheathing.

Advanced-level Questions

How would you treat these lesions?

Therapy with intravenous ganciclovir or foscarnet is given lifelong to protect unaffected areas but does not restore functional areas already affected. The optimal treatment for patients with AIDS, normal renal function and CMV retinitis is foscarnet plus an antiretroviral nucleoside such as zidovudine. For similar patients with impaired renal function, ganciclovir would be the drug of choice, perhaps with an antiretroviral agent such as didanosine that has few overlapping side-effects. Late retinal detachment occurs despite therapy in one-fifth of these patients.

What do you know about ganciclovir?

It is a derivative of acyclovir. It can cause bone marrow depression and hence should not be administered simultaneously with zidovudine.

What do you know about foscarnet?

It is an organic analogue of inorganic pyrophosphate. Its side-effects include renal impairment, electrolyte imbalance and seizures. It can be safely administered with zidovudine.

What are the other retinal manifestations in patients with AIDS?

- Toxoplasmosis retinochoroiditis – usually nasal to the disc, characterized by extensive whitish infarction and inflammation, with minimal associated intraretinal haemorrhage.
- *Pneumocystis carinii* choroiditis – characterized by scattered nodular yellowish lesions deep in the retina.
- Acute retinal necrosis syndrome – with severe peripheral retinal infarction and retinal vasculitis. Atrophic retinal holes appear later in these areas.
- Progressive outer retinal necrosis syndrome – characterized by diffuse whitish opacification of the retina beneath the retinal vessels and a cherry-red spot in the fovea. It is associated with herpes zoster and the prognosis for visual acuity is dismal.
- Ocular presentations of syphilis include anterior and posterior uveitis, retinitis, retinal vasculitis and papillitis.
- Acute syphilitic posterior placoid chorioretinitis – large placoid yellowish lesions at the level of the retinal pigment epithelium in the posterior retina with inflammation of the vitreous and loss of vision.

What diagnostic tests would you perform to detect retinal manifestations of AIDS?

- Careful clinical observations.
- Serology.
- Culture.
- Retinal biopsy by pars plana vitrectomy.
- Testing of ocular fluid by polymerase chain reaction.

Mention some ocular non-retinal manifestations of AIDS.

- Optic neuropathy.
- Kaposi's sarcoma of the conjuctiva.
- Orbital lymphoma.

Reference

Studies of Ocular Complications of AIDS Research Group and AIDS Clinical Trials Group (1992) Mortality in patients with acquired immunodeficiency syndrome treated with either foscarnet or ganciclovir for cytomegalovirus retinitis. *N Engl J Med* **326**: 213–220.

CASE 249 Retinal Detachment

Instruction

Examine this patient who complained of a dark curtain progressing across the visual field.

Salient features

- The retina has lost its pink colour and appears grey and opaque.
- When the collection of subretinal fluid is large, the retina shows ballooning detachment with numerous folds.

Proceed as follows:

- Tell the examiner that you would like to:
    Examine visual acuity and visual fields.
    Check urine for sugar.
    Check the blood pressure.
    Comment on any walking aid for the registered blind.

Diagnosis

This patient has neovascularization and retinal detachment (lesion) due to underlying diabetes mellitus (aetiology). She has a walking aid for the registered blind (functional status).

Advanced-level Questions

What is the pathology of retinal detachment?

It is a separation within the retina between the photoreceptors and the retinal pigment epithelium, characterized by collection of fluid or blood in this potential space.

What are the types of retinal detachment?

Rhegmatogenous retinal detachment is defined as the presence of a hole or break in the retina that allows fluid from the vitreous capacity to enter the subretinal space. It usually occurs spontaneously in those who have a predisposition to it following trauma to the eye or after intraocular surgery. Most of these patients develop symptoms. A break in the peripheral retina is associated with a sudden burst of flashing lights or sparks that may be followed by small floaters or spots in the field of vision. When the retina detaches, the patient perceives a dark curtain progressing across the visual field, and when the fovea detaches central vision is abruptly diminished.

It is treated surgically with a scleral buckling procedure where all retinal breaks are localized and adhesions between the choroid and retina are performed around the break with diathermy or a cryoprobe. After draining the subretinal fluid, the detached portion of the retina is indented towards the vitreous cavity by a scleral implant or explant. This results in pushing the retina towards the vitreous causing closure of the retinal break (by the buckled sclera and choroid) and release of traction of vitreous.

Traction retinal detachment is that in which the intact retina is forcibly elevated by contracting membranes on the surface of the retina or by vitreous traction on areas of retinal neovascularization. Causes include diabetes, intraocular foreign body, perforating eye injuries and loss of vitreous following cataract surgery. These retinal detachments are difficult to treat and pars plana vitrectomy is the only way to treat these lesions.

Secondary retinal detachments occur secondary to systemic disorders including hypertension, toxaemia of pregnancy, chronic glomerulo-nephritis, retinal venous occlusive disease and retinal vasculitis. Treatment is directed towards the underlying cause as these detachments are not amenable to scleral buckling surgery.

CASE 250
Age-Related Macular Degeneration (Senile Macular Degeneration)

Instruction

Look at this patient's fundus.

Salient features

- Drüsen.
- Disruption of pigment of the retinal pigment epithelium into small areas of hypopigmentation and hyperpigmentation.
- Choroidal neovascularization.

Proceed as follows:

- Comment on the white walking aid by the bedside, which indicates the patient is registered blind.
- Tell the examiner that you would like to check visual acuity and visual field (in most patients there is loss of central vision and maintenance of peripheral vision).

Remember that age-related macular degeneration is now the commonest cause of registrable blindness in the United Kingdom.

Diagnosis

This patient has senile macular degeneration (aetiology) and is registered blind, as evidenced by the white walking aid (functional status).

Questions

What are drüsen?

Drüsen are pale yellow spots that occur individually or in clusters throughout the macula. They consist of amorphous material accumulated between the Bruch's membrane and pigment epithelium. Although the exact origin is not known, it is believed that drüsen occur due to the accumulation of lipofuscin and other cellular debris derived from cells of the retinal pigment epithelium that are compromised by age and other factors.

Advanced-level Questions

What do you know about neovascularization in these patients?

Substantial visual loss occurs as a result of it. Choroidal vessels proliferate across the Bruch's membrane under the retinal pigment epithelium and, in certain cases, continue their extension into the subretinal space. Substantial leakage from these neovascular membranes can result in retinal detachment. The most devastating consequence is haemorrhage, which resolves forming a disciform scar.

How does this condition manifest?

- Often visual loss is detected when one eye is covered for testing visual acuity.
- Decrease in visual acuity.
- Metamorphosia (distortion of the shape of objects in view).
- Paracentral scotoma.
- Variable visual loss due to atrophy of a large area of retinal pigment epithelium involving the fovea.

What investigations are performed to detect choroidal neovascularization?

- Rapid-sequence fluoroscein angiography.
- Retinal angiography using indocyanine green and infrared photography.

How is the neovascularization treated?

- Laser photocoagulation of regions outside the foveal avascular zone.
- Subfoveal neovascularization when photocoagulated is associated with a treatment-induced visual loss immediately but in the long term is found to be beneficial. Treatment may have to be deferred in those with good initial visual acuity because a large scotoma occurs as a result of treatment.
- Interferon α is currently being evaluated.
- Surgical removal of subfoveal choroidal neovascularization has been reported to be useful but the results are not as good as laser photocoagulation.
- Zinc – the use of zinc as a therapeutic agent for macular degeneration has not been evaluated in a rigorous trial.

What is the difference between krypton and argon laser photocoagulation?

The krypton red photocoagulator is useful to treat when the neovascular-ization is closer than 200 μm but not under the fovea, because of its ability to spare the inner retina by its virtual lack of absorption by haemoglobin (unlike the argon laser). The conventional argon laser has blue and green wavelengths. The green wavelength is absorbed by haemoglobin and thus may damage the retina, whilst the blue wavelength is absorbed by the macular xanthophyll and results in foveal damage.

Mention some drugs that can cause maculopathy.

Chloroquine, thioridazine, chlorpromazine.

INDEX

Numbers in **bold** refer to main reference